# CLEANSE & PURIFY THYSELF

"... and I will exalt thee to
the throne of power."

**BOOK 1.5**
**1998**

**A method of achieving self-healing,**
**exceptional health, and**
**unconditional Love and Joy**
**Mother Nature's Way:**
**through**
**Advanced Intestinal Cleansing and**
**Mental and Physical Rejuvenation**

**RICHARD ANDERSON, N.D., N.M.D.**

# Foreword

*"This book here, in reaching out to our full potential, is one for an awakening. It is one which shows that we have an upbuilding path before us. Damaged, deteriorating tissue demands the stopping of old ways of doing things and requires bringing in the new. Toxic tissues need elimination. We find out that repair and rebuilding cannot take place unless we have the proper foods to go with it. This is why I believe that this book could be one of the finest assets in a person's home; it provides current information on these issues.*

*There are many forms of healing, many forms of elimination, many building programs. Once we learn about it all, then it is a matter of sitting down and finding how we can grow out of our misery, out of our disease, and find a place in life where we find good health, where we find contentment, where we find what relationship the mind has to the body, and what relationship the body has to the mind. We cannot expect sweet thoughts on a sour stomach, but we have to recognize that the brain is the one that controls every activity in the body. To put it under control and to make the proper play at the proper time, with the knowledge that we have, is the thing that will keep us in good health. And above all, to start the moral path, as suggested in this book, is one that is needed so much.*

*Whether this book meets the needs of a few, or many, it makes no difference. I am acquainted with Dr. Anderson, the author, and he is one who wants to be of help, spreading good cheer, good health among those he meets. He deserves a lot of credit, for this is one of the most difficult jobs that we have today: to get the blind to see and the deaf to hear. But after all, we find out, aren't we all a little deaf, a little blind, and also, aren't we all just a little ignorant and in need of just a little of the intelligence that maybe someone like him can spread out before us to give us a life that is really worthwhile living."*

*Sincerely,*

*Dr. Bernard Jensen*

## Acknowledgments

A very special thanks to Judith Brewer, Renee Getreu, Avona L'Carttier, Marguerite Ogle, and Jonni Sue Perlman, for all the encouragement, support, advice, organization, patience, kindness, and editing. Their incredible joyful and loving attitudes made all the work fun. Thanks to Michelle, and all our illustrators and photographers for their wonderful graphic additions to the book. And a great big thanks and hugs to all the people who accomplished the Cleanse Thyself Program and sent me their testimonies.

I wish also to thank the medical libraries of the University of Arizona, the University of California at Berkeley, the University of Washington, and the University of California at Stanford, as well as the National Library of Medicine, the Southern Oregon University Library, and the College of the Siskiyous Library for all their assistance.

**Illustrators**

Michelle Fridkin
Tucson, Arizona
(pg. 3-51; 3-52; 3-53; 3-61;
6-138; 8-187; 9-221)

Nadine Aiello
Mt. Shasta, California
(pg. 1-19)

Dr. Leonard Mehlmauer, H.P.
Camarillo, California
(pg. 8-184)

**Photographers**

Pierluigi Marignani, M.D.
Associate Clinical Professor
of Medicine, Yale University
School of Medicine.
New Haven, Connecticut
Office: Ansonia, Connecticut
(pg. 3-88 — 3-94)

Dr. Richard Anderson
Mt. Shasta, California
(pg. 3-58; 3-59; 3-60;
3-85; 8-185)

**Final Editing by G. Renee Getreu**

Published by Triumph
P.O. Box 901
Mt. Shasta, California   96067

# Dedication

This book is dedicated to God; the Creator, the Sustainer and the Source of All Life, and to all the Sons and Daughters of God who have purified themselves before us and have come back to help us do likewise. Also, to all the strong, wonderful souls who are willing to purify themselves so that they too can become effective instruments in assisting all life everywhere in obtaining the greatest achievement of all, UNCONDITIONAL LOVE FOR EVERYONE AND EVERYTHING.

This book contains information gathered from my many years of research in the medical and health field, along with related experiences in the realms of the mind, emotions, and the unexpected. It reveals experiences that touch the hem of our fullest potential.

The purpose of this book is to encourage you to clean yourself out and to cultivate the attitudes and habits that allow you to achieve health and joy. This is not medical advice, nor a prescription, just good sense. You clean out your home, you clean out your car, but it is far more important and helpful to your well-being to clean out yourself. To do so involves your consciousness: your mind, emotions and how they manifest in your body.

This book offers powerful tools for cleansing the obstructions that interfere with the natural flow of the greatest and most powerful healing force in existence, the universal energy of Love and Joy. When this force is fully cultivated within us, it opens us into unlimited happiness, abundance, health, strength and peace.

Note: To the very best of my ability, every experience recounted in this book is absolutely true and accurate.

Publication or duplication of this book is prohibited. However, short excerpts of this book may be used without permission from the author. I hope you do use it and help get people healthy!

An important note: To those who have a serious degenerative disease, such as cancer or leukemia, I wish to issue a warning. When people have a disease that can shorten life, it is imperative not to postpone treatment. I have seen people with these kinds of diseases follow an effective cleanse program and have incredible changes in their lives. Their energy increases, pain goes away, and they often feel well, or at least much better. But that does not mean they are well. I have seen some of these people, who then had a wishbone confidence instead of a backbone confidence, postpone the other treatments they so desperately needed. This can be a very deadly mistake. Other treatments may be necessary to go along with it, as well as strict diets and nutrition. The Cleanse Thyself program is not the complete answer to overcoming these deadly diseases although, in my opinion, it may be the most important for a large number of people. The Cleanse Thyself Program is NOT a cancer treatment, it is merely an effective method to help remove toxins from the mind and body.

People with these so-called terminal conditions need to act quickly and never back-slide for a moment. They must be willing to change their lifestyles completely, eat properly, and be on an exact nutritional program. They must be willing to cleanse very deeply on mental and emotional as well as physical levels, and do whatever is necessary to win this difficult battle. They should learn relaxation, and how to direct the mind, body, and emotions. But, probably most important of all they must remove old negative emotions.

I firmly believe that a degenerative disease can be the greatest blessing a person has ever had. **To do whatever is necessary to be victorious over any disease, can greatly assist in the development of the mind and spirit.** To do whatever is necessary to win, can propel that person into an entirely different world of joy, adventure, awareness, and Love. Many people who are in pain and at the threshold of death, and then go on to conquer their disease, become exceedingly grateful for their frightening experience, for they find a completely new way of life. This new life brings them the greatest happiness and peace they have ever known.

**Please consult a qualified physician if you have any serious, chronic or degenerative disease.**

# CHAPTER 1

# CHAPTER 2

## CHAPTER 3

## CHAPTER 4

## CHAPTER 5

# CHAPTER 6

## CHAPTER 7

## CHAPTER 8

# CHAPTER 9

# CHAPTER 10

# CHAPTER 11

# CHAPTER 12

# CHAPTER 13

# CHAPTER 14

# CHAPTER 15

# APPENDICES

**Chapter 1**

# UNIVERSAL REMEDY: PURIFICATION AND LOVE

*"Accept nothing that is unreasonable; discard nothing as unreasonable, without proper examination."*

- Buddha

## The Real Source of Health

The real source of health is the Divine Source, and that source is essentially, LOVE! What holds the atom together? Love. Love is far more than a feeling; it is the cohesive power of the universe. That is why when there is Love, there is birth, growth, construction, healing, and life. Where Love is not, there is destruction, deterioration, decay, and death. Every molecule and every cell is perfect if the feelings penetrating it are Love, joy and delight. Thoughts and feelings less than Love are mutations of the perfect design or the perfect potential. Although this book deals primarily with the physical body, the real causes of disease are negative thoughts and feelings created by a struggling soul. Indeed, our earth is a training ground for aspiring souls. And, the foundations of perfect health are the positive thoughts and feelings, saturated with love, automatically expressed by those who have conquered fear, doubt, and judgment.

We live in a universe that is ruled by exact Law. One of these laws is: the infallible law of cause and effect.[1] In terms of recorded history one of the first to teach this law was Buddha, later Jesus Christ, and many others and on to Isaac Newton who declared it scientific. How does this law apply here? Our thoughts and feelings are potent instruments in the manifestation of specific conditions in our lives. To what part of our lives do these conditions apply? Every part of our lives. In fact, in my opinion, every single thing in existence is a manifestation of thoughts and feelings.

---

[1] That which we sow, is that which we shall reap. For every action, there is an opposite and equal reaction. One of the most serious problems of this world is that people have failed to realize that this law applies to consciousness as well as to the physical.

As sound is solid enough to impress itself upon our ear drums to hear, and light to impress the retina to see, so are thoughts and feelings real and solid within their own octaves, and never fail to impress their energies upon the creative membrane or film of our bodies. They do not dissipate after they are created. Thoughts and feelings seep into the etheric and emotional vehicles of our bodies and then solidify not only into our worlds as conditions or things, but also solidify into our bodies and minds as vibrant health or disease.

**Mind is the Master Power**
that molds and makes.
And man is mind
and forevermore he takes
his tools of thought
and shaping what he wills-
brings forth a thousand joys,
a thousand ills.
He thinks in secret,
and it comes to pass.
Environment
is but his looking glass.

- James Allen, *As a Man Thinketh*

Consider the words of the Master Jesus: "Ye shall pay even the last penny." "That which you sow shall you also reap." "According to your faith it is done unto you." Most of us are affected more by the past than by the Now. Thoughts and feelings of the past constantly seep into our brains, bodies, and environments, producing the cause behind the apparent cause. Man may be unjust, but Nature (God) is not. Through the invisible realms of Spirit, man receives his just rewards. But the good news is, if we are not satisfied with our minds, bodies, and conditions in our worlds as they are, we can choose to "cleanse and purify", think new thoughts, and come into alignment with the divine order of the universe. The key is to remove the old patterns and their manifestations and replace them with patterns of unconditional love towards everybody and everything. The results of such is unending joy, vibrant health, and even bliss. And, achieving this remarkable state of consciousness is within the reach of every single person on earth who is willing to make the choice to do so.

# An Ancient Point of View

## Man, The Son of Mother Earth

I quote from *The Gospel of Peace of Jesus Christ* by the disciple John:[2] Keep in mind that this was written almost 2,000 years ago by one of great wisdom. When it talks about the "Mother," it is referring to Nature and the spiritual forces behind Nature that give life to the earth. It refers also to certain basic laws which mankind has almost entirely forgotten in our modern civilization.

> *"I tell you truly, you are one with the Earthly Mother; she is in you, and you in her. Of her were you born, in her do you live, and to her shall you return again. Keep, therefore, her laws, for none can live long, neither be happy, but he who honors his Earthly Mother and does her laws. I tell you truly, should you fail to keep but one only of all these laws, should you harm, but one only of all your body's members, you shall be utterly lost in your grievous sickness and there shall be weeping and gnashing of teeth.* **I tell you, unless you follow the laws of your Mother, you can in no wise escape death. And he who clings to the laws of his Mother, to him shall his Mother cling also.** *She shall heal all his plagues, and he shall never become sick. She gives him long life, and protects him from all afflictions; from fire, from water, from the bite of venomous serpents. For your Mother bore you, keeps life within you. She has given you her body, and none but she heals you. Happy is he who loves his Mother and lies quietly in her bosom. For your Mother loves you, even when you turn away from her. And how much more shall she love you, if you turn to her again? I tell you truly, very great is her love, greater than the greatest of mountains, deeper than the deepest seas. And those who love their Mother, she never deserts them. As the hen protects her chickens, as the lioness her cubs, as the mother her*

---

[2] The American version is called, *The Essene Gospel of Peace*. The original Hebrew and Aramaic Texts were translated and edited by Edmond Bordeaux Szekely. He had found this ancient manuscript in the secret archives of the Vatican. It is an exceptionally beautiful book to read. It is a story about Jesus and John when they went into the hills and found a group of very sick people. Instead of healing them, he taught them how to heal themselves, what to eat and what not to eat, and just what to do to be well.

*newborn babe, so does the Earthly Mother protect the son of Man from all danger and from all evils."*

## Slaves of Desire and Attachments

How firmly attached are we to our desires - our desires for food, drink, entertainment, and social life? How firmly are we attached to relationships, moods, fear, anger, guilt, or anything that might distract us from living the laws of life, including Love, non-judgment and trust, that bring us health, happiness, and success? Listen to these words of wisdom and perhaps we can also call them prophecy. For very few have escaped from experiencing the following:

*"For I tell you truly, evils and dangers innumerable lie in wait for the Sons of Men. Beelzebub[3], the prince of all devils, the source of every evil, lies in wait in the body of all the Sons of Men. He is death, the lord of every plague, and taking upon him a pleasing raiment, (which may be hamburgers and coke) he tempts and entices the Sons of Men. Riches does he promise, and power, and splendid palaces, and garments of gold and silver, and a multitude of servants, all these; he promises renowned glory, fornication and lustfulness, gluttony and wine-bibbing, riotous living, and slothfulness and idle days. **And he entices every one by that to which their heart is most inclined.**"* (Oh, did he get us on that one!)

## The Wages of Attachments are Death

*"And in the day that the Sons of Men have already become the slaves of all these vanities and abominations (slaves to our own thoughts, lusts, desires, appetites, fears, self-pity, resentments, hates, and other habits), then in payment thereof he snatches from the Sons of Men all those things which the Earthly Mother gave them so abundantly. He takes from them their breath"* (smokers beware), *"their blood"* (cancer & leukemia and other blood disorders), *"their bone"*

---

[3] Beelzebub, may be a word describing the attachment of desires. It could also be defined as judgement based upon selfish desire, fear, or lack of trust in the Divine. Can you see the association of each of these concepts and how they all corrupt?

*(arthritis & osteoporosis), "their flesh" (eczema, rashes, leprosy), "their bowels" (ulcers, constipation, colitis, and cancer of the bowels, etc.), "their eyes and their ears" (Know anyone who wears glasses or hearing aids - is blind or deaf?). "And the breath of the Son of Man becomes short and stifled, full of pain and evil-smelling, like the breath of unclean beasts." (What is your breath like in the morning? - use mouth wash? Can you run without getting out of breath?) "And his blood becomes thick and evil smelling, like the water of the swamps; it clots and blackens, like the night of death."[4] (Most people are shocked to see their blood under a microscope.) "And his bone becomes hard and knotted;" (Mother, listen, it's your arthritis.) "it melts away within and breaks asunder (osteoporosis), as a stone falling down upon a rock. And his flesh waxes fat and watery;" (Who's overweight in America?) "it rots and putrefies, with scabs and boils that are an abomination. And his bowels become full with abominable filthiness, with oozing streams of decay; and multitudes of abominable worms have their habitation there." (And they knew about it way back then - think about it! Why haven't medical doctors learned about this? Too bad they didn't have the Cleanse Thyself Program 2,000 years ago!) "And his eyes grow dim, till dark night enshrouds them, and his ears become stopped, like the silence of the grave. And last of all shall the erring Son of Man lose life. **For he kept not the laws of his Mother**, and added sin to sin. Therefore, are taken from him all the gifts of the Earthly Mother: breath, blood, bone, flesh, bowels, eyes and ears, and after all else, life, with which the Earthly Mother crowned his body."*

Could this have been a prophecy of the 20th century?

---

[4] If you want to see what eating flesh does to the blood, see the video, *Diet For a New America: Your Health, Your Planet*, hosted by John Robbins. 1 (800) 765-7890. A man ate a hamburger. Afterwards a sample of his blood was put into a vial and left to set for several hours. It turned thick, icky yellow, and oily. Get the video and see it for yourself.

# The Way Out

*"But if the erring son of Man be sorry for his sins and undo them,"* (to undo them is to cleanse and purify the thoughts, emotions, habits, and our bodies) *"and return again to his Earthly Mother; and if he do his Earthly Mother's laws and free himself from Satan's clutches"* (the activities of negative thinking, feeling and habit - the human ego), *"resisting his temptation,* **then does the Earthly Mother receive again her erring Son with love and sends him her angels that they may serve him. I tell you truly, when the son of Man resists the Satan that dwells in him and does not his will, in the same hour are found the mother's angels there, that they may serve him with all their power and free utterly the Son of Man from the power of Satan."*

Could it be that "Satan" refers to mankind's misuse of his/her creative power of thoughts and feelings, all based upon the attachments of selfish desires?[5] And that the "Mother's angels" are the healthy use of mankind's creative power of thoughts and feelings? Be it symbolic as I have suggested, or actually an evil or Divine being, matters little - the results are the same.

*"For no man can serve two masters. For either he serves Beelzebub and his devils or else he serves our Earthly Mother and her angels. Either he serves death or he serves life. I tell you truly, happy are those that do the laws of life and wander not upon the paths of death. For in them the forces of life wax strong and they escape the plagues of death."*

# Today's Reality

**Our bodies are supposed to be the temples of the Living God. Instead they have become seething, smelly cesspools that house fermenting, putrefying, rotting death.** There are two main causes: 1) the negatively-charged energy of our thoughts and feelings which physically solidifies in the cells of our bodies in the form of toxins, and 2) energy draining "dead" and toxic foods and drink we have taken which reflect and

---

[5] When you stop and really think about it, almost everything that has been said about Satan can be applied to the human ego. It is the human ego that truly competes with God and says; "My will be done." It is the thoughts of ego that create the desires and attachments that get us into trouble.

reinforce negative thought and feeling. You may prove this to yourself as you cleanse your body. For the deeper you cleanse the toxins from your body, the more memories, thoughts, feelings, desires, tastes, and smells from the past come to your awareness. Some remembrances will come back very vividly even though you had totally forgotten them. Many times when I would be giving talks to groups, I ask those who have accomplished my cleansing program to raise their hand if they had experienced old memories, thoughts, and feelings surfacing while cleansing. Better than 80% of the cleansers raise their hands.

The standard American diet, followed by a large percentage of Americans, is deficient in critical electrolytes as well as trace minerals. Due to this, plus emotional and environmental factors, most Americans today have become so over-acid, as a result of electrolyte deficiencies, that their bodies have been forced to create massive amounts of mucus as protection against the acids, especially in the intestines. In many cases, this mucus, and the poisons contained within it, have been there since they were children - in some cases, babies. **As this old substance breaks up, you may recall incidents that occurred a long time ago.** Many temporarily feel the emotions they were feeling when they ate something years ago. How many people do you know, who, when emotionally upset, "pigged out" on ice cream, candy, or foods they knew were not good for them, etc.? I wish we could all remember exactly what we ate during these periods of extreme stress. **All my research indicates that as long as the vibratory energy vortices of negative emotions, thoughts, or desires are still within us, our minds and bodies will be patterned by them.**

Almost every basic science course demonstrates the geometric patterns of vibration. Placing black sand upon a plate and then subjecting the plate to any constant vibration, the sand takes on specific geometric patterns. **Change the frequency of the vibration and the geometric patterns of the sand change with it.** It is nothing but the natural physical expression of energy and vibration. **Similarly, our thoughts and feelings emit specific waves (like radio waves) of energy and vibration that influence the patterns within our bodies.** The patterns of negative thought and feeling automatically create physical patterns that result in disease. **The patterns of love and joy automatically create physical patterns that result in health, strength, and vitality.**

**Like energized recorded tapes, capable of sending out messages over and over again, thoughts and feelings remain within our minds and bodies, and attract the substances which store the patterns that accurately reflect those messages.** It is only a matter of time and these messages manifest in our physiological structures. If they are positive, helpful, strengthening, vitalizing, then let us keep them and reinforce them. However, if they are negative, weakening, de-vitalizing, and disease-causing, then let us remove them or transform them into patterns that help bring us the goals we desire. This is what this book is all about: **to help you see how you can remove these disease-causing patterns.** Many therapists attempt to help their patients to remove negative patterns via the mind, and it is a long and difficult process that seldom produces the desired result, because they fail to remove the thoughts and feelings that are stuck at the physical level. Hence, neurotic[6] people fight a tough battle if they never cleanse; but once the substance anchoring those emotions is removed, many have testified that the old emotions do indeed lose their power.

*"At the end of the Power Phase, after releasing feet of accumulated "Dark Green Rubber" and years of held in stress and emotional pain, I feel ready to really live. Thank you!" - Genevieve Gowman, San Francisco, CA*

To a certain degree, emotions are stored in cell tissue throughout every area of our bodies, but I believe a major amount of negative consciousness is stored in the unnatural mucin accumulations (mucoid plaque) in the stomach, small intestine, and the colon. Fortunately, this mucoid plaque is the easiest to extract. After we have cleansed out the plaque from the digestive tract, it comes more easily within our reach to release negative consciousness from the rest of the body. Then the potential of becoming "super-human" beings may also come within our reach.

# A Problem With Eating Meat

You may now have an insight about benefits gained by the great spiritual geniuses of antiquity through their committed practice of fasting. It was by intelligent design that Jesus, Buddha, and others fasted for 40 days and more before they obtained the awareness and ability to accomplish their work. As long as the accumulated negative consciousness remains within, heavy burdens hold us low. Perhaps herein is also the key to why no great spiritual genius would eat meat - it would stand to reason that

---

[6] W. R. Hensyl, ed., *Stedman's Medical Dictionary*, 25th Edition, (Baltimore, MD: Williams & Wilkins, 1991) : "**Neurosis**: Emotional maladjustment that may impair thinking and judgment but causes minimal loss of contact with reality." "**Obsessive-compulsive neurosis**. Disorder marked by the persistent intrusion of unwanted ideas and the compulsion to perform repetitive acts." I doubt if there is anyone on this planet who hasn't had these troubles to some degree or another. Some degree of sickness is a way of life for most people, but restoring health is possible.

negative feelings of fear, hate, resentment, and death vibrate throughout the animal as it is being murdered.  Who would want to assimilate that?

It took one year after I quit eating meat and several fasts before I could rid myself of subtle,  but disturbing negative feelings and the seeming inability to find peace within.  After that I steadily became more and more aware of many things, which previously I could not perceive.  This should make obvious why we should never eat when our negative feelings are stirred up.  Refuse to do so from here on out!  If you're still a meat-eater and think you are happy, give up meat-eating for a year-and-a-half, cleanse or fast a few times, and you will find a peace and happiness you never knew existed.  But even more than that, many people find that their perceptional awareness expands beyond anything they previously experienced.  Not only that, but many will learn more about how to love, for **the willingness to murder the innocent for the unnecessary gluttony of animal flesh ingestion and for the selfish appeasement of habits and appetite, is in direct opposition to a loving heart**.

The kind of love I am talking about is not what is commonly thought of by most people.  The Hindus have studied this subject in depth and have identified over 500 different kinds of love.  I am not talking about the love someone has for a delicious meal, or the lust one may feel for any physical pleasure.  More like the love we have for our children;  an unconditional love that sweetens everything in our lives.  Imagine the love you feel for your most favorite person,  perhaps your mate, parent, or dog. Now imagine how you would feel if you were able to double the intensity of your love.  Imagine how you would feel if you could feel that way towards everyone you met, everything you saw, and even every situation you experienced.  Now increase it all by ten.  Can you imagine the ecstatic bliss this would bring you?  Imagine how people, animals and other life forms would respond to you.  Every problem, every ache and pain, would be smothered into insignificance by this overwhelming love, and this love is what heals.  This is what I am taking about and it is within the reach of every intelligent person on this planet.  There is a way to allow this to happen, and the main purpose of this book is to give you tools that will help you achieve this incredibly lofty state.

Consider the many ways we block the experience of unconditional love - often unconsciously.  For example, **how can we ever expect healing or continued health when we willingly choose to steal the life of another creature for our own selfish gain, for indeed, we reap what we sow - for every action there is an opposite and equal reaction**.  It is through loving acts that we can optimally sustain and enhance our own life force.  It is only through an abundance of love that the Universe can flow through us, and truly heal us.  St. Paul said; "The last enemy to overcome is death."[7] He points the way. Love. "Love thine enemies as thyself, and bless them that curse you. Thou shalt love thy neighbor as thyself." Indeed, incredibly potent Biblical guidelines serve as a gauge revealing to us just how close we are to freedom, joy, and perfect health. The teachers of every great religion say the same thing. Yet, most people can't even love their own selves. When we truly know what the self is, we will find it includes all life - even animals, for we are life and that life will move us to honor itself, in every form. **Love is giving, not stealing. Love is assisting, not murder, and love should be for all life, not just humans**. It is the only thing that can give us freedom from our own self-created limitations.

Two cells, one from mother and the other from father, connect during conception and thus begins the magic of birth. Contained within those two cells is the Divine Intelligence which governs all the anatomical, physiological, chemical, and psychological processes that produce these incredible bodies. Love is the essence of Divine energy. Always contained within that same energy that built our bodies is the same intelligence which knows how to sustain our bodies. Not only that; it automatically purifies, heals, strengthens, protects and perfects everything that is open to it.

# Mind, the Great Governor of Health and Disease

*"Disease will never be cured or eradicated by present materialistic methods, for the simple reason that disease in its origin is not material. Disease is in essence the*

---

[7] *The Holy Bible*, Corinthians 15:26. (King James Version)
Scientifically, death by old age is a mystery. Our bodies replace injured and dying cells very rapidly. Within one year more than 90% of all our cells have been replaced with new ones, so why do we age? Evidence that physiological deterioration is under the direction of the mind and feelings is becoming stronger all the time. The reason that people scoff at the possibility of overcoming death may be nothing but a programming of society. There are many historical references to people who lived to be several hundreds of years old and maintained perfectly healthy bodies. There are forces that have a major influence upon the general public and upon Christianity that try to deny this reality. And these forces do not want people to think about these things. However, the knowlege of how death can be overcome - its exact procedure - is available to those who search deeply enough. Accomplishing it is another story.

*result of conflict between Soul and Mind, and will never be eradicated except by spiritual and mental effort."*

- Edward Bach, M.B., B.S., D.P.H., Creator of Bach Flower Remedies.

Conflict is an activity of separation from the oneness of life, wherein judgment, criticism and fear replace love. It is always associated with not trusting that the Infinite (God) is in control. It is the automatic result of doubt and fear acting instead of trust and love. It is a confirmation that "Thy will be done" has been replaced with "my will be done" - an act that gets us in trouble every time. For when there is only love, there is harmony, peace, joy, power, and trust.

## Modern Evidence of the Body-Mind Connection

*A clinical study: Scientists took the saliva from a man who was in a rage and had it analyzed in a lab. The analysis revealed the composition of his saliva matched the composition of a rattlesnake's venom. Then they took the saliva and injected some of it into small animals, and each one died.*[8]

---

[8] Hal Huggins, D.D.S., M.S., ed., *The Price of Root Canals*. This book is available from Dr. Huggins office at (719) 522-0566 in Colorado Springs, CO. See the section on research by Winston Price, D.D.S. Dr. Price, head researcher for the American Medical Association for more than 17 years, did a similar thing with root canals. **He would take root canal teeth out of a patient's mouth and place them just under the skin of rabbits. Interestingly, they either died within 48 hours or they would develop cysts around the tooth.** Later, he would use only a very tiny piece of the tooth so it wouldn't kill the rabbit, and **the rabbits would take on the same exact diseases the tooth donor had.** One example was with Doctor Price's own son. After his son had died of a heart attack, Dr. Price removed the root canal tooth and placed part of it under the skin of 30 different rabbits. Each of them died of a heart attack. Later he found that deadly bacteria lives in the dentum of teeth that have root canals. A living healthy tooth is able to resist the bacteria, but when the tooth dies, as in a root canal, the tooth environment changes and is no longer able to resist the bacterial growth. Could these bacteria cause various diseases throughout the human body? The key here is the lack of life force in the tooth. When any animal body dies, it rapidly decays and is 'dissolved' by bacteria. What's the difference between a dead body and a living body? Life force energy. Life force may be the most critical factor in vibrant health and disease-free living.

Every single thought and feeling has an effect upon the chemistry of all our glands, hormones, nervous system. There is no question whether this is true or not, the only question is, to what degree? Is it possible that our emotions can trigger glands to modify hormones in such a way that they can alter the chemistry of our saliva, or other bodily fluids in a way that creates deadly poisons?

*Psychologist **Daniel Goleman** studied a child named **Timmy who experienced about 11 separate personalities**. One of these personalities was allergic to orange juice and would break out in hives after consuming orange juice. If Timmy (main personality), drinks orange juice there is no problem. However, if Timmy drinks orange juice and the personality who is allergic to it takes over the body while the juice is still being digested, then hives develop quickly. Now get this, if Timmy comes back while the allergic reaction is present, the itching of the hives will immediately cease, and the blisters will begin to subside.*

Studies with Multiple Personality Disorders (MPD) patients reveal more belief shattering facts. It was found that with patients who experienced multi-personalities that each personality expressed different physiological responses and traits even though they all shared the same body.

*For an example one personality, sharing the same body, has diabetes, another does not. When one personality with diabetes is in control, the body chemistry reveals this serious disease.[9] When another personality without the consciousness that produces diabetes takes over, then all chemical and psychological symptoms disappear within minutes.*

What's the significance of the above cases? **The same body demonstrates startling physical changes when the only changed factors are differences are in attitudes, feelings and beliefs. One set of emotional profiles allows health, the other creates disease.**

---

[9] Deepak Chopra, D.M.D., *Quantum Healing*, (New York, NY, Bantam Books, 1989), pg. 122-123. Is diabetes really a serious disease? Tibetan doctors apparently do not think so. They never give their patients insulin. Going to the doctor once is all that is necessary, for they are given herbs, told how to change their diet, and if they follow these directions, they get over it. For more information, see the video, *Tibetan Medicine*. May be ordered (or special ordered) from Greenleaf - (800) 905-8367. They must order from the wholesaler: New Leaf.

**Sir William Osler**[10], a famous Canadian doctor and medical historian, said that **the outcome of tuberculosis had more to do with what went on in a patient's mind** than what went on in his lungs.

*I am reminded about the **first "documented AIDS survivor"**. He was told by his friendly, good-intentioned medical doctor, that he would die in 6 months. He **chose** to feel depression and hopelessness. Almost immediately after he **chose** to feel negative emotions his body developed Kaposis Sarcoma.[11] However, he began to meditate and practice visualization, and he went on and survived.[12]*

Have you ever heard of **psychological dwarfism**, seemingly caused by parent hostility? This is a condition where growth of a child has been severely stunted. The hostility causes the child to feel rejected, which then develops into "little" self esteem. It was found that **this variety of stress shuts off the growth hormone**[13], **somatotropin**,[14] **produced by the pituitary gland.** Not only does this variety of stress inhibit natural growth, but it also causes unusual behavior problems such as: bizarre eating habits[15], depression, self-mutilation, sleep disturbances, lack of response to pain, enuresis, encopresis, and poor performance on cognitive tests. This condition seems to be related to a negative mother-child

---

[10] Bernie Siegel, M.D., *Love, Medicine and Miracles*, (New York, NY: Harper and Row Publishers, 1986), pg. 2.

[11] *Stedman's Medical Dictionary:* "Kaposis Sarcoma: A multifocal malignant neoplasm (cancer), occurring in the skin and sometimes in lymph nodes or viscera. Most common in men over 60 and with AIDS patients."

[12] Siegel, pg. 39-40.

[13] D. Skuse, A.. Albanese, R. Stanhope, J. Gilmore, L. Voss, "A New Stress-related Syndrome of Growth Failure and Hyperphagia in Children, Associated with Reversibility of Growth Hormone Insufficiency," *Lancet*, 1996; Vol. 348(9024), pg. 353-356.

[14] S. E. Mouridsen, S. Nielsen, "Reversible Somatotrophin Deficiency (Psychological Dwarfism) Presenting as Conduct Disorder and Growth Hormone Deficiency," *Developmental Medicine and Child Neurology*, 1990; 32(12), pg. 1093-1098.

[15] I've noticed over the years that when people become emotionally imbalanced, they tend to eat food that is not good for them. Knowing the standard American diet, it makes one wonder if most Americans are emotionally imbalanced.

relationship.    Fortunately, however, positive changes in the child's environment will usually correct all the symptoms, even the IQ deficits and delayed puberty.

Experimental evidence reveals that **emotions such as grief, guilt, feelings of failure, resentment, and suppressed anger produce** *oversecretion* **of the same hormones that suppress the immune system.** Can we reverse this by activating emotions of joy, forgiveness, success, love, etc.?

*Shlomo Brezntz[16], a psychologist at the Hebrew University in Jerusalem, proved that positive and negative expectations have opposite effects on blood levels of two hormones (cortisone and prolactin) that are important in activating the immune system.*

Is everyone who has a dysfunctional immune system harboring negative expectations, perhaps subconsciously? Probably.

*A cancer patient who was expected to die within 6 months had dropped to 95 pounds. He was taught how to visualize his white blood cells eating his cancer. This visualizing activity has several benefits.   1.   It stimulates the most powerful immune builder known: hope!   Hope is a very positive expectation and this activity leads to a second benefit, as follows.   2.   Hope stimulates the exact hormones which activate the immune system.   In 30 days he was completely free of cancer.*

It is a known fact that **depressed men are twice more likely to get cancer than happy men.** It is known also that cancer is associated with grief and depression, as well as with a lack of emotional expression or "holding it all in," as in cases of suppressed anger.

A medical doctor visited me in my office a few months ago. Somehow we got on the subject of breast cancer. He was telling me how he has seen so many **women with breast cancer take both hands, hold them out just in front of their breasts, and as they were saying: "I just hold everything in"**, they would draw their hands out in front of them as though they were grabbing something and then pulling it towards their breasts. He said that he has talked with other doctors who said the same

---

[16] Siegel, pg. 29.

thing. Interestingly, last week I just saw another woman with breast cancer do the very same thing.

> *M. R. Jensen found that breast cancer spread fastest among women who had repressed personalities, felt hopeless, and were unable to express anger, fear, and other negative emotions. Similar findings have emerged for rheumatoid arthritis, asthma, etc.*

Studies have shown consistently that emotional trauma exists behind every disease, even with children.

> *A study done by Albert Einstein College of Medicine revealed 31 of 33 leukemia children had experienced a traumatic loss or move within 2 years of getting leukemia.*

Every cancer patient that I have associated with has proven to have serious, deep-seated, unresolved emotional patterns. Often it can be traced back to childhood experiences, or to a divorce, or long term emotional suppression. Animals also appear to be affected by emotions similar to humans.

> *One study revealed that lab rats who were prematurely separated from mothers were found to be more susceptible to cancer. Another clinical study on mice proved interesting.* **Researchers had developed specially bred mice to be susceptible to breast cancer and they were able to vary the rate of cancer 7 to 92% by controlling their stress levels.**

Suppose we learned to control our stress levels? Could it be that we would stop the disease process or even reverse it? Could we even slow down the aging process?

**Dr. Deepak Chopra, M. D., said; "We are the only creatures on earth who can change our biology by what we think and feel."[17]** If we change our thinking, can we un-create disease? That is not exactly the way it works. But, if we change the way we feel and think, and eliminate the negative consciousness that is stuck at the cell level, *that* may work! There is no doubt that we can un-create disease. And if we can un-create disease, then certainly we can create or mold our bodies and minds into achieving perfect or at least better health.

---

[17] Deepak Chopra, M.D., *Ageless Body, Timeless Mind*, (New York, NY: Harmony Books, 1994), pg. 4.

Chopra also noted: **"If you want to change your body, change your awareness first."**[18] "Belief creates biology."[19] **"We are no longer in doubt about the fact that invisible wisps of thought and emotion alter the fundamental chemistry of every cell."**[20] Did we hear that right? Thoughts and emotion alter the fundamental chemistry of every cell! Things are changing. Highly intelligent and empathic M.D.s are beginning to speak out. This awareness opens the door of new possibilities. We need to learn the fundamentals of saturating our bodies with love.

Bernie Siegel, M.D. was also convinced that changing the mind changes the body through the central nervous system, endocrine, and immune systems. He said that **the most fundamental problem most patients have is the inability to love themselves.**[21]

*Bernie Siegel, M.D. points out in his book, **Love, Medicine and Miracles**, that women with advanced breast cancer doubled their survival time by using group therapy and auto hypnotic techniques.*[22,23]

An important guideline to gauge how much we love ourselves is to ask ourselves how much we really love others. If we do not love others, it is impossible to love ourselves, and if we cannot love ourselves, we really do not know ourselves.

*The USA and Japan have been conducting research on spontaneous cures of cancer. It is a known fact that **both small and extremely large masses of tumors can disappear and have disappeared virtually overnight.** Researchers have found that **just before the cure appears, almost every patient experiences a dramatic shift in awareness.** That shift in awareness reveals itself as a knowing for certain that they will be healed. Achieving this state is one of the major keys in*

---

[18] Chopra, pg. 37.

[19] Ibid., pg. 56.

[20] Ibid., pg. 118.

[21] Siegel, main premise of the book.

[22] Ibid., pg. XI.

[23] If these same people had deeply cleansed their bodies, eaten a perfect diet and used powerful, natural supplements, they might all be alive today!

*achieving spontaneous healing. Its success depends upon: 1) removing the negative thought forms, patterns, emotions, and habits, and 2) replacing them with attitudes of success, confidence, joy, love and trust, etc.*

Our own research indicates that love is the great key. When we understand that love is the natural state of our beings and **when love is not flowing through our beings every moment, then some other emotion or concept is interfering.** These interferences are usually emotions of great intensity or some quirk in our point of view, such as the habit of judging conditions, things or people in negative ways, and most of the time they are unconscious. One of the activities we all need to initiate, is to **remove these conscious and unconscious negative emotions so that love may flow freely through us.** Herein lies one of the most important points in this book.

There is a residue, a substance that attaches itself to our cells and organs and causes malfunctions. I will call it "emotional plaque". It is not visible to physical sight, and we cannot see it under the microscope, but it is there nevertheless.[24] **It is like a magnet, in that it attracts toxic physical substance to it which appears to be the physical cause of disease.** But the main point is, **mucus and toxins are held in place by this undetected residue created by negative consciousness.** This emotional plaque contains consciousness in the form of unconscious memories, attitudes and feelings. Like a radio wave, it continues to send out messages, and draws to itself conditions similar to its own nature. Create enough of these and you will have habits. Habits create consistency and consistency creates persistent manifestation. **The greatest downfall in medicine is the failure to recognize this emotional plaque and the lack of knowledge of how to remove it.** And how do we remove it? By first eliminating judgment, refining true discernment, focusing on the beauty in life, practicing gratitude, appreciation, kindness and love, while at the same

---

[24] Chinese acupuncturists have mapped energy meridians in the human body. They use needles to help unblock the energy meridians that have become blocked. Scientists and doctors have learned the effectiveness of their techniques. There isn't any doubt about it, it works! But medical science has not discovered any physiological evidence as to why. *Yet, in my opinion, the effects have proven to be so obvious, that there is little doubt that acupuncture theories are true.* What is this substance that blocks the meridians? I assert that it is "emotional plaque" stuck in the etheric body. How do I know? There are those who have the sight to see it. When several people have this ability and they all see the same thing independently, you can learn to identify what it is, where it is, where it comes from, and then remove it.

time cleansing the body and feeding it pure foods. These are the fundamental techniques required. As we practice them, we will discover further techniques which will carry us to our goal. For the more love that flows through us, the more intelligence that also flows through us, and the more energy and life force that flows through us. Developing greater awareness allows us to pick up on the intelligence of love and use it.

**It is the power of love that strengthens, heals, and maintains**. It is this emotional plaque residue that blocks our natural flow of love. **Anything less than love needs to be released, and transformed into love. The most powerful immune systems will always be in bodies flowing with love.** On the contrary, the weakest immune systems are in bodies overloaded with hurts, hates, fears, guilts, resentments, angers, etc.

## How the Mind Influences our Chemistry

Everything we see, feel, touch, hear, experience, think, interpret, respond to, or judge, causes glands to secrete hormones and nerves to be stimulated. How does all this work? How does the body respond to our interpretation of events and environmental inputs? Here is the scientific explanation.

Science considers **nerves to be electrical messengers and hormones to be chemical messengers of the body.** They transmit information necessary for the regulation of the metabolic functions of all organs and cells. Through the hypothalamus, thoughts and feelings stimulate nerves and glands in specific ways. The ear drum receives vibrations of sound and transmutes the sound into mental awareness. Similarly, light vibrations are transmuted into mental images by the retina of our eyes. We can think of the hypothalamus as delicate membranes similar to those in the retina and ear drums, but with a much more intricate activity. Here mental and emotional vibrations affect the hypothalamus in a manner that causes hormonal secretions and nerve stimuli. The degree of feeling and variety of thought, determines how much and what variety of hormones will be produced. It has become obvious that our minds can alter hormones. Yes, **we tailor-make our hormones; they are perfectly designed by the intensity and types of thoughts and feelings that we create.** Nerves stimulate glands and organs in specific ways, and glands create hormones in specific ways which alter fluid chemistry and **virtually control every physiological activity in our bodies**. It has been proven on a scientific level that our bodies are indeed, an extension of our consciousness.

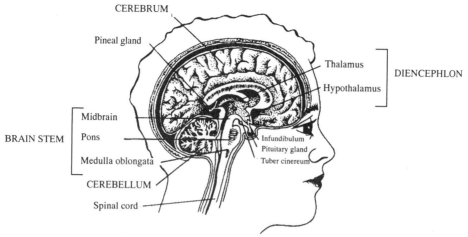

CEREBRUM

Pineal gland

Thalamus

DIENCEPHLON

Hypothalamus

Midbrain

BRAIN STEM    Pons

Infundibulum
Pituitary gland
Tuber cinereum

Medulla oblongata

CEREBELLUM

Spinal cord

MEDIAL ASPECT OF THE BRAIN IN SAGITTAL SECTION

## Attention is the Key

When we understand the degree to which our thoughts and emotions affect our bodies, we begin to understand how critical it is to focus our mental and emotional attention in a manner that is life supporting or at least favorable to our goals in life.

*We become that upon which we put our attention.*
*"...God if thou seest God, dust if thou seest dust."*

- Anonymous

You can see that what we have been conditioned to believe about our bodies and ourselves is not a reality. **We have been programmed** into believing that our bodies become diseased, usually by outside enemies known as germs. **Many medical doctors tell their patients that their disease is not their fault and is not their responsibility.** It is a clever and subtle programming, adopted by society and those who seek to manipulate and control. The impact of this programming is to **cause us to deny our own potential**. It proclaims that we are not in control but that we are victims of uncontrollable situations and invisible organisms. **It denies our own innate ability to correct our lives and heal ourselves.** This is the exact opposite of what the patient needs to hear.

For if we believe that we are not responsible and that we had **nothing to do with acquiring the disease, then we automatically proclaim that we have no power to change it; therefore why bother to try** - and that is the downfall of millions of people. The truth is, we are responsible and just as we created an undesirable condition we can also un-create it and make it better. For **it is consciousness - our personalities,**

1-19

the beliefs we hold about ourselves, our basic mental points of view, our emotional habits, which govern our physiology. Germs and disease are automatic results of inner causes. It is this consciousness that we have created that controls every chemical action inside and outside of every cell in our bodies. All we need to do is learn the *Laws Of Life*, practice using the *Laws Of Life*, and Cleanse and Purify ourselves, and we will alter not only our bodies, but everything in our lives as well. And there are ways to greatly speed this process up.

This book takes us to the first step in dramatically and rapidly changing our lives for the better. I hope to show you what you can do to begin eliminating the negative conditions you've created in the past and to begin to reprogram your habits, thoughts and feeling states to achieve the health and happiness you deserve.

# Seven Keys to Overcoming Disease

## Mental Keys

### KEY 1: Stop the Energetic Cause of Disease

The **first KEY** in overcoming disease is to *put a stop to its cause*. This should always begin **by eliminating the source of the habits and acts of creating negative thoughts and feelings which are the original cause of disease.** It is simply a choice, but most of us acquired habits based upon the influence of others which became the way of least resistance. Unfortunately, we've all created strong habits following the course of least resistance and because of this, it is more difficult to change. The decreasing health of our bodies and the undesirable experiences in our lives begin with thoughts and feelings such as hate, anger, criticism, condemnation, judgment, blame, self-pity, jealousy, resentment, depression, and guilt. Each of these feelings and their related thoughts have specific influences on our glands and nerves which result in the production of poisonous chemical compounds. Who can afford to have such degraded poisons in their lives? Good health requires not only the practice of abstaining from negative emotions, but also continual cultivation of joyful thoughts and loving feelings. This does not mean that we should suppress or deny our emotions; it means to root out their causes and replace them with new archetypes that produce Love.

## KEY 2:  Practice Appreciation and Trust

The **second KEY is ESSENTIAL, and that is to seriously and enthusiastically practice appreciation, joy** *and Love* **- for all life unconditionally.**  Love, peace, harmony, gratitude, and praise trigger positive hormonal and nerve influences - expanding the life, energy, and light in the body; bringing vitality and happiness.  **For these states of consciousness purify and strengthen the life force within us.  We will also greatly benefit by practicing trust:  trust and faith in ourselves, trust in the laws of life, and in the Divine Intelligence which flows through us and everything else in the Universe.  Anyone who doubts in the Divine Intelligence obviously has been searching in the wrong places, or listening to the wrong words.  Ask to be shown the truth and prepare for the avalanche of unending knowledge which opens one door after another.**[25]

## Physical Keys

*"Disease symptoms are an effort of the body to eliminate waste, mucus, and toxemia. This system assists Nature in the most perfect and natural way. Not the disease but the body is to be healed; it must be cleansed, freed from waste and foreign matter, from mucus and toxemia accumulated since childhood." - Professor Arnold Ehret.*

## KEY 3:  Remove Congestion and Toxins

The third KEY toward overcoming disease is to *remove congestion and toxins from the body, mind, and emotions.  Many toxic substances have lodged deep within our bodies.*  Some health professionals choose to address the local area of obvious trouble alone (symptoms).  But, as Dr. Bernard Jensen likes to say, "If you step on a cat's tail, it's the other end that yells!"  For there is no single part of the body that is not affected by the other parts.  Intestinal cleansing is perhaps one of the most important systems for healing and bringing energy back into our minds and bodies, for not only is it the fastest and safest way to remove massive amounts of

---

[25] Ask, and it shall be given you; seek, and ye shall find; knock, and it shall be opened unto you. From: *The Holy Bible*: Matthew 7:7.  But don't settle for anyone else's opinion. Go deep, deep within. Demand to know the truth. Demand proof! And then prove it.

toxins and poisons from our bodies, giving rapid relief to vital organs and body elements, such as the liver, kidneys, heart, the blood, lymph, nerves and glands, but it is a method that can greatly assist in removing old negative and suppressed emotions as well. So, all congestion and toxins must be removed and it begins with a change of the mind and heart.

## KEY 4:  Stop Eating Harmful Foods

The **fourth KEY** toward perfect health of the body is to *stop eating "foods" that are dead, deficient, processed or toxic*, for they cause mucus, excess acid, more toxins, and congestion (especially congestion of the intestinal tract). More on this later.

## KEY 5:  Supply Needed Elements

The **fifth KEY** toward lasting health is to *supply the body with the needed elements of organically grown foods,*[26] *clean air, pure water,*[27] *alkaline minerals, and massive doses of Love and joy.*

---

[26] Tests have shown that organically grown foods have twice the nutritional elements as the foods in regular supermarkets. Source: Robert F. Heltman, "Organic Food Is More Nutritious," *Townsend Letter for Doctors & Patients*, 1997; Nov.; Issue # 172; pg. 12. I do not believe that it is possible to maintain good health when eating the commerically grown foods people buy at regular supermarkets. Purchasing organically grown produce is essential, but better than that, eat organically grown produce out of your own garden. There is a major difference.

[27] Water without chlorine, fluoride or other poisonous contaminants. Chlorinated water is assocated with cancer of the gastrointestinal tract and urinary tract. M. Koivusalo; Rev. T. Vartianinen, "Drinking Water Chlorination By-Products and Cancer," *Environmental Health,* 1997; Apr-Jun; 12(2), pg. 81-90. Chlorine has also been linked to breast and colon cancer, low sperm counts, decreased testosterone levels and libido, suppression of the immune system, thyroid dysfunction, diabetes, birth defects and other cancers. See "Chlorine, Human Health and the Environment: The Breast Cancer Warning," A Greenpeace report. 1436 U Street NW, Washington DC 20009, (202) 462-1177.

## KEY 6: Rebuild Organs and Glands

The **sixth KEY** is to *rebuild the body's organs and glands*. This means to rebuild the digestive function after we have cleansed it, and to cleanse and rebuild the liver, kidneys, spleen, and the glandular system. It means also to strengthen the heart, lungs, and muscles. However, this cannot be successfully accomplished unless we first transform suppressed emotions and have made progress in removing the toxins and congestion from the bowel and the rest of the body.

## KEY 7: Exercise

The **seventh key** is to *exercise* on a regular basis. This means to exercise hard enough to sweat and pump the lungs and heart vigorously at least two times a week or more.

> The degree to which we follow these seven KEYS will be reflected in our health, vitality, success, and happiness.

# A Departure from Nature

Isn't this sensible? This logical process (the above seven keys) is Nature's own remedy. It's within the grasp of each one of us, yet it is almost entirely neglected by health professionals and their patients. This neglect explains their innumerable failures, for even when there is success in curing one ailment through the use of drugs, radiation, scalpels, supplements, herbs, and diet, it is rarely more than a brief time before the patient develops another ailment. This is because the symptoms alone were treated, not the cause. The medical world claims no cure for cancer and, what's more, no one else can either. **In America it is against the law to treat cancer in ways that eliminate the cause.**[28] The effectiveness of

---

[28] Chemotherapy, radiation, and surgery, the standard cancer treatments of modern medicine, do nothing to correct pH, emotional disturbances, nutritional depletions, immune weakness, congestion, toxic accumulations, intestinal problems, nor weakness of specific organs. On the contrary, the standard medical treatments contribute even further towards the destruction of these valuable organs. For example:
* Liver toxicity is common with certain doses of chemotherapy. When using total-body radiation and chemo, close to 50% of patients are affected, and liver failure occurs with one-third of these patients. T.

some banned cancer therapies far surpasses conventional medical treatments for cancer. Helmut Keller, M.D. of Germany states that his Carnivora treatment has achieved a 98% cancer remission rate for patients with early malignancies who did not have any "noxious therapies," such as chemotherapy or radiation.[29] Other highly effective cancer therapies such as 714X, known to be about 70% effective against some cancers, are also illegal in the United States. When we understand the causes, we also understand the proper treatment. **But to admit true cause compels the true solution, and there isn't any profit in it for the medical industry.**

Disease is never acquired. It is always earned. **Disease is a natural result obtained from an unnatural lifestyle.** Disease is not a question of exposure. It is an internal development which can lead to exposure susceptibility. The survival of every animal, bird, fish, plant, and germ whether it be bacteria, viruses, fungus, or protozoa, depends entirely upon the environment. **Disease occurs only when one's internal environment is favorable for disease growth. We create our internal environments.** Yet we have been programmed to believe that people are constantly "catching" the flu or catching a bug from someone else. I hope that I have made it clear; about 99.9% of the American population have created a polluted internal environment capable of catching or *creating* just about any disease. We attack our own bodies principally by eating the wrong foods and by generating stressful emotions which alter our internal environment. **As you never see flies in a clean garbage can, you also never see disease in a completely pure being.** Disease seldom, if ever, can occur in a clean, healthy, loving body. In fact, it may be totally impossible; but we don't know for sure because there probably isn't anyone pure enough to test.

For decades people have rid their bodies of cancer while intelligently practicing the Seven Keys, Nature's own remedy. But, these days, a doctor takes terrible risks if he or she uses the effective treatments that work on cause rather than the ineffective treatments that work on symptoms. This is why so many doctors have gone to other countries to do their work. To think that there are those who can cure cancer and other terrible diseases such as AIDS, but are not legally permitted to even try! What a crime against our people! **Therefore, I hereby announce that I**

---

Yamada, ed., *Textbook of Gastroenterology*, (Philadelphia, PA: J.P. Lippincott Co., 1991), p. 901.
\* Chemotherapy has caused toxicity in over 80% of the patients and this apparently caused serious damage to the liver, bile ducts, stomach, and duodenum. Ibid., p. 1804.

[29] Norton Walker, D.P.M., "Medical Journalist Report of Innovative Biologics," *Townsend Letter for Doctors and Patients*, 1977; October; pg. 86.

**do not claim that my program will cure cancer or any other disease**. Should you find your cancer, AIDS, and other diseases disappearing when you use this system, I will not accept responsibility. You'll have to take the credit yourself.

I had better be careful here. I had better not say that all diseases can be cured. No disease is curable if the patient's attitude will not permit healing or if they are unwilling to make changes within themselves. But based on the people I've known of who have conquered cancer, heart disease, diabetes, HIV, and leukemia; and based on the numerous books I've read and health professionals I've talked to, as well as clinical studies I have read, the following is undeniably true: **America must look to other healing methods if it wants to return to the healthy nation it once was. We must return to Nature's ways - to that which is natural; to that which is of God, not man!**

# Facts of Medical History

The U.S. Public Health Service revealed the rate of health deterioration of the American people. Out of 100 participating nations of the world, America **was** the healthiest in 1900. In 1920, we dropped to the second healthiest nation. During World War II, we went back to number one - that's when sugar and meat were hard to get, family vegetable gardens were common, and many doctors were out of town (in the army). But after the war, Americans adopted SAD, the Standard American Diet (high protein, processed foods, excessive salt, alcohol, sugar, dairy products and chemicals in food and water). In 1978, we dropped to 79th. In 1980, we were 95th! About 1990, we hit rock bottom - that's number 100 on the list. Yet we are said to be the wealthiest nation in the world. Who, or what, is responsible?[30]

Since 1900, the basic, sensible theories of health care have changed dramatically. The major change was the shift from Nature, or natural healing methods, to drugs, especially antibiotics[31] and vaccines.[32] The

---

[30] The US Public Health Service. Quoted in "Health Realities," by Queen and Company. Also: Victor Earl Irons, Sr., *The Destruction Of Your Own Natural Protective Mechanism*, (Kansas City, MO: V.E. Irons, Inc., 1995). They may be reached at (800) 544-8147.

[31] "The End of Antibiotics," *Newsweek*, 1994; March 28. Science thought it had vanquished infectious diseases. But now the bugs are fighting back. This article explains that antibiotics have caused a mutation of bacteria into super bacteria that are resistant to any known antibiotic. The article explains that medical science has announced that **an increase of deaths is occurring due to strains of bacteria that have**

prescribing of drugs and use of surgery has gotten terribly out of hand. **In America, the leading cause of death is heart disease, the second is cancer, and the third is - are you sitting down? Get ready! Medical drugs!** Let's continue. Next follow stroke, lung disease, accidents, pneumonia/influenza, and then - get ready! **Medical doctors!** Yes, they are killing the Americans so fast that they are responsible for the eighth largest fatality rate. Tens of thousands of people are dying prematurely and millions suffer because of medical doctors and their disease-causing drugs. They even have a name for it - Iatrogenic disease. Iatrogenic disease means disease caused by doctors and their treatments. This is not to say that we should never use drugs or surgery, but that we should use them *only* with great discretion, only when we are certain that nothing else can work: this would be rare. Dr. Yamada, physician-in-chief, University of Michigan Medical Center, explains in his book that **there is NO EVIDENCE that chemotherapy prolongs survival, even with patients whose tumors did respond to treatment.**[33]

In my opinion, as long as the approach to healing (except in rare cases) involves the use of drugs, chemicals, radiation, and scalpels, it will never be successful in the long term. And I am not alone. If we sincerely want to bring the American people back to health, or if we personally wish to reclaim our own perfect health, we must stop using drugs and chemicals that suppress, pollute and weaken our bodies. Let us use the more natural sciences of chiropractic, homeopathy, acupuncture, herbology, and/or other effective and safe methods of healing. It is imperative that we return to Nature and follow Her ways: by removing any mental/emotional causes within that interfere with our full expression of Love, and by using herbs, fresh living foods, and other natural methods that cleanse, purify and strengthen the body.

---

**been created by antibiotics**. The article implies that there is nothing they can do about it, and they fear major epidemics of uncontrolled bacteria. This has now occurred, for in 1996, more than 150,000 American patients who entered hospitals without any infection, died as a result of acquiring one at the hospital.

Another result of antibiotic use, recently recognized, is that many people develop various diseases as a result of the destruction of their friendly bacteria by the antibiotics. If the friendly bacteria are not replaced, serious physiological problems may develop.

[32] Vaccines are not what we have been programmed to believe. Some doctors believe that vaccines are related to the massive epidemics of disease, such as cancer, in the Western World. For a list of books about vaccines, see the section on Suggested Reading in the back of this book.

[33] Yamada, ed., p. 1803.

In addition to the shift in health care which evolved after 1900, came the increasing use of preservatives and chemicals which are taken into our bodies through food, commercially grown produce (using pesticides, herbicides, toxic fertilizers, etc.), polluted air, synthetic fabrics, and electronic poisoning. And perhaps most important of all has been the substantial increase in the use of meat, dairy products, sugar, salt, alcohol, and processed foods. This unnatural approach to life has had a profoundly detrimental effect not only upon the American people, but the entire world.

# Must Seek The Cause to Heal Disease

Most people never stop to ask if chemotherapy or radiation therapy will remove the cause of disease? Emphatically no! Positively not! Never! After these severe and brutal treatments, the body is greatly weakened. Energy and other reserves which could have been available to fight the cancer or other diseases are greatly diminished by the immense effort required to protect the body from the abusive treatments. Chemotherapy and radiation destroy many essential enzymes and **severely damage the immune system** almost every time. The liver is the most important organ in the battle against cancer. Yet, it is severely challenged and often damaged beyond repair after the use of chemotherapy.[34] The body becomes so weak it can barely survive, much less heal itself. When on chemotherapy, some people have died because they had a cold and no immunity left to fight it. **Chemotherapy actually destroys or damages the immune system, and a fully functioning immune system by itself is capable of eliminating all cancer.**[35] Does it make any sense at all to destroy one of the most vital mechanisms within the body that is capable of solving the primary problem. I wonder if it has ever occurred in the minds of these doctors to strengthen the immune system. Many people die of complications related to the extreme toxicity of chemotherapy.[36]

---

[34] Liver toxicity is common with certain doses of chemotherapy. When using total-body radiation and chemo, close to 50% of patients are affected, and liver failure occurs with one-third of these patients. Yamada, ed., pg. 901. Chemotherapy has caused toxicity in over 80% of the patients and this apparently caused serious damage to the liver, bile ducts, stomach, and duodenum. Yamada, ed., pg. 1804.

[35] I recommend that people get a list of Chemotherapy Drugs that any doctor wants you to use and look each one up in the Edward Every, ed.,"Physician's Desk Reference," (Oradell, NJ: Edward Barnhart Publishers, 1988). I have provided some examples which you can find in the Appendix on Chemotherapy.

[36] Richard Lee, M.D., Thomas Bithell, M.D., John Forester, M.D., John Athens, M.D., John Lukens, M.D., Wintrobe's Clinical Hematology, (Philadelphia, PA: Lea & Febiger, 1993), pg. 1744. Here it explains that

When a person gets a tumor cut out or burned out by radiation and if by rare chance the tumor is completely, 100% gone, the chemical and the emotional profile that caused its development in the first place is still there, isn't it? The radiation didn't do a thing to change the body chemistry that caused it. The intestinal tract is still unhealthy and even worse off because the body is now weaker and more toxic. The blood is now more toxic because it is full of radiation. The glands are still sickly, the liver and kidneys are even more sluggish, and even more electrolyte minerals have been depleted.[37] The toxic body becomes much more toxic and depleted. The ingestion of toxic foods and drinks is still continuing, and negative thoughts and feelings are still present or laying beneath conscious awareness. How can anyone think for a moment that the cause disappeared with treatments such as radiation, drug therapy, or surgery? Yet this is precisely what they want people to think and as illogical as it is, many doctors do think that way.

One prominent cancer researcher, Dr. Hardin Jones (University of California) said, "My studies have proved conclusively that **untreated cancer victims actually live up to four times longer than treated individuals...** Beyond a shadow of a doubt, radical

---

the use of chemotherapy for several diseases has caused serious and often fatal results. These diseases include: polycythemia vera, all childhood diseases, non-Hodgkin's lymphoma, as well as carcinoma of the breast, ovary, gastrointestinal tract, and lung. They even explain that **the "major risk" is the treatment rather then the disease. Imagine if you will, having a serious disease that has a high percentage of fatality, and then getting treated with chemicals that have an even higher fatality rate than the disease.** Now does that make any sense at all? This is what we can expect when we are treated by conventional medicine. I remember reading about the first successful heart transplant. The patient died, but the doctors were thrilled that they had succeeded with the transplant. The conclusion they came to, however, was that nobody should receive a heart transplant unless they are in good health. Do you really think that anyone in good health should have a heart transplant? Perhaps my concept of good health, is quite different from those doctors.

Can chemotherapy cause disease? After doctors thought that chemotherapy was successful in treating Hodgkin's disease, the survivors later developed leukemia. And they called it a triumph! This is an example of the "time bomb effect" of drugs and medical thinking.

[37] Based upon my own observations and the many people I have tested, I believe that close to 100% of people who have cancer are deficient in electrolytes. And no one can get well if they are electrolyte deficient.

**surgery on cancer patients does more harm than good."**[38] *Dr. Jones advocates less surgery and less chemotherapy.* According to Edward Griffin, author of **World Without Cancer**, (a fantastic book that I urge everyone to read) *the average long term cure rate of cancer is only 7.5%. And that figure includes patients who survive without treatment of any kind! This means that the rate of those who survive with the commonly used conventional medical treatments is even less.*[39] Would you take your car to a mechanic if he claimed a mere 7.5% success rate for repair of transmissions? It is time to consider other methods.

There are many practitioners who know how to take care of cancer, but who will not take a patient who has had chemotherapy because they feel that person is a lost cause. Except in some extremely rare situations, chemotherapy and radiation are never a part of wisdom. I remind the reader that cancer victims live, on an average, four times longer if they do not get regular medical treatment for their cancer.[40] Now we have a better idea why.

A few years ago I was talking to a Registered Nurse. She said, "I think your program is great, but how many people are strong enough to use it?" I could only nod my head as I replied: "Indeed, many are called, but few are chosen." Many believe that this potent body cleansing program is **the most efficacious healing program available**. When used with other healing methods it is incredible. But **full use requires strength of the soul and the spirit**. Many, maybe most, people are so afraid, weak, or should I say, so conditioned and out of control, that they have become totally governed by the momentum of their own bad habits or the influence of others. In that state many people feel as if they are unable to change the habits that are leading them toward disease or death. **Since then, I have found ways to make the cleanse easier and more gentle so now anyone can accomplish it, and get a head start on changing old patterns.**

---

[38] Hardin Jones, "Report on Cancer," March 7, 1969. Available at the University of California Bancroft Library. (510) 642-6481. Found in the Manuscript Collection: Hardin Blair Jones Papers, 1937-1978." Request call number: BANC MSS 79/112C. (Found in Carton #4.)

[39] G. Edward Griffin, Edward Griffin, *World without Cancer*, (Denver, CO: Nutri-Books, 1974), pg. 228.

[40] I firmly believe that chemo should be outlawed. But instead, treatments that often work without toxic side-effects are outlawed and some patients don't know that they have a choice in the matter. I believe that anyone who could survive chemo, would have survived with holistic natural methods far better, with very few exceptions. I also believe that many of the people who died from that treatment would have survived had they not taken it. See Appendix on Chemotherapy.

For the true cause of disease is negative consciousness. As I said, this negativity gradually seeps into the etheric structure which the physical body reflects. The energy meridians become congested and here is where toxins settle. Negative attitudes are like putting slimy and sticky tar-like substance upon the electronic parts of your body components. The life-force energy and nerve energies become short circuited. As our life-force body becomes more and more congested with our negative thoughts and feelings, the nerves and fluids of our physical body also become more congested and slower. Electrical pathways in our cells and organs can become sluggish and sometimes short-circuit. Mucus and toxins accumulate and disease begins to appear in the forms of symptoms. Work on the symptoms with drugs etc., and the toxins remain. Force the symptom to disappear with drugs or surgery and soon you will have another disease somewhere else. Only this time you have the added toxin from the drug, and weaker organs. **Drugs and radiation suppress the body's toxin and emotion-releasing activity. If we want true healing, we must allow all toxins to surface and be released.** [41]

I know many very good doctors who really care about their patients and have the greatest intentions. But I have learned that "truly good doctors" keep on learning after medical school. They have open minds; they seek, they search, they discover. These kinds of doctors change, and they work with cause. They stay away from the drug scene as much as possible, and they use alternative methods.

I bow before these great people - the doctors of courage who know right from wrong and put their patients above their own concerns. They are the material that can make a nation great. They have great courage. I pray for their success and survival, and I suggest that you do the same. For the truth is that the medical industry is far less than optimal. It is basically controlled by those who support the drug companies. The drug companies are owned by those who control the banking industries. They manipulate nations and war. Enough said. If anyone does not believe me, I say: **Seek the truth with an open mind and you will find all the proof of that which I have said.** We all need to know the truth and the sooner the better, if we want to save the freedom and health we still have.

---

[41] **See "Cleansing Reactions" in Chapter 9.**

# Chapter 2

# HOW WE MUTATE OUR INTERNAL ENVIRONMENT, DESTROY OUR DIGESTIVE SYSTEMS, DRAIN OURSELVES OF MINERALS, AND CREATE MUCOID PLAQUE

*"The gods are innocent concerning the sufferings, and all diseases and pains of the body are the products of extravagances."*

- Pythagoras

I have noted the close tie between negative thoughts, feelings, and disease. Now I will address the physical conditions that relate to both health and disease.

## Understanding pH - the Acid/Alkaline Balance

**Every breath we take, and even the beating of our hearts depend upon our bodies maintaining a precisely balanced pH in the blood, and in other critical body elements.**[42] Every enzyme system and the entire electrical functioning of our bodies are dependent upon electrolytes. (The levels of electrolytes are reflected in the body's pH.) This means that without proper pH, cells cannot receive the nutrients and energy they need to stay healthy.[43] As cells weaken, they cannot perform

---

[42] "pH" is a symbol used to measure acidity or alkalinity. pH means potential hydrogen. The more hydrogen ions, the more acid. Regulation of pH is an activity of controlling the hydrogen ion concentration. Anything from 0 - 6.9, indicates acidity. The lower the number, the greater the acid level. Anything from 7 - 14, indicates alkalinity. The higher the number, the greater the alkaline level. To a large degree, the body uses electrolyte minerals to control pH.

[43] A. C. Guyton and J. E. Hall, *Textbook of Medical Physiology*, 9th

well. If this persists, tissues and whole organs begin to malfunction. This then impairs the functioning of whole body systems, and serious disease begins to evolve. Excluding accidents and genetic weakness, disease most often begins to occur after we have altered our normal pH balance by becoming deficient in minerals, especially electrolyte minerals[44]- **not minerals from rock, but minerals from organic matter** (plants).[45]

Anytime our pH is off-balance even to a small degree, it is usually a sign that we have depleted ourselves of valuable electrolyte minerals. **A lack of organic minerals anywhere in the body means a decrease in enzyme function, and a corresponding deterioration in cell health**. When this occurs, many organs and glands may be under great stress, for **only slight changes in pH from normal levels can cause extreme alterations in the rates of chemical reactions - inside and outside the cells**. Some cells will be depressed; others will be accelerated. This is why the regulation of pH is one of the most important physiological functions in maintaining homeostasis. When people become too acidotic they are likely to die in a coma, and when they become too alkalotic they are likely to die of tetany or convulsions.[46] At a certain point between the two, we have health, but if the pH of any organ or cell moves toward one of these extremes, dysfunction is *always* the result.

**Most people in America have already lost this delicate balance and are moving towards these extremes**.[47] However, long before they

---

Edition, (Philadelphia, PA: W.B. Saunders Company, 1996), pg. 385.

[44] An electrolyte is any compound that, in solution, conducts electricity, and is decomposed by it. Sodium, potassium, calcium, magnesium, lithium and phosphorus are the primary electrolytes that the body needs.

[45] The body cannot efficiently use rock minerals. It must use the minerals that have passed through the plant kingdom. Minerals from the plant kingdom are rock minerals that have been chelated to a protein molecule by the magic of photosynthesis.

[46] A. C. Guyton, *Textbook of Medical Physiology*, 7th Edition, (Philadelphia, PA, W.B. Saunders Company, 1986), pg. 438.

[47] The standard American diet places heavy emphasis on acid-forming foods. These foods force our bodies to use precious electrolyte reserves to balance the excess acidity they create. As long as adequate mineral reserves are present, health is maintained. However, once the reserves are depleted, acid-forming foods destroy the body's delicate pH balance, resulting in poor function and disease. Heart disease, cancer, AIDS, diabetes, and bowel problems are all associated with electrolyte deficiencies.

come close to death, they usually have contracted various disease conditions which most people are totally unaware of until the disease has advanced into pain, tiredness, or some other symptom.

# Digestion and pH

The main causes of mineral depletion in the Western world today are the consumption of excess amounts of acid-forming foods, and too much stress.[48]  If we eat a diet high in acid-forming foods, we can become deficient in many minerals including sodium, calcium, magnesium, potassium, phosphorus and sulfur.[49]  These six minerals are the most important, for they have a direct impact upon maintaining proper pH, fluid viscosity, tissue softness, cell function, and bowel chemistry, as well as being the most common minerals found to be deficient in people today. An exact pH is necessary for blood purity, enzyme activity, and full immune potential.

The further we deplete our minerals and move towards greater acidity, the more our bodies lose control over pH, and the more the liver and all organs are impaired.  From this depletion of minerals and development of acidity, *our immune systems become depressed, we can lose the ability to create hydrochloric acid, the bile turns acid, our normal friendly bacteria mutates, and we may become susceptible to infiltration of "germs"* - various bacteria, viruses, fungus, yeast, and perhaps protozoa. Both minerals <u>and</u> the harmonious feelings of enthusiastic love, joy and inner peace are essential in maintaining this delicate pH and metabolic balance.  In summary, we can lose this balance as a result of:  1) taking drugs (either medicinal or recreational), which can cause metabolic stress,[50]

---

[48] Acid-forming foods are meat (including fish and birds), most dairy products, grains, processed foods such as coffee, pop, cereals, donuts, etc., and foods that are grown in mineral deficient soil (includes commercially grown produce), as are found in most super markets.

[49] Guyton and Hall, pg. 11.

[50] Example:  Antibiotics cause extreme stress upon the metabolic function of our bodies.  Stress is always very acid-forming.  However, even more important than that is after the antibiotics have destroyed most of the friendly bacteria in our bodies, more often than not, acid-forming bacteria take their place.  This may last a lifetime.  Acid-forming bacteria can slowly deplete our bodies of the main electrolyte minerals which can eventually be responsible for creating life-threatening disease. Perhaps the medical community has often not noted this because it

2) being stressed, for emotional stress drains electrolytes just as if we were eating acid-forming foods, or 3) eating acid-forming foods. In the Western world all three are prevalent; the latter two are the most common. Less common causes of electrolyte depletion may include: strenuous exercise; illness and infection; and cleansing and fasting.

When we eat, we chew the food and it goes into the stomach. Here it is saturated by hydrochloric acid (HCL) which activates pepsinogen enzymes. This results in creation of a proteolytic enzyme known as active pepsin. This enzyme helps digest protein. **It is important to remember that all foods, except oils, have protein.** When the stomach has completed its job it releases the entire mass through the pyloric valve and the food, now very acid from the HCL, enters the duodenum. Here it is saturated by large amounts of alkaline fluids from the Brunner glands, the bile, and the pancreatic juices. This is absolutely essential, for **the pancreatic enzymes can only function optimally in a pH above 7.** And not only that; before the body can absorb the food into the bloodstream and use it, the pH of the food must be 7.4.

### pH of Body Fluids

| | |
|---|---|
| Saliva | 6.0 - 7.0 |
| Gastric | 1.0 - 3.5 |
| Brunner's Glands | 8.9 - 9.1 |
| Bile | 4.5 - 8.6 |
| Pancreatic | 8.0 - 8.3 |
| Small Intestine | 7.5 - 8.0 |
| Large Intestine | 7.5 - 8.0 |
| Blood | 7.35 - 7.45 |

Keep in mind that it is very essential for our bodies to maintain a perfect pH balance. As long as they are able to do so, we have a very good chance of maintaining health all through our lives. But if this balance is lost, it is impossible to maintain good health. My estimation is that more than 90% of the American population has lost this balance. Our bodies have several incredible control mechanisms to maintain this delicate balance of pH. One process is called the buffer system or the regulation of acid-base balance. By eliminating complex explanations, we can say that the first step is for the body to buffer the acids by absorbing the acid with sodium bicarbonate. Each time an acid is buffered by the sodium, the pH rises. In

---

takes so many years for symptoms to appear that seldom does anyone ever consider looking for the cause and trace it back to the drug.

this process, the body brings the acids to a level in which it can safely remove them out of the body through the kidneys and increase the pH of the food so that it can be assimilated.[51]

This may bring more clarity. When we eat alkaline-forming foods, there are more than enough electrolytes to buffer whatever acids were in the food and the remainder is an excess of electrolytes. When we eat acid-forming foods, there are not enough electrolytes to buffer the acids and what remains is an excess of acids or a depletion of electrolytes. The body then has to deplete its own alkaline reserves (also needed for exercise, illness and stress) to handle these acids.

## Organic Sodium

We have heard a great deal about calcium and potassium deficiencies, but we never hear about sodium deficiencies. Yet **sodium deficiency is the number one mineral deficiency**. How can this be when everyone eats so much salt? Sodium chloride (table salt), cannot be used by the body because the sodium and the chloride are held together by ionic bonds. This form of salt is toxic, can increase blood pressure (which proves it's toxic), and cannot be used in the buffer system. The body can only efficiently use sodium that has been chelated to a protein molecule which can only occur as the salt passes through the plant kingdom. This form of salt is covalently bonded, meaning the bonds are easily broken down and utilized.[52]

Though the conventional medical profession does not acknowledge that sodium chloride cannot be used by the body, it is quite obvious to some doctors, and it has been proven by clinical studies. One such study has shown that **when sodium chloride was given to certain people, their blood pressure rose, but when *organic* sodium was given to these same patients, blood pressure moved towards normal.** (See footnote at end of paragraph.) It was also found that **sodium chloride induced the body to lose calcium, whereas organic sodium induced a decrease in calcium loss.** The reason for this is that when organic sodium is unavailable to be used to buffer acids, calcium may be used in its place. The reason that table salt (sodium chloride) induces the body to lose calcium, is that sodium chloride cannot be used as a buffer because it is not in the organic

---

[51] Guyton, pg. 439-441.

[52] M.T. Morter, Jr., B.S., M.A., D.C., "Correlative Urinalysis - The Body Knows Best," (Rogers, AR: B.E.S.T. Research Inc., 1987), pg. 43-44.

(chelated to a plant protein) form that the body requires. In fact, sodium chloride actually causes an increase in acidity which can further deplete calcium. However, when organic sodium is provided to the body, it can use that as a buffer against acids, and losses of calcium will decrease. Another interesting fact arose in this study that completely baffled the researchers. Whenever sodium chloride was given, the body did all it could to rid itself of it. However, when organic sodium was given, the body held on to it. It did not release it. Why? By now you should have the answer. The body could not use the sodium chloride and wanted it out as quickly as possible, because it is toxic. But it needed the organic sodium and kept it.[53]

Organic sodium is used for many things in the body such as keeping calcium from hardening, conducting electrical currents, and it is one of the main electrolytes used in the buffer system. The sodium buffer can bring acid fluids up to 6.1. Then other buffers bring the fluids up to 7.4. The body knows exactly what to do. However, the problem is that if we keep eating acid-forming foods, we can *use up* our stores of sodium and other electrolytes and deplete our body of the precious minerals used in the buffering process. **When the body becomes low in its supply of an electrolyte such as sodium, it will go to other parts of the body and take it from wherever it can extract it, to maintain critical pH factors.**

# How Disease Relates to Mineral Deficiency

**When, due to a deficiency, organic sodium may be removed from the stomach, hydrochloric acid (HCL) production will be reduced or stopped entirely.** For sodium is needed in the stomach to serve as a buffer against the acids it creates through the parietal cells. Contrary to popular belief, the stomach cells are not acid. Even when the stomach lumen[54] has a pH as low as 2, the epithelium[55] cells are near 7.[56]

---

[53] Theodore W. Kurtz, M.D., A. Hamoundi, Al Bander, M.D., R. Curtis Morris, Jr., M.D., "Salt-Sensitive Essential Hypertension In Men," *New England Journal Of Medicine,* 1987; Vol. 317(17), pg. 1043-1048.

[54] Lumen: The cavity within a tubular structure..., Ruth Koenigsberg, ed., *Churchill's Illustrated Medical Dictionary,* (New York, NY: Churchill Livingstone, Inc., 1989).

[55] Epithelium: The cellular covering of the skin and mucous

If this were not so, ulcers would develop. Yes, it is the organic sodium that prevents ulcers. Therefore, a lack of sodium in the stomach usually means a shut down of acid production which means that pepsinogen cannot be activated.[57] Effective digestion is greatly inhibited by lack of hydrochloric acid and pepsin enzymes. Not only that, but a lack of the normal acid in the stomach allows potential pathogenic bacteria, parasites, and yeasts to enter the gastrointestinal tract.[58] This allows the entire body to become exposed to these microorganisms. So you see, hydrochloric acid has at least two very important functions. It protects us from harmful microorganisms and helps digest our food. **When hydrochloric acid is unavailable, we become more vulnerable to disease and digestion becomes inefficient, and then even good food can become toxic.** This is a very serious problem affecting the health of a large percentage of the population in the Western World.

A few years ago, when the two children died from *E. coli* poisoning from eating a hamburger at one of the fast food chains, it was very likely that they had been depleted of organic sodium and had little or no hydrochloric acid production.[59] Otherwise, the hydrochloric acid would have eliminated the *E. coli* while still in the stomach. And even if a few *E. coli* survived the stomach, they would have been challenged and most likely eliminated by the friendly intestinal bacteria. We can be sure that most of the people who eat at such places are also lacking in hydrochloric acid and have become depleted of electrolytes. These two children were likely to have been extremely depleted. How many other children and adults that day ate the same meat that contained *E. coli*? Probably hundreds or even more. But only these two children were ill and died. People who suffer from so called food poisoning have the same problem. They lack organic sodium and hydrochloric acid production is inefficient. It is common with those who eat the Standard American Diet.

---

membranes..., Ibid.

[56] Yamada, ed., Vol. 2, pg. 109.

[57] Guyton, pg. 775.

[58] Yamada, ed., Vol. 2, pg. 97.

[59] They probably also lacked proper bacteria in the gut, which, had it been present could have handled the *E. coli*. I would be willing to bet that these children had a history of eating acid-forming foods and drink, and antibiotics treatment which destroyed their normal intestinal bacteria. If this is true, we might consider what really killed them; the *E. coli*, their diet and lifestyle or the antibiotics?

**When organic sodium is removed from the joints, which is common, then arthritis, osteoporosis, and other bone problems may occur.** When sodium is removed from the muscles, the muscles become weak and flabby. When organic sodium is removed from the liver, the liver becomes weak and inefficient. Many serious difficulties can develop such as skin problems, headaches, pains, poor eyesight, depression, mental problems, sugar problems, allergies, blood sugar problems, tiredness, cancer, digestion weakness, poor memory, digestion weakness, etc. When the body becomes deficient in organic sodium, its partner, potassium, can become deficient. **A lack of sodium automatically depletes potassium.**[60] Potassium is abundant in most foods, especially fruits and vegetables. It is almost impossible to be deficient in potassium unless: 1) you don't eat, 2) you can't digest food, or 3) you are deficient in sodium.

When the body is deficient in potassium, heart disease, muscle aches and pains, mood swings, depression, weakness, fears, cynicism, sagging organs, edema, etc. may develop.[61]

Evidence also indicates that when organic sodium and organic potassium deficiencies occur, that organic calcium and magnesium may be used to replace sodium and potassium. This then can develop into calcium and magnesium deficiencies.[62]

The healthy body has several good store houses of organic sodium - the liver, joints, bile, and the stomach mucosa. As indicated above, if normal sodium reserves are deficient, the body can extract what it needs

---

[60] Why do we lose potassium when sodium is low? The body demands a specific ratio of sodium and potassium. When sodium is low, the body secretes the hormone aldosterone. **Aldosterone triggers the body to try and reabsorb sodium, but when there is not enough sodium to reabsorb, aldosterone forces the body to release potassium into the urine, thereby achieving the proper ratio.** In this way the body attempts to maintain the proper sodium/potassium ratio even when the body is deficient in sodium. See Guyton, pg. 434.

[61] One or more of the following symptoms may mean a potassium deficiency: Mood swings, depression, fears, sucidal impulses, cynicism, sagging organs, heart problems, sunken eyes, feels like sand in eyes, swollen ankles, dry skin, gastritis, muscular atrophy, bowel problems, eye problems, sore knees, shallow breathing, skin erruptions, liver problems, cracked lips, nerve problems, and muscle weakness.

[62] Professor C. Lewis Kervran, *Biological Transmutations,* (Magalia, CA: Happiness Press, 1988), pg. 20.

from various sources, however, the easiest, safest, and most likely the first source for the body to extract sodium from is the bile. **When the sodium is removed from the gall juices (bile), a chain reaction occurs that will affect the entire body.** As sodium is removed from bile, the bile pH is lowered. In a healthy person, bile pH should be as high as 8.6.[63] In an unhealthy person, the bile may be as low as 4.5.[64] The healthy person has a high supply of minerals and especially sodium, and the bile pH will be near 8.6. The unhealthy person may have a bile pH between 4.5 and 8. The pH of the bile is controlled by organic sodium. The less sodium in the bile, the more acid it becomes. The more acid it becomes, the more likelihood there will be gallstones forming.

We find that gallstones are formed as a result of sodium and potassium being removed from the bile.[65,66] It has been found that the highest rates of gallstone formation are in countries where diets are high in animal protein foods.[67] The lowest gallstone rates are in countries where diets are mostly vegetarian.[68] **Medical science is very aware that gallstones are related to acid conditions,[69] but until they accept the fact that our bodies cannot use inorganic minerals, they are unlikely to accept that high protein diets and stress cause the formation of**

---

[63] Tortora and Grabowski, *Principles of Anatomy and Physiology*, 7th Edition, (New York, NY: Harper Collins College Publishers, 1993), pg. 792.

[64] Guyton and Hall, pg. 386.

[65] By taking the composition of bile and the composition of cholesterol gallstones, we find that the only difference between the two, is that gallstones lack sodium and sometimes potassium as well. Everything else is the same. We also know that in the presence of sodium, calcium (which is in bile) remains soft, but without sodium, calcium hardens. There may be other contributing factors, but this appears to be the most logical explanation. "Composition of Gallstones," in Howard M. Spiro, *Clinical Gastroenterology*, 3rd Edition, (New York, NY: McGraw Hill, 1983), pg. 873-888.

[66] Morter, pg. 69.

[67] Guyton and Hall, pg. 29.

[68] Yamada,ed., Vol. 2, pg. 1967.

[69] "Gallstone patients are known to have a defect in the normal pH of their gallbladder bile." Yamada, ed., pg. 1971.

**gallstones because of sodium deficiency.** If a person has a low bile pH and consumes large amounts of sodium chloride (table salt), their bile pH will drop further. If that same person consumes large amounts of organic sodium (from vegetables or fruits), their bile pH will move towards normal. The same shifts are reflected in the urine and saliva pH readings. Therefore, both urine and saliva pH readings may be used as an effective indicator of the body's electrolyte reserves. [70]

In a healthy person, the alkaline fluids from the Brunner's glands, bile and alkaline pancreatic juices flood the duodenum shortly after food passes through from the stomach into the duodenum. These highly alkaline fluids saturate the acids from the stomach and raise the pH up to alkaline levels, thereby allowing the perfect environment for the pancreatic enzymes to optimally digest food. Pancreatic enzymes can only function optimally in a pH above 7. [71] As long as the body is able to do this, then a good digestive system will continue throughout the life of that body. However, after the bile turns from alkaline to acid, and the body is unable to correct the acid fluids, a very serious condition occurs in the duodenum. When the acid foods pass into the duodenum and when the bile has turned acid, then the food is unable to be fully alkalized. When this occurs, the enzymes from the pancreas are unable to function properly and digestion may be greatly inhibited.

## Results of Prolonged Mineral Depletion

If diet and lifestyle are consistently acid-forming, then minerals continue to be depleted, the bowel may be unable to correct the bowel pH with its other mechanisms, and the entire bowel may be affected. As this becomes more and more out of control, a chain reaction of pathogenic conditions continues:
♦ Digestive ability declines.
♦ Friendly bowel bacteria may be destroyed or mutated into undesirable species. (pleomorphism).
♦ The bowel's resistance to bacteria, viral, and parasitic infection is reduced.
♦ Bile acids irritate mucosa and mucoid plaque is created in the gut as a protection.

---

[70] **See Appendix I: How to Do the pH Test.**

[71] Guyton and Hall, pg. 826.

- ♦ Various toxins and pathogens increase and unnatural growths begin to develop.
- ♦ Constipation, diverticula and other bowel disorders begin to develop.
- ♦ Liver and kidneys are challenged.
- ♦ B vitamin (including B12) and amino acid production is reduced or eliminated.
- ♦ Nutritional deficiencies begin at the cell level.

As these conditions advance, constipation and/or diarrhea often develop. The bowel then becomes extremely toxic and may allow toxic particles to enter the blood, forcing the liver and kidneys to handle the toxic overloads. Too much toxicity and acids from the bowel will eventually weaken the liver, and gut lining. Leaky bowel syndrome develops and then the liver, kidneys, spleen, and other organs are even more challenged. Toxins from the blood may contaminate the hereditarily weak and injured areas of the body first. On and on it goes until every organ and gland is affected. How rapidly will these conditions develop? This depends upon the constitutional weakness of the body, attitudes of the mind, and upon the degree of indulgence in acid-forming food and highly processed foods. It also has to do with the quality of fruits and vegetables that are eaten (organically grown versus the mineral-deficient commercially grown produce), and most of all, with the ways we think and feel.

## MINERALS - Important Key to Health

From this explanation, it is easy to see how we create our own disease. It also explains how important it is to eat a diet of mostly alkaline-forming foods (at least 80% alkaline-forming and 20% acid-forming) that are grown on soil that has an abundant supply of minerals and other nutrients the plants need. **Eating only organically grown produce is the only way we can be confident that we are receiving an adequate supply of minerals, since commercially grown produce is usually deficient in minerals.**[72, 73]

---

[72] Robert F. Heltman; "Organic Food is More Nutritious," Townsend Letter for Doctors & Patients, 1997; Nov; Issue #172, pg. 12.

[73] Even eating organically grown food is no guarantee that we will receive all the minerals. Eating food grown out of our own garden and orchard is by far, the best thing we can do.

**Every function of the body is dependent upon an adequate supply of minerals.** It is critical to have enough of the right kind of minerals to even stay alive, not to mention being healthy!

## Minerals are Essential for the Following:

Enzyme function
Maintaining proper pH
Growth
Cell function
Electrical potential
Oxygen transport
Every physiological activity of our bodies.

There, does that make it clear? Our bodies are totally dependent upon the right amount of minerals and in their perfect combination. Whenever our bodies go "hay-wire", minerals are usually involved. With every case of chronic or degenerative disease, the mineral supply has become deficient and the pH of body fluids abnormal. **Adequate healing cannot occur until we have replenished our mineral supply and brought our bodies into the proper pH.** The worst mistake made by doctors is when they fail to put their patients on a diet that consists of at least 80% alkaline-forming foods. In my opinion, any doctor who fails to do this, especially when treating chronic or degenerative disease, should not be a doctor.

## How We Deplete Ourselves of Minerals

Of many ways that we deplete ourselves of minerals the most important include:

Negative emotions
Poor digestion and assimilation
Excess stress
Medical drugs
Eating foods from inadequate soil - commercially
grown foods[74]

---

[74] Do not expect good health if you eat commerically grown produce you find at the average supermarket. Two reasons; first, they lack sufficient minerals. Commerically grown tomatoes have been tested for mineral content. One test revealed only 8 minerals. Tomatoes should have over 50 minerals. Tests were conducted on carrots. Some carrots were found with no calcium. Robert F. Heltman, "Organic Food is More Nutritious," *Townsend Letter for Doctors & Patients*, 1997; Nov; Issue # 172, pg. 12. The second reason is: pesticides. The primary poison found on commerically grown produce is arsenic. Do you want arsenic and other

Malnutrition
Eating too many acid-forming foods
Dysfunctional adrenals or kidneys
Bacteria and parasite infections
Shallow breathing.

### Ways to Maintain Better Health and Build our Mineral Reserves

Breathe deeply
Think positive thoughts
Eat wholesome organically grown fruits
 and vegetables
Get plenty of rest and exercise
Avoid drugs and other toxins
Cleanse & Purify the entire body
Rebuild the digestive system and other organs

# How Chronic and Degenerative Diseases Develop

As we can now see, over a period of years, the average person may eat so much acid-forming food and think so many acid-forming thoughts or eat excessive amounts of mineral-deficient foods, etc. that organic sodium and other minerals can become very deficient in the body. Sodium is such an important factor that we cannot live without it. As we become "too" depleted, the body will leach sodium and other minerals from other parts of the body for the critical purpose of maintaining proper blood pH. This presents the cells with even more serious levels of deficiency; deterioration sets in, toxins build, and the stage is set for disease to flourish.[75]

---

chemicals in your body, or in the bodies of your children?  Robert Berkow, M.D., ed., *Merck Manual of Diagnosis and Therapy*, 15th ed., (Rahway, NJ: Merck Sharp and Dohme Research Laboratories, Division of Merck and Company, 1987), pg. 2548.

[75] See Chapter 8: How to Determine if You Need a Cleansing Program, under "Reading the Eye: Iridology."

# How Common is Bowel Distress?

Now, how common is Bowel Distress? Merck's Manual explains that around age 40, almost every person in the U.S. is rapidly developing ulcerative bowels or diverticuli. And if they lived long enough, the manual projects that all Americans would develop this disease.[76] However, my observation is that this applies mostly to meat eaters. I estimate that more than 90% of those who do my full cleanse program eliminate mucoid plaque and little, yellow-white popcorn-like objects. These are polyps or pieces of fibrous substance which are caused as a result of too much acid. They are a sign that the bowel is already in serious trouble. Not all polyps are a sign of cancer, but some are. Deaths caused by cancer in the digestive system rank third only to heart disease and lung cancer. **Cancer of the digestive system has sharply increased over the last few years and appears that it will exceed lung cancer in a few more years.** The Japanese have the highest death rates in the world from stomach cancer. (They also eat the most salt.) It is almost eight times higher than in the United States. But, we surpass them with cancer of the colon and rectum. What a contest!

The majority of people who do my cleanse are already on a path of improvement. Yet most of us started out on the standard American diet (SAD) and damaged ourselves while still young. Some of us have changed to an almost perfect raw food diet, but due to the fact that the plaque is still in there, even ideal diets have not repaired the damage done.

We have had many people say that "there is no way that this plaque can still be in me. I have been on raw foods for 10 years and have fasted many times". The typesetter of our first publication thought this, but after a few days on the cleanse, however, he found out that it was still in there. After the cleanse, he said that he had never felt so good in all his life.

The strengths and genetic weaknesses of the body along with habits and attitudes, determine the potential threat of an overly acid bowel and mucoid accumulation. Crohn's disease is very common among meat-eaters, but is very rare among people in countries where vegetarian diet predominates.[77] Why will one person get colitis, or Crohn's disease, and another person get some other bowel disease, when dietary habits are very similar? I believe there is just enough difference in chemistry because of varying habitual thought and emotional patterns to create the variety of diseases we observe.

---

[76] Ibid., See: "diverticulitis" in the Index.

[77] B. C. Morson, *Color Atlas of the Gastrointestinal Pathology*, (London, England: Harvey Miller Pub., W. B. Saunders, 1988), pg. 120.

It is a known fact that individuals who have had extensive ulcerative-colitis have a risk of developing colon cancer 10 times greater than the general population. Deaths from cancer of the lower bowel are still rising! Medical survival rate is shamefully low. Even in cases where surgery removes 100% of the cancer, one third of the patients will find cancer recurring.[78] It is almost unbelievable that a surgeon can cut out a piece of the colon or whatever and think that the patient is cured of cancer. **What did cutting out the cancer do to the cause? Did it improve the diet; did surgery give the patient minerals, antioxidants and other needed nutrients; did it cleanse the toxins out of the body that are responsible for the cancer; did it rebuild the digestive system and liver?** Cutting out the colon would be like going to your auto repair shop and asking the mechanic to cut off the exhaust pipe because there is black smoke coming out. When they found a tumor in the lungs of John Wayne, doctors cut it out and did nothing for the rest of his body. Three months later they found a tumor in his stomach, cut it out and again did not treat the cause. Three months later they found more tumors in his bowel, but apparently there were so many that they couldn't cut them all out, so he died. He probably would still be alive today if he had consulted someone who understood that **there are causes to disease**.

In the *American Journal Of Gastroenterology*, December 1990 issue, page 1629, an article about polyps was presented. It revealed that "the detection rate of gastric polyps during routine endoscopy has been much higher, gradually increasing from 1.4% in 1967 to 8.7% in 1979. That is an increase of more than six times in just twelve years." I'd be willing to bet that it's far worse than that by now. I also question how often they can even be seen, because I think that most of the time they are covered with a thick lining of mucoid plaque, and when they do find them, it is usually because inflammation, due to excessive acidic conditions, which has burned away the mucoid plaque - or the polyp was immense.

As a rule, medical doctors know almost nothing about nutrition and cleansing the body, unless they learned it outside of medical school. There are 125 medical schools in the United States. Only 30 of them have any training in nutrition and of those 30, nutrition amounts to less than 3 hours of training.[79]

People must awaken to the fact that disease has become an industrial by-product. Though on the surface it appears that everything is being done to find the cures to disease, below the surface everything is

---

[78] Yamada, ed., pg. 1801.

[79] John Robbins, *Diet For A New America*, (Walnole, NH, Stillpoint Publishing, 1987), pg. 150.

being done to suppress the cures.  The cures, in terms of treatments, have been discovered, and rediscovered, many times.  It is well known among those who investigate the medical system, that to give out effective cures is a very dangerous thing to do.[80]

## The Good Doctor Who Interrupted My Lecture

One evening many years ago, I was giving a lecture to a group of people at a health food store.  About twenty minutes into the lecture, someone slipped me a note which said, "There is a medical doctor in the audience.  Maybe you should be a little more tactful."  About an hour went by, then the doctor stood up and asked if he could say a few things.  I was thinking fast, for I knew most medical doctors know absolutely nothing about the subject of my lecture and most of them are against holistic practitioners.

After he gave a list of rather impressive credentials,  he said,  "I have spent nearly twelve years working in the field of post-mortem diagnosis.  I have seen many thousands of dissected cadavers.  I have seen thousands of colons and intestinal tracts of all types of people and I want all of you here tonight to know that what Rich Anderson is telling you ..."  (About this time I began to sweat.  I wondered what he was going to say.  I was fully aware that in America, whenever there is a conflict between truth and credentials - credentials always win, and his credentials were more impressive than mine.)

He continued, "What Rich is telling you is the absolute truth.  Everybody has it in there.  We have a way of attaching a hose to the upper intestines and with the aid of powerful chemicals, we literally blow that "stuff" right out of the intestines.  I have seen the heavy "beer belly" and so-called fat people lose all that bulk in five minutes.  It wasn't fat.  It was the mucoid layers that Rich is talking about and in that filthy substance were all sorts of worms, bacteria, fungi, and many unidentifiable things.  It is almost unbelievable that people can live with that filth in them.  All these people were dead, of course, and it wasn't hard to see why.  You had better listen to what Rich is saying, and if you follow his program you will certainly be glad you did."

I could hardly believe my ears.  A medical doctor who knows about these things!  He sat down and I said with a great big smile, "Would you like to come to all my lectures?"  Later I invited him over to my

---

[80] **See "Medical Conspiracy" under the Suggested Reading List at the end of this book.**

house. He said he came to listen to me, but I wanted to listen to him. He was full of impressive information. He should be writing a book, especially about what medical science has done to people. It was almost unbelievable. He had information about cancer cures that could shake the very foundation of those who believe in conventional medicine. But, of course, those in power would never listen. He functioned under a low profile, never letting anyone fully realize what he does or knows.

# Chapter 3

# MUCOID PLAQUE

*All truth passes through three stages. First, it is ridiculed; second, it is violently opposed; third, it is accepted as being self-evident."*

## - Schoepenhauer

Author's Note: This chapter contains some very technical information. If it seems too difficult to read easily, I suggest you read only the highlights and go back to it later when you are ready for more detailed information.

# What is Mucoid Plaque?

## Definition

The phrase "mucoid plaque" is a coined term that I developed to describe complex glycoproteins secreted by the goblet cells[81], which create a gel-like, viscous and slimy mucus that forms as a layer or layers covering epithelium (inner lining) cells in various hollow organs, especially all the organs of the alimentary (digestive) canal. These include the stomach, small intestine and colon. Mucoid plaque appears to develop in the presence of acids, wherein the mucus is secreted and coagulates. It can then compound with other elements, forming an increasingly firm substance. For those who have followed the standard American diet which is acid-producing, it is common for mucoid plaque to form a continuous cover, arranged in layers,[82] over the glycocalyx[83,84,85] of the small intestine, as well

---

[81] For a description of the goblet cells, see later in this chapter under: "Understanding Mucosa and the Intestine."

[82] J. R. Forstner, "Intestinal Mucins in Health and Disease," *Digestion,* 1978; 17(3), pg. 234-263.

[83] "Glycocalyx: A thin layer of acid polysaccharides, particularly sialic acid, adherent to the outer surface of many cells. It may be the site of

as in the stomach and the large intestine. In most cases, this layer or layers has become intermingled with a variety of damaging toxic constituents. These may include: drugs, noxious fecal compounds, heavy metals, pesticides and more, depending on what the person eats.

Considering the potentially toxic composition of mucoid plaque, it is not surprising that people sometimes respond miraculously to the removal of mucoid plaque. The hundreds of testimonies I have received clearly indicate that mucoid plaque contributes towards a high percentage of pathological problems, as well as premature death. Is it any wonder that the greatest healers in the world have always insisted upon cleansing and rebuilding the digestive tract?

"**Mucoid**" is a general term for mucin, mucoprotein, or glycoprotein, which is the primary substance of mucoid plaque. My choice of the word "**plaque**" is based on Webster's definition; a film consisting of mucus. Mucins or glycoproteins are produced and secreted by the salivary glands, the esophagus, stomach, small and large intestine, gall bladder and pancreatic ducts.[86,87] Clinical and anatomical studies from many papers and textbooks have demonstrated that mucoid plaque exists in the alimentary canal, and that its thickness can be measured with phase contrast microscopy. Later in this chapter I will explain in detail some of the research that has been done in viewing the **many different stages of mucoid plaque as it transforms or alters into disease forms**. Medical science has many words to describe each of these conditions, but there has been no effective term which consolidates them all under one category. Hence, I created the term 'mucoid plaque' which has been readily accepted by tens of thousands of people.

Medical doctors, and surprisingly, many gastroenterologists, are not trained in school about the difference between mucoid plaque and

---

intense enzyme activity and also contains the surface antigens of the cell. Also 'fuzzy coat'. *Churchill's Illustrated Medical Dictionary.*

[84] The glycocalyx is designed to lubricate the structured fibrillary network of microvilli (the brush border), and allows for assimilation of nutrients. A continuous cover of mucoid plaque over the glycocalyx would obviously inhibit nutrient assimilation.

[85] Later in this chapter, see the section titled: "Understanding Mucosa and the Intestine" for more on the glycocalyx.

[86] Glenn R. Gibson and George T. Macfarlane, ed., *Human Colonic Bacteria, Role in Nutrition, Physiology, and Pathology*, (Boca Raton, FL: CRC Press, 1995), pg. 175.

[87] Guyton, pg. 772.

glycocalyx, nor about the early stages of mucoid plaque development. They are, however, aware of the many altered forms that mucoid plaque transforms into, but have failed to recognize that **the advanced stages of bowel diseases, such as diverticulitis, polyps, atrophic gastritis, cystic fibrosis[88], malignancy, inflammatory bowel disease, peptic ulcers, intestinal metaplasia, dysplasia, bowel cancer, and others, are in fact, actual transformations of mucoid plaque or are associated with contaminated mucoid plaque.**[89,90] If allopathic doctors (M.D.s) were more concerned about the prevention and causes of disease, and the importance of cleansing the body, rather than just treating symptoms with highly toxic drugs, they would have long ago delved into this extremely important subject. Those who have been seriously involved with cleansing the body report almost unbelievable amounts of mucoid plaque being released from the body. Medical scientists should have looked into this about 50 years ago, because **its existence is so blatantly obvious and because its removal produces such incredible benefits for the body and mind.**

Mucoid plaque can line the entire alimentary canal, from the tip of the tongue to the anus. **If the abnormal bile acids or other conditions which usually stimulate mucoid plaque production continue without reprieve, the mucoid substance seems to build and become thicker, firmer, and more widespread.**[91] Clinical studies have shown this to be true, and most people who have used our cleansing program are often astonished to see just how much is removed in just a few days of cleansing. The accumulated mucoid plaque may be several inches thick but, in most areas of the gut, it is probably less than 1/4" thick. Since this plaque occurs in the stomach as well as the entire length of both the small and large intestines, it is important to cleanse the entire digestive tract. Yet,

---

[88] Cystic Fibrosis (or Mucoviscidosis): A congenital metabolic disorder, inherited as an autosomal trait, in which secretions of exocrine glands are abnormal; excessively viscid mucus causes obstruction of passageways (including pancreatic and bile ducts, intestines and bronchi). *Stedman's Medical Dictionary*, under "Mucoviscidosis."

[89] S. Thiru, G. Devereux, A. King, "Abnormal Fucosylation of Ileal Mucus In Cystic Fibrosis: I. A Histochemical Study Using Peroxidase Labeled Lectins," *Journal of Clinical Pathology*, 1990; 43, pg. 1014-1018.

[90] R. Whitehead, ed., *Gastrointestinal and Oesophageal Pathology*, 2nd. Edition, (New York, NY: Churchill Livingstone, 1995), pg. 45, 47, 73, 80.

[91] J. Rainier Poley, "The Scanning Electron Microscope: How Valuable In The Evaluation of Small Bowel Mucosal pathology In Chronic Childhood Diarrhea?" *Journal of Pediatric Gastroenterology and Nutrition*, 1991; May-June; 7(3), pg. 386-394.

even those health care professionals who are enlightened as to the benefits of internal cleansing, generally consider only the first four to six feet of the colon. However, it is more important to work on the 20+ feet in the small intestine, because that is where our food is digested and our nutrients absorbed.

## The Digestive System: How It All Fits in the Body

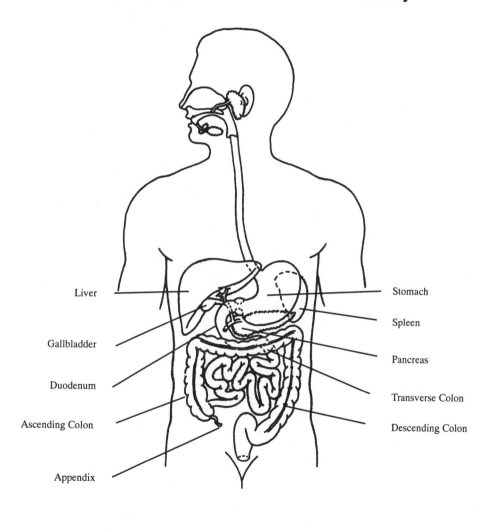

Liver

Gallbladder

Duodenum

Ascending Colon

Appendix

Stomach

Spleen

Pancreas

Transverse Colon

Descending Colon

# Anatomy of a Digestive System

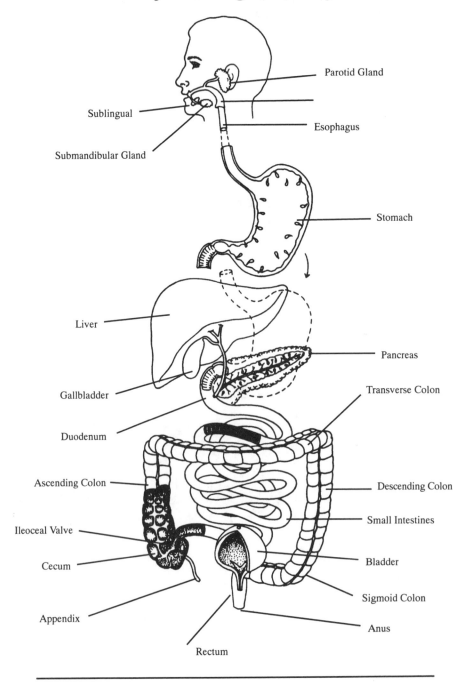

# How The Digestive System Works

Food enters the mouth. Salivary glands secrete alkaline saliva (8.0 ph) containing enzymes to mix with food.

Hydrochloric acid (0.8 pH) created by parietal cells activates pepsinogen enzymes and mixes with food.

Food passes through the pyloric valve and moves past the highly alkaline Brunners glands (8.9 pH) and into duodenum. Here the alkaline pancreatic juices (8.3 pH), full of enzymes, enter the duodenum along with alkaline gall juices (bile)(8.6 pH). With a healthy person, the food mixture (chyme) now becomes alkaline.

Liver provides alkalinity for saliva and creates bile. All food that is assimilated will go through the liver and the liver will detoxify harmful substances and produce the final preparations for use throughout the body.

Bile is stored in the gall bladder. If necessary the body will extract organic sodium from the bile and use it in other areas. The bile pH will drop when this occurs and gallstones may be formed.

Small intestines produce even more alkalinity from the crypts of Lieberkuhn and more than 22 other enzymes gradually mix with the food, if the guts are clear of mucuoid plaque. Then the small intestines gradually assimilate digested food.

Food moves out of the small intestines through the ileocecal valve and into the cecum. This is a sight where many parasites dwell in unhealthy people. Then the food moves up through the ascending colon, through the transverse colon and down the descending colon, past the sigmoid, rectum, and out the anus. The sigmoid and rectum are among the most common sites of cancer and other bowel diseases in constipated individuals.

Because most people in the Western World are in the habit of eating toxic, processed and high-protein foods (which are acid-forming foods) with, and often in between every meal, bowel problems and mucoid plaque development are epidemic, along with gallstones, calcium problems, heart disease, cancer, chronic fatigue, mental and emotional problems, and related disorders. It is important to know that mucoid plaque seems to be the forerunner of many disease conditions. And these diseases are not just in the bowel, but throughout the entire body. This is an extremely important subject. Therefore, I will provide documentation to back up this theory in this chapter and in Chapter 6. Continuous use of harmful, so-called "foods", causes a gradual increase of mucoid plaque, which can become so thick and adhesive that the reversal of this condition seldom, if ever, occurs in an entire lifetime. However, **with the use of specific herbs in specific combinations, the body can shed the mucoid plaque, layer after layer. Even people who have changed their diets and eat only raw fruits and vegetables still retain the plaque in their bowels until they take effective steps to remove it.**

As these mucoid accumulations build, the peristaltic action in the intestines may become  less and less effective, and one form or another of constipation or diarrhea often develops. **A gradual weakening of the body's immune system may also occur after long term toxic bowel environment destroys the natural bacterial growth, weakens the liver, and interferes with nerve meridian points related to hundreds of other parts of the body.** As bowel problems advance, disease conditions also advance, seemingly in direct proportion to electrolyte deficiencies and the disintegration of digestive processes. For those who truly care about their health, the following statement should be emphasized and placed upon the top of their list of health concepts: **The bowel feeds every organ, every tissue, every cell in our bodies. When the quality of that feeding is contaminated or inadequate, the cells and organs in the rest of the body will reflect that poor quality. A toxic bowel means toxic blood and lymph, toxic organs and cells, and distortions of DNA and body function.**

Some doctors believe that excess mucoid plaque is naturally removed by either bacteria or enzymes.[92] **In a normal bowel, about one percent of the bacteria are known to possess all of the enzymes necessary for the degradation of mucin.[93] Unfortunately, they also eat the epithelium wall, as seen in colitis, ulcers, bowel inflammation, and Crohn's disease.** It is possible that when the body loses its natural balance of healthy bacteria that these microorganisms severely contribute

---

[92] Forstner, pg. 234-268.

[93] A. P. Corfield., et al., "Mucus Glycoproteins and Their Role in Colorectal Disease," *Journal of Pathology*, 1996; Sept.; 180(1), pg. 14.

towards many diseases. It has been suggested that enzymes can remove mucoid plaque. Possibly, if our bodies produced enough pancreatic enzymes. However, this does not appear to be the case with more than 98% of the people, as indicated by the percentage of people who remove mucoid plaque when cleansing. I have conducted more than 26 experiments using various enzymes, bacteria, and other substances to determine what will dissolve mucoid plaque. I never found anything, including enzymes, that made a dent on any fresh mucoid plaque. (However, I also was not able to exactly duplicate the bowel environment in these experiments.)

Until I developed my cleanse program, no one knew how to extract the mucoid plaque from the stomach and small intestine. Indeed, **the entire gastrointestinal tract and stomach must be cleansed of toxic and/or altered mucoid plaque if we want to truly rebuild our digestive systems and revitalize our bodies and minds.** Healthy digestion, a full reserve of minerals, and **efficient nourishment of all organs are essential for long-lasting health.**

### Exactly What Is Mucoid Plaque & Why Is It Created?

Mucoid plaque is primarily composed of glycoproteins called mucin. More specifically, mucin contains more than 50% carbohydrates and more than 20 amino acids.[94,95,96] Mucin is associated with normal epithelium as well as with carcinomas of the lung, breast, ovary, and gastrointestinal tract.[97] Other ingredients found mixed in with the mucin include water, electrolytes, sloughed off epithelial cells, bacteria and bacterial by-products, digested food (fecal matter), plasma proteins, bile salts, pancreatic enzymes, and most all other constituents normally found in

---

[94] J. Holland, R. Bast, Jr., D. Morton, E. Freil III, D. Kute, R. Weichselbaum, *Cancer Medicine*, Volume 1, 4th Edition, (Baltimore, MD: Williams & Wilkins, 1997), pg. 228.

[95] John B. West, *Physiological Basis of Medical Practice*, Twelfth Edition, (Baltimore, MD: Williams & Wilkins, 1990), pg. 652.

[96] *Stedman's Medical Dictionary* describes "mucin" as a secretion containing carbohydrate-rich glycoproteins such as that from the goblet cells of the intestine, the submaxillary glands, and other mucous glandular cells; it is also present in the ground substance of connective tissue, especially mucous connective tissue, is soluble in alkaline water, and is precipitated by acid.

[97] Holland, Bast, Morton, Freil, Kute, & Weichselbaum, Volume 1, 4th Edition, pg. 228.

the intestinal juice.[98,99] Mucoid plaque is created by the body to protect itself when it is under attack by acids, or toxic compounds such as drugs (esp. aspirin & alcohol), salt[100,101,102,] heavy metals, toxic chemicals, antigen-antibody complexes, microbial activity, the toxins produced by bacteria, yeast, and parasites[103,104,105,106] as well as solutions resulting from incomplete digestion and absorption of carbohydrates.[107] And all of these substances have been found in mucoid plaque. In addition, evidence now indicates that the long term use of *acidophilus*, due to its creation of lactic acid, may also contribute to mucoid plaque development and other disorders.[108,109,110]

---

[98] Forstner, pg. 234-263.

[99] A. Allen, et al., "Studies on Gastrointestinal Mucus," *Scandinavian Journal of Gastroenterology*, Supplements, 1984; 93, pg. 101-113.

[100] For pictures of the villi damaged by salt, see H. W. Davenport, *Physiology of the Digestive Tract*, Vol. 4, (New York: Yearbook Medical Publisher and Digestive Disease and Sciences, 1980), pg. 162. For alcohol, see *Digestive Disease and Sciences*, 1980; July; Vol. 25, No. 7, pg. 513.

[101] A. Allen, A. Bell, and S. McQueen, "Mechanisms of Mucosal Protection of the Upper Gastrointestinal Tract," *Mucus and Mucosal Protection*, (Philadelphia, PA: Raven Press, 1984), pg. 317.

[102] Lindsay H. Allen, Ph.D., E.A., Oddoye, Ph.D., and S. Margen, M.D., "Protein Induced Hypercalciuria; A Longer Term Study," *The American Journal of Clinical Nutrition*, 1979; April; Issue 32, pg. 741-749.

[103] Guyton and Hall, pg. 847.

[104] Allen, Bell, and McQueen, "Mechanisms of Mucosal Protection of the Upper Gastrointestinal Tract," *Mucus and Mucosal Protection*, pg. 201.

[105] J. Rainer Poley, ed., "Chronic Nonspecific Diarrhea in Children: Investigation of the Surface Morphology of Small Bowel Mucosa Utilizing the Scanning Electron Microscope," *Journal of Pediatric Gastroenterology and Nutrition*, 1983; 2, pg. 71-94.

[106] Glenn R. Gibson, George T. Macfarlane, *Human Colonic Bacteria; Role in Nutrition, Physiology, and Pathology*, (Boca Raton, FL: CRC Press, 1995), pg. 179.

[107] A lack of sucrase, lactase, and maltase enzymes may prevent proper digestion of certain carbohydrates. Some medical scientists have considered that mucoid plaque may prevent these enzymes from reaching the carbohydrates and thereby prevent proper digestion and assimilation. See Poley, "Chronic Nonspecific Diarrhea in Children."

After a meal, the body naturally attempts to digest and assimilate food. However, mucoid plaque may inhibit this process. For it stands to reason that the body will attempt to assimilate anything in the bowel, even mucoid plaque. One study revealed that when the body absorbs mucins into the bloodstream, it can cause hypercoagulability and venous thrombosis (blood clots).[111] When the body attempts to absorb food but there is only mucoid plaque which acts as a barrier to the food, then mucoid plaque and whatever elements it contains are likely to enter the bloodstream. Therefore it stands to reason that if we have contaminated mucoid plaque in our bowels, our blood will be toxic as well.

**Mucoid plaque found in the bowel is *not* equivalent to the natural healthy gastric and intestinal mucosa.** I want to point this out because many doctors, when viewing the inside of the intestines, believe that they are seeing the normal mucosa, when they are actually seeing mucoid plaque. This is discussed later in this chapter under the section, "Why Most Surgeons are Unaware of Mucoid Plaque." My research indicates that in fact it would be very rare to see normal mucosa because the layer or layers of mucoid plaque that cover the entire intestinal tract are so common. The natural mucosa is beneath the glycocalyx and is meant to serve as the necessary buffer for the gastrointestinal wall, and as a lubricant for peristalsis - but cannot when it is covered by mucoid plaque.[112,113] Hence mucoid plaque is usually associated with some degree of constipation as well as various other bowel irritations and problems. **Many doctors who are unaware of mucoid plaque believe that the mucoid plaque is the normal mucosa. This is not true.**

---

[108] The lactic acid created by *Lactobacillus acidophilus* has a pH of 4.5, and sometimes less. John G. Holt, Noel R. Krieg, *Bergey's Manual Of Systematic Bacteriology*, Vol. 2, (Baltimore, MD: Williams & Wilkins, 1984), pg. 1212.

[109] Joseph T. Thurn, Gordon L. Pierpont, Carl W. Ludvigsen, John H. Eckfeldt, "D-Lactate Encephalopathy," *The American Journal of Medicine*, 1985; Dec.; Vol:79, pg. 717-720.

[110] Lawrence Stolberg, Rial Rolfe, Norman Gitlin, Jeffrey Merritt, Louis Mann, Jean Linder, Sydney Finegold, "D-Lactic Acidosis Due to Abnormal Gut Flora," New England Journal of Medicine, 1982; Vol. 306, #22, pg. 1344-1347.

[111] Forstner, pg. 254.

[112] Guyton and Hall, pg. 837.

[113] Ibid., pg. 846.

# Mucoid Plaque is Real

*From Colon*

*From upper ileum*

*From colon*

*From colon*

*From colon*

*From colon. When we see mucoid plaque from the colon, we can know that we may be removing blockages to major lymphatic drainage areas. The colon can affect many areas of the body. For example, bowel pockets in the ascending colon can affect the heart. A bowel pocket in the cecum can affect the right kidney, etc.*

# Understanding Mucosa and the Intestine

The mucosa is a mucous membrane consisting of four distinct anatomical sections, the serosa, muscularis, submucosa, and mucosa. On the lumen side of the mucosa is the glycocalyx, which covers the mucosa and serves as a protection for it. The mucosa is the gateway that allows all nutrients from the bowel into the blood and lymph as well as the rest of the body. It also serves as a barrier to anything that should not enter the inner sanctum of our precious bodies. The surface cells, next to the lumen, are known as epithelial cells. The epithelium consists of absorptive cells, secretory cells, mucus-secreting cells (goblet cells), and possibly, endocrine cells. **These epithelium cells renew themselves every 4 to 7 days.**[114]

## Cross Section of the Gut

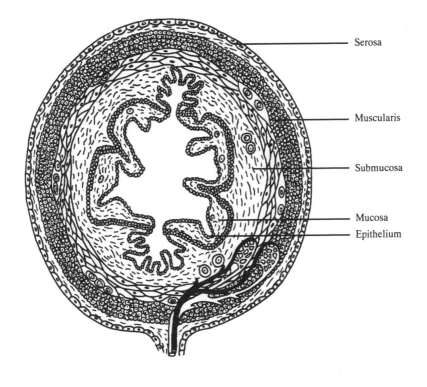

Serosa

Muscularis

Submucosa

Mucosa
Epithelium

---

[114] Yamada, pg. 266.

The wall of the small intestines has extensive folds called plicae circularis. **These folds give the mucoid plaque its unique shapes and markings you see when mucoid plaque sections are removed.** They also serve to churn up the food so that all food stuff has the opportunity to touch the "brush border" enzymes along the epithelium/glycocalyx wall. These folds expand the surface area by 3 times. Each fold contains numerous macroscopic structures called villi, which expand the surface area another 10 times. Each villi consists of a single layer of surface epithelial cells and covers an inner core of tiny blood and lymph vessels, nerve fibers and smooth muscle cells. In a healthy individual, each epithelial cell of the villi project approximately 1000 microvilli.[115] These microvilli, expand the surface another 20 times. **Altogether, the plicae circularis, the villi, and the microvilli increase the absorptive surface by six hundred-fold, providing an area the size of a tennis court for nutrient absorption.[116]**

On the surface of the microvilli is a very important substance called *glycocalyx*. Glycocalyx is a carbohydrate-rich substance consisting of proteins, lipids, and some glycoproteins and **is negatively charged, which gives most cells a negative surface charge that repels other negatively charged objects.[117]** As I said, most doctors are unaware of the difference between this normal protective layer called glycocalyx, and the mucoid plaque. In fact, very few clinical studies have discussed this important difference. It was not until biopsies were studied with the electron microscope that a clear understanding was reached. The glycocalyx is a microvillous membrane which contains many of the enzymes, receptors, and carriers necessary for final digestion and absorption. In fact, more than 22 enzymes, such as the disaccharide, alkaline phosphate, and peptide enzymes abide here.[118] Also at this site, in healthy individuals, are large volumes of alkaline buffering agents that protect the bowel wall from invasions of acids, toxins and microorganisms. The epithelium cells produce glycocalyx. Glycocalyx is amazingly durable. It cannot be removed by saline washes, mucolytic and proteolytic enzymes, by EDTA,[119] or by fasting.[120] The glycocalyx is readily permeated by water

---

[115] Guyton and Hall, pg. 837-838.

[116] Wynn Kapit, Robert I. Macey, Esmail Meisami, *The Physiology Coloring Book*, (Cambridge, MA: Harper Collins Publishers, 1987), pg. 74.

[117] Guyton and Hall, pg.13 -14.

[118] Yamada, ed., pg. 1414.

[119] EDTA: ethylenediaminetetraacetic acid. From *Churchill's Illustrated Medical Dictionary.*

ions and small molecules, and appears to be a major barrier to keep bacteria and other particulate matter from direct contact with the microvilli.

Some have speculated that mucoid plaque may serve as a barrier against pathogenic microorganisms. Although this is probably true with transient bacteria, evidence indicates the exact opposite with non-transitory microorganisms. **Mucoid plaque actually *protects pathogens* from whatever medications or herbs we may take in the effort to eliminate them.** Clinical studies have shown that **pathogenic bacteria, such as E. coli, actually hide underneath the mucoid plaque and are completely separated from luminal contents.**[121,122] E. coli are also known to stimulate mucin release.[123] Not only that, but in animal experiments, it has been shown that **bacteria actually penetrate the mucoid plaque within two hours after infection.**[124] In fact, mucoid plaque actually helps to promote the growth of certain bacteria. To some extent, therefore, mucoid plaque determines the bacterial flora, especially in the colon.[125] **There is evidence that various parasites and yeasts also find a safe environment in the mucoid plaque.** Not only that, but the **mucoid plaque may actually serve as a "culture medium" for some human pathogens** and may serve as a food source for anaerobic bacteria. In other words, **the greater the mucin secretion, the greater the microbial invasion.**[126,127] It stands to reason that the type of microorganisms that live in or beneath the mucoid plaque have a major impact upon the intestinal environment and our internal environment: the blood, the lymph, glands, organs, etc. And further, it follows that **the species of microorganisms are dependent upon the degree of purity or toxicity within the mucoid plaque - and the rest of the bowel environment.**

---

[120] J. Rainer Poley, "Loss of the Glycocalyx of Enterocytes in Small Intestine: A Feature Detected by Scanning Electron Microscopy in Children with Gastrointestinal Intolerance to Dietary Protein," *Journal of Pediatric Gastroenterology and Nutrition,* 1988; 7, pg. 836-394.

[121] Gibson, and Macfarlane, pg. 184.

[122] Poley, "Chronic Nonspecific Diarrhea in Children," pg. 71-94.

[123] Forstner, pg. 234-263.

[124] Gibson and Macfarlane, pg. 184.

[125] Forstner, pg. 234-263.

[126] Ibid., pg. 252.

[127] Allen, Bell and McQueen, "Mechanisms of Mucosal Protection of the Upper Gastrointestinal Tract," *Mucus and Mucosal Protection,* pg. 101.

Contained within this entire system is a rather incredible and very impressive protective mechanism known as the bowel immune system. It comprises one of the largest immunologic and essential systems in the body. **This mucosal immune system allows nutrients to cross bowel barriers unimpeded and yet prevents entry of injurious agents.**[128] **A strong healthy bowel immune system may be capable of eliminating any known pathogen from living in the bowel,** for it is fully capable of mounting an intense, protective inflammatory reaction in response to infectious agents or injurious substance, such as bacteria, viruses, and parasites.[129] This extremely valuable immune function appears to have become very weak and ineffective with the vast majority of people today.

It is very important to understand that the small intestine is designed to churn and mix the food in such a way that all of the food touches the brush border of the microvilli as it passes through the small intestines. This is essential, because **the food must make contact with the 22 or more digestive enzymes that extrude from the brush border cells/epithelium and out through the glycocalyx.**[130] **However, this is not happening with the vast majority of people in the Western World, because of the layer or layers of mucoid plaque.**[131,132]

On the surface of the epithelium glycocalyx is the area that generates mucoid plaque, via the secretion of the goblet cells through the crypts of Lieberkuhn. Evidence indicates that **"mucoid plaque", with the possible exception of the stomach, is *unnatural* to a healthy body and is found only after the body has moved out of perfect health and descended towards dis-eased states.** It is a natural protection from an unnatural toxin. This evidence includes: 1) Tens of thousands of people have dramatically improved their health when they began to remove the mucoid plaque by intestinal cleansing; 2) Medical studies have shown that mucoid plaque can interfere with digestion, assimilation, and protect pathogenic microorganisms from being eliminated via medicines and/or mechanical means; 3) Studies have shown that mucoid plaque can transform into a variety of disease conditions, some of which are deadly serious, as will be shown **later in this chapter.**[133]

---

[128] Yamada, ed., pg. 85.

[129] Yamada, ed., pg. 85-99.

[130] Poley, "Loss of the Glycocalyx of Enterocytes in Small Intestine," pg. 386-394.

[131] Poley, "Chronic Nonspecific Diarrhea in Children," pg. 71-94.

[132] Poley, "The Scanning Electron Microscope," pg. 386-394.

As indicated above, mucoid plaque is undoubtedly created as a protective mechanism against acids and other toxic substances. It appears that the primary caustic substance is bile acids. Bile, as a result of organic sodium deficiency, can become extremely acid, and due to the acid-forming diets of most people, acidic bile can be relentless. Until the cause of acid bile is remedied, mucoid plaque will be created and the bowel will remain vulnerable to a large variety of bowel disorders, including cancer. The source of bile is the liver and **more than 80% of patients who die of metastatic colorectal cancer suffer from hepatic (liver) involvement.**[134] Abnormal liver function is considered a common finding in cancer patients.[135] Not only that, but a large percentage of the population have gallstones, and as disease states advance, the number of gallstones increase. These are important clues that bile may have become abnormal. For, if the liver and gallbladder cannot function properly, how can we expect the bile to be the right composition when it is made by a dysfunctional liver, and is stored in an abnormal gallbladder environment?[136] It has also been shown that acid bile, especially in the form of deoxycholic acid, increases cellular proliferation and is suspected to be a cause of bowel cancer.[137]

**As long as the gut remains acid due to electrolyte deficiencies and acid bile, mucoid plaque is a necessary protection.** It will also continue to be created as long as there are pathogenic microorganisms present.[138] Diet is undoubtedly the key, for the wrong foods contribute towards electrolyte deficiencies, the decrease of hydrochloric acid, calcium deficiencies, enzyme dysfunction, and the feeding of pathogenic microorganisms. It stands to reason that **after continual abuse, large amounts of mucoid plaque may be formed.** It has been shown that the **thickness of mucoid plaque increases with age** and **is surprisingly thick even in some children who are experiencing bowel disorders.**[139] Mucoid plaque thickness varies from person to person and **can be as much**

---

[133] **See the sections titled: "Mucoid Plaque Mutates," and "Mucoid Plaque and Cancer."**

[134] Yamada, ed., pg.1804.

[135] Holland, Bast, Morton, Freil, Kute, and Weichselbaum, Volume 2, 4th Edition, pg. 3225.

[136] It is also an important clue that the liver is involved with cancer and should be considered an important organ that needs to be purified and strengthen when treating cancer patients. Why is this completely ignored by allopathic doctors?

[137] Yamada, ed., pg.1776

[138] Poley, "Chronic Nonspecific Diarrhea in Children," pg. 71-94.

[139] Poley, "The Scanning Electron Microscope," pg. 386-394.

as ten times greater in one person compared to another.[140] Abnormal build-ups of mucoid plaque have been identified with pathogenic bacteria, and various bowel diseases, including cancer.[141,142]

One thing that is surprising is the tenacity of mucoid plaque to remain in the gut. **It sticks tenaciously to the epithelium or glycocalyx, which is why it takes the form of the epithelium wall.**[143] This is very apparent when the plaque is removed via intestinal cleansing. Every successful experienced cleanser knows what I mean. The mucoid plaque coming out of our bodies takes on every shape, fold, bump, striation, and crease that the gut wall had when the plaque was formed. Mucoid plaque is not easily removed except with certain herbal formulas and as I explained, can become a hindrance to metabolic bowel functions and it may provide a sanctuary for many pathogenic substances.

# Old Mucoid Plaque:  Barrier to Assimilation, Pre-cursor to Disease

Mucoid plaque tends to remain in the system even when it is no longer needed for protection, and after a period of time, **contributes towards toxicity, by binding toxic matter from food, fecal matter, bacterial and parasite by-products, as well as their dead bodies. This profile weakens intestinal function, causes interference of nerve meridians, and development of bowel disease.** Even a small layer of mucoid plaque, especially when adhering closely to the mucosal surface, appears to **function as a barrier to membrane digestion and absorption, and may cause protein and carbohydrate intolerance.**[144,145]

---

[140] Gibson, and Macfarlane, pg. 178.

[141] Joseph B. Kirsner, M.D., Ph.D., D.Sc. (Hon.), and Roy G. Shorter, M.D., *Inflammatory Bowel Disease*, (Baltimore, MD: Williams & Wilkins, 1995), pg. 143.

[142] Whitehead, pg. 81, 82, 85.

[143] Poley, "Loss of the Glycocalyx of Enterocytes in Small Intestine," pg. 386-394.

[144] Poley, "The Scanning Electron Microscope," pg. 386-394.

[145] Jack D. Welsh, J. Rainer Poley, Jess Hensley, and Mira Bhatia, "Intestinal Disaccharidase and Alkaline Phosphatase Activity in Giardiasis," *Journal of Pediatric Gastroenterology and Nutrition*, 1984; 3(1), pg. 37-40.

It is considered by almost every gastroenterologist and physiologist, that the secretion of mucin (mucus), which is the source of mucoid plaque, is a very important function of the gastrointestinal epithelium.[146] But what many doctors fail to realize is that in most people today **mucoid plaque is not released out of the body once it has served its purpose.** What may appear as normal mucosa is far from being normal, especially in a bowel that has cancer.[147]

**There are transforming substances, such as lectins, that have the capacity to alter mucoid plaque (mucin) into various disease states.**[148,149] Lectins are a type of glycoproteins that are found in plant seeds.[150] They bind to specific types of human cells, particularly immature, transformed or tumor cells. This binding can result in cell toxicity leading to cellular damage and ultimately, an increase in cell turnover. **White sugar, soft drinks, wheat products, rancid, spoiled food, table salt, hormones, antibiotics found in animal products, abnormal bile salts, and especially prescription antibiotics, are all suspicious compounds in their ability to transform mucoid plaque into disease profiles.** By-products of microorganisms and negative (acid-forming) thoughts and feelings also belong on the list. Certain drugs may also alter the mucoid plaque, and, as I said, especially antibiotics, particularly penicillin. It has been shown that the fungus, *penicillium commune*, from which penicillin is derived, "develops pleomorphic giant cells packed with minute rods, unlike anything known in classic colonies of this mold".[151] Though mucoid plaque is not the same thing as mold, it is possible that mucoid plaque may contain molds or other elements that contribute towards the transformation of normal mucoid plaque into diseased states. Molds contain plant proteins as do lectins, which are known to cause mutations of mucins.[152]

---

[146] Whitehead, pg. 73.

[147] Ibid., pg. 45.

[148] Ibid., pg. 73-91.

[149] J. R. Poley, "Scanning Electron Microscopy of Soy Protein-Induced Damage of Small Bowel Mucosa in Infants," *Journal of Pediatric Gastroenterology and Nutrition,* 1983; May; 2 (2), pg. 271-278.

[150] Whitehead, ed., pg. 576.

[151] Lida H. Mattman, *Cell Wall Deficient Forms, Stealth Pathogens,* 2nd Edition, (Ann Arbor, CRC Press, 1993), pg. 241.

[152] Lectin: A protein of primarily plant (usually seed) origin that binds to glycoproteins on the surface of cells causing agglutination, precipitation, or other phenomena resembling the action of specific antibody; lectins

# Mucoid Plaque and Cancer

Clinical studies have shown that intestinal mucins are frequently altered in such a way as to trigger the evolution of epithelial cells into cancer cells.[153] Studies also show that altered mucins or altered mucoid plaque, can develop into intestinal metaplasis, then into dysplasia, and finally, into adenocarcinomas. This process may take as long as 20 years.[154] Gastric carcinomas have also been shown to develop from intestinal metaplasia that has mutated from mucoid plaque.[155,156] It has been shown that most adenocarcinomas secrete a small or moderate amount of mucin. 10 to 20% of tumors may be described as mucinous or colloid carcinomas on the basis of their more prodigious production of mucin. It has also been shown that these mucinous tumors of the bowel are associated with a poorer survival rate than non-mucinous tumors.[157] Indeed, there are many levels of mucoid plaque degradation and each level is a sign of a pending disease state.

The big question is: How can mucoid plaque, composed primarily of mucins and lacking cells, become cancerous? It can't; but it may be able to stimulate the conditions necessary for cancer growth and become intermingled with it. **The development of cancer and other diseased and unnatural growths in the bowel appear to be associated with increased cell proliferation. In fact, this is generally considered to be the cause of cancer.**[158] So the logical question is: What causes increased cell proliferation?

There are many elements that can cause increased cell proliferation and generally, they are toxic substances called carcinogens. Some of these

---

include plant agglutinins (phytoagglutinins, phytohemagglutinins), plant precipitins, and perhaps certain animal proteins; some have mitogenic properties. Source - Stedman's Medical Dictionary.

[153] Whitehead, pg. 73-91.

[154] Ibid., pg. 80.

[155] P. Sipponen, K. Seppala, E. Varis, et al., "Intestinal Metaplasia With Colonic-Type Sulphomucins In the Gastric Mucosa, Its Association With Gastric Carcinoma," *Acta Pathologica Microbiologica Scandinavica*, 1980; 88, pg. 217-224.

[156] J. R. Jass, M. I. Filpe, "Sulphomucins and Precancerous Lesions of the Human Stomach," *Histopathology*, 1980; 4, pg. 271-279.

[157] Yamada, ed., pg. 1786.

[158] Whitehead, pg. 108, 111.

elements include pesticides and other man-made chemicals, burnt materials, bile acids, hormones, drugs, sodium chloride, chlorine from water, alcohol, microorganisms, etc. Basically, **anything that causes cell damage can cause excess proliferation and, if certain other factors are present, this proliferation of cells can initiate carcinogenesis.**[159] Obviously, the above elements can cause cell damage, so the next question is, what are the other factors?

**Important factors that encourage the development of cancer include**: nutritional deficiencies (vitamins, minerals, fatty acids, antioxidants, amino acids, etc.), a weak liver, a weak immune system, high levels of toxicity throughout the body, pathogenic bacteria, a diet high in animal products, constipation, an over-acid system, acid bile, a lack of electrolytes, suppressed emotions, etc. Now, how does mucoid plaque contribute towards cancer and other bowel diseases?

This is an area of mystery in medical science and there is a great deal of speculation. Hypothesis and theories abound as scientists frantically search for reasons. Yet, because most of them have become so 'conditioned,' they fail to put it all together and don't see the picture clearly. I believe that there are several ways that mucoid plaque is associated with diseased conditions in the bowel. **One way is that mucoid plaque could contribute towards a lack of normal circulation or enhanced viscosity, and block the normal out-flow of lymph and mucin drainage.**[160] In any area of the body, **when there is a lack of circulation, *toxins accumulate* and normal *oxygen levels decrease*. Both of these conditions are associated with cancer.** Photographs of intestinal metaplasia biopsies reveal what appears as plugs in the crypt openings. On the top of these "plugs" is a layer of mucoid plaque resting on the epithelium wall.[161]

**Another possibility is that because mucoid plaque binds toxins to one locality, a condition of continuous cell irritation and damage is created.** When under attack from toxins, the body purposely initiates the secretion of mucus and other substances and according to its specific chemistry, can form cyst-like barriers that help to protect the tissue from the toxins. **Some toxins, such as heavy metals, can be stored in the body for 25 years or longer. Because they are so toxic, the body would rather bind them in one location rather than risk greater damage in the removal process.** If these toxins remain at one particular site long enough and are associated with the epithelium cells, they could

---

[159] Ibid.

[160] Ibid., pg. 84.

[161] Ibid., pg. 80-81.

cause continuous cell irritation, dysfunction, and damage. Imagine if the plaque held some pesticides or heavy metals in one spot and the epithelium was constantly attacked. This certainly could force cell proliferation. Evidence supports this theory in that adenomas (non-malignant bowel cancers) are often adjoining extra thick mucoid plaque.[162]

**A third possibility is that mucoid plaque layers could cause pressure upon the epithelium wall and actually force mucins back into the epithelium wall.** Using light microscopy, researchers can show photos of the epithelium wall. Many photos reveal backed up mucin, or congestion, both inside and outside the epithelium wall. **Most of these photos also show a thick layer of mucoid plaque on the epithelium (gut) wall.** This may be what happens with intestinal metaplasia and diverticulitis.[163] Based upon the chemical profile of the mucoid plaque, a variety of disease states could induce this type of pressure.

There are basically two kinds of mucin found in the bowel. One is acid mucin and the other is neutral mucin.[164] Both are involved with the development of cancer. My studies indicate, however, that the acid mucin seems a more likely trigger mechanism that could cause cell proliferation and the neutral mucin may be an attempt to buffer a toxic element. Mucins are generally secreted in response to something toxic and irritating. It is also possible that the cells themselves secrete mucin in an attempt get rid of something toxic. Even cancer cells secrete mucins.[165] Why? In order to remove toxins? Ideally, the bowel would carry the toxin, bound in mucin, out of the body. Unfortunately, for most people, however, mucins seem to remain in close proximity to the source of irritation for decades, binding toxins to that locality. I believe that this occurs as a result of an extremely toxic and nutritionally deficient bowel.

**Note:** I believe that it is possible that **the development of cancer, and any other diseases involving cellular deformity, anywhere throughout the body, may very well be caused by a lack of nutrients.** In fact, **cancer is a disease in which the host often dies of starvation** because the cancer cells rob the rest of the cells and ultimately, the whole body, of nutrients. **A cell must have its full range of nutritional elements or it will not be able to effectively handle a toxin that it normally could, hence the proper diet is always essential in the overcoming of disease.** Imagine the construction of a building in which the cement was lacking

---

[162] Ibid., pg. 85-86.

[163] Ibid., pg. 80-81.

[164] Ibid., pg. 74.

[165] Ibid., pg. 84.

certain compounds that are necessary for its strength and integrity. How long would it stand? Even mild rain water could break down its structure. Wouldn't it be shocking to learn that cancer was nothing but a nutritional deficiency? After all, how can our cells have strength and integrity if they do not have all the nutrients they need. I believe that cancer and most other diseases, as well, are associated with nutritional deficiencies. If this is true, **there would be only three primary causes: a nutritionally deficient diet, an inefficient digestive system, and congestion in the system. Any of these can block nutrients from reaching all of our cells.**

## Mucoid Plaque Mutates!

There are many different names used by medical scientists and authors to describe the mucus development in the gut.[166,167] Not only that, but there are many other medical terms that describe the various diseased states into which mucoid plaque can mutate. A partial list includes: atrophic gastritis, polyps, intestinal metaplasis, dysplasia, cystic fibrosis, as well as the various cancers.[168] Not only that, but **gastroenterologists have studied mucoid plaque mutations as possible clinical markers to help predict potential disease crisis.**[169,170,171] One of these methods is based upon a theory called "Transitional Mucosa".

Transitional mucosa (TM) is a medical term that describes **the alteration of normal mucosa combined with mucoid plaque into**

---

[166] Other authors and scientists have described this "mucoid plaque" substance as "mucoid matter," "mucoid material," "mucoid," "mucoid layer," "mucoid pseudomembrane," "mucosal barrier," "mucus barrier," "layer of mucus," "transitional mucosa," "mucous glycoproteins," and "surface mucin."

[167] There are more than 45 different medical descriptions of the phenomenon I refer to as mucoid plaque.

[168] Whitehead, pg. 45, 47, 73, 80.

[169] Kirsner and Shorter, pg. 316.

[170] C. F. A. Culling, P. E. Reid, J.D. Burton, and W.I. Dunn, "A Histochemical Method Of Differentiating Lower Gastrointestinal Tract Mucin From Other Mucins In Primary or Metastatic Tumors," *Journal of Clinical Pathology*, 1975; 28, pg. 656-658.

[171] H. C. Cook, "Neutral Mucin Content of Gastric Carcinomas as a Diagnostic Aid In the Identification of Secondary Deposits," *Histopathology*, 1982; 6, pg. 591-599.

**disease patterns.** This term was introduced in 1969 to describe the **zone of transition from normal mucosa to carcinoma.** It is characterized by "abnormal mucin secretion". There has been a great deal of controversy concerning this theory. The theory of TM offers a method to identify potential cancer growths by viewing the **alteration of mucoid plaque.**[172] It has been recognized that **TM (sialomucins) - another form of mucoid plaque - is adjacent to 98% of bowel carcinomas and is seen in only 13% of non-adenocarcinoma tumors.** Another very interesting point is that there is a gradient of increased proportion of sialomucins from right to left colon (where mucoid plaque becomes thicker). This is where the incidence of carcinoma is higher. And there is no such gradient in normal colorectal mucosa.[173,174] TM is also associated with various kinds of polyps (juvenile, inflammatory, metaplastic), non-adenocarcinomatous neoplasias of the colorectum. **Excess acid mucin, which is a TM indicator, is also associated with diverticular disease, Crohn's disease, colonic inflammation, ulcerative-colitis, solitary ulcer syndrome, dysplasia, larger polyps, and possibly, other disease states as well.**[175]

The important point is that **mucoid plaque, under certain unknown conditions can transform and contribute toward pathogenesis.** It has been suggested that a genetic defect in mucoid plaque or mucoid plaque production, when combined with something toxic in the diet, or from bacteria, or altered immunity, triggers the mutation factors.[176] **Investigation of the changes of mucoid plaque patterns have been conducted in the attempt to diagnose and detect early malignant transformation.**[177]

---

[172] Whitehead, pg.85.

[173] Whitehead, pg. 86.

[174] M. L. Filipe, "Transitional Mucosa," *Histopathology,* 1984; July; 8(4), pg. 707-708.

[175] Whitehead, pg. 86.

[176] Ibid., pg. 89.

[177] M. L. Filipe, "Histochemical Characteristics of Mucins in the Small Intestine. A Comparative Study of Normal Mucosa, Benign Epithelial Tumors and Carcinoma," Histochemical Journal, 1979; 11, pg. 277-287.

# Electrolytes and Bowel Disease

It is interesting that when mucoid plaque has a neutral pH, the mucosa appears normal,[178] but when the mucoid plaque becomes acid, then it is more likely to mutate into one of the aforementioned disease profiles. Sialomucins, or transitional mucosa, and sulphomucins are both acidic mucins and have been associated with disease states including cancer.[179,180,181] **This supports my theory that most bowel diseases are associated with electrolyte deficiencies.** The variance in the pH of mucins also may be associated with electrolyte deficiencies. When medical researchers finally realize that there is a vast difference between organic sodium and sodium chloride, and that sodium chloride cannot be used efficiently by the body, research will take an entirely new course. I say this because none of the researchers in this arena has considered the difference.

One clinical study found that **when the mucoid plaque became more alkaline, the viscosity of the plaque decreased and became more fluid**. It was even suggested that a low luminal pH may contribute towards conditions such as cystic fibrosis. Further, **when the intestinal environment became more acid (4.5 or lower), the normal viscosity of the mucoid plaque became more firm and formed a dense white precipitate**. It was even suggested by the author conducting this study that **an acid intestinal environment** and/or **increased intestinal serum proteins** might cause mucoid plaque to undergo a pathological transformation into either a more dense gel or an insoluble precipitate.[182] Numerous people using my cleanse program have seen some of their mucoid plaque come out so hard that they could not cut it easily with a knife. Sometimes the plaque was so hard and stiff that it stuck out like a piece of wood. Excessive acids caught in various bowel pockets may have been the reasons for these bizarre mutations. Strong **acid producing bacteria may also contribute towards these conditions**.

As you can see, there may be a great advantage in removing the mucoid plaque. Some people may think, however, that we should just leave it alone. They think that it was put there for a purpose and maybe if we remove it we will become more vulnerable to attack. Many doctors believe that mucoid plaque is needed for lubrication and protection of the

---

[178] Whitehead, pg. 79.

[179] Ibid., pg. 74.

[180] Ibid., pg. 82.

[181] Filipe, "Transitional Mucosa," pg. 707-708.

[182] Forstner, pg. 234-263.

mucosal surface. Most of these doctors are unaware that the activities of the glycocalyx naturally include these important functions. In other words, **glycocalyx is the normal mucus barrier that lines the epithelium wall, not the mucoid plaque**. In fact, most doctors do not even know the difference between mucoid plaque and glycocalyx. However, unless we are in perfect health, and all pathogenic microorganisms have departed, and the natural, normal intestinal biological terrain established, it's probably impossible to remove all mucoid plaque through bowel cleansing because it would just keep being recreated. The body can produce the mucins that form mucoid plaque within minutes.[183] Even if the body does reproduce plaque immediately, I still believe it is very beneficial to remove the old mucoid plaque before it begins to mutate into diseased states. To not want to remove it is like not wanting to remove Giardia, E. Coli, or cancer. After all, these things get into people for a reason as well. For people who are concerned about losing mucoid plaque which they feel the body may need, they can rest assured that given an over-acid condition (from eating poorly or being stressed) which would require the formation of mucoid plaque, the body will quickly and easily produce more as long as it has an adequate electrolyte supply. **So, for people who still consume acid-forming foods, cleansing simply removes old, contaminated mucoid plaque, allowing the body to replenish new, *clean* mucoid plaque as needed.**

# Facts Supporting Acid Bile and Mucoid Plaque Theory

It is a well known medical fact that acids induce physiological responses.[184] The *Textbook of Medical Physiology* by Guyton[185] describes the various buffer systems that protect the body against acids. The Textbooks of Gastroenterology by Yamada and Clinical Gastroenterology by Spiro, describe the damages caused when bile becomes unnaturally acid. **Both of these authors have described that cancer of the bowel is often associated with bile that has become too acid**. Mucin and mucus, are natural protective liquids that are excreted by the mucous cells and goblet cells throughout the stomach and intestines to help protect the delicate mucosal membranes from acids and toxins. Guyton explains that: **"Even the slightest irritation of the mucosa directly stimulates the mucous**

---

[183] Ibid., pg. 108.

[184] Spiro, pg. 254.

[185] Guyton, pg. 438 - 450.

**cells to secrete "copious quantities of this thick, viscid mucus".** This in turn forms a gastric barrier that prevents the digestion of the gastric wall and also greatly reduces the absorption of food substances by the gastric mucosa."[186]

Another interesting and well known fact is that 90% of the ulcers which develop in the human body are found in the duodenum.[187] This occurs primarily in an area of the duodenum where the Brunner's glands are located. Normally the Brunner's glands secrete a large amount of alkaline mucus which naturally protects the body from the large amounts of acids that are released from the stomach through the pyloric valve into the duodenum. This is normal, and when the body has abundant electrolytes, it can easily handle the job. **Ulcers develop after the body has lost its ability to create *alkaline* mucus.**

Doctors cannot figure this out because they fail to see the difference between organic sodium and inorganic sodium. The fact that medical science does not recognize that most people are deficient in sodium (which is the primary buffer of acids), causes them to fail in the realization that the primary problem is that patients have a defect in their ability to buffer the acids. There simply isn't enough sodium to go around and the body has to prioritize its use. Handling an ulcer may be a lower priority than keeping the body alive. Acids can severely damage the gastrointestinal tract and the normal method of defense is to create alkaline mucus. If it cannot create the alkaline mucus due to a severe shortage of organic sodium, ulcers, Crohn's disease, colitis, etc., may be the outcome. Abnormalities in colonic mucin glycoprotein are considered as potential clinical markers for ulcerative-colitis and possible other bowel diseases.[188]

As indicated above, various bowel diseases occur after the bile has become too acidic. Bile is created by the liver and flows to the gall bladder. All the bile which flows from the liver to the gall bladder should have a pH from 7.6 - 8.6.[189] But **sometimes the bile can become very acid, even as low as 4.5.**[190] Many people, in fact, most people, are rapidly moving towards disease states[191] and one step towards disease occurs

---

[186] Guyton, pg. 776.

[187] Kapit, Macey and Meisami, pg. 78.

[188] Kirsner, M.D., Ph.D., D.Sc. (Hon.) and Shorter, M.D., pg. 316.

[189] Tortora, and Grabowski, pg. 792.

[190] Guyton and Hall, pg. 386.

when they have lost the ability to maintain alkaline bile and acid bile develops. Under these conditions, the body is forced to secrete abnormal amounts of mucus to protect itself from the acids. This mucus, when it remains in the system, becomes mucoid plaque.

Even though I have shown through documented medical literature that **mucoid plaque is a normal by-product of unnatural acid stimulation**, it would mean very little if we could not demonstrate its existence by removing it from the bowels. We can show from hundreds of testimonies that the elimination of that which we call mucoid plaque is common among those who have used our cleansing program.

**At least 90% of the people who use our program have found mucoid plaque being eliminated from their bodies and most of them have improved their health, increased their energy, and eliminated a large spectrum of disease conditions.** This indicates that the elimination of the substance called mucoid plaque, and the general cleansing that takes place with our cleansing program removes a debilitating level of toxicity closely associated with the loss of vitality and chronic disease. Countless written testimonies and verbal statements of people who have done the cleanse provide strong evidence of the value and validity of this program and its association with the removal of mucoid plaque.

Medical scientists have clearly stated that they do not have all the answers. There is a great deal of guessing, and current concepts are in a constant state of flux. **Most medical scientists avoid the word normal, because "normal" implies that they know what normal is and what it is not.** The truth is they really do not know.[192] I have developed a system of cleansing the entire digestive tract that has assisted thousands of people in achieving better health. Other doctors such as Dr. Bernard Jensen and V.E. Irons have also developed good programs for cleansing the bowel. For many years, I have attempted to find out what the anatomical, physiological and chemical reasons for our success are. I believe that I have been able to successfully fill certain gaps in the field of Gastroenterology and some other fields of science. Although some of my concepts appear to be new and challenging to the average medical doctor, most of them are not new and make a great deal of sense. Indeed, much of my work is involved with finding the most sophisticated and current medical research available.

I previously stated that bile acids can stimulate mucosal and cell proliferation and that the main reason that bile becomes too acid is related

---

[191] More than 50% of the American population will have heart problems; more than 33% will have cancer before they die. See further statistics. From: Vital Statistics http:\\www.cdc.gov\nchswww\

[192] Yamada, ed., pg. 532.

to dietary ingestion of acid-forming foods or to an emotional condition.[193] Yamada has supported these concepts clearly, especially in relation to fats.[194] Yamada explains that the mechanism by which a high-fat diet enhances tumor production appears to be directly related to bile acids. He explains that an increase of animal fat in the diet, produces a significant increase in total fecal bile acids.[195] This is significant information, but there is one very important fact missing in all the studies I have seen about cancer and fats. **It is not just fats that are causing cancer! It is high-protein foods, especially meats - all meats, chicken, fish, and animals. For they all drain electrolytes and force the bile to become more acid.**

Constipation is associated with bowel problems. **Constipation is also associated with a poor diet;**[196] the same acid-forming diet that creates the conditions that force the bowel to defend itself against acids and toxins, by creating the protective mucus. Constipation is common in the majority of patients who have Irritable Bowel Syndrome.[197]

For anyone who still doubts the mucoid plaque theory, the normal colon is composed of a series of folds, saccules or pouches called haustra. A healthy colon, when using endoscopy, would show haustras and blood vessels. Between page 616 and 617 of *Clinical Gastroenterology* by Howard Spiro, there are several color photos revealing recognizable mucoid plaque in the stomach, duodenum, and colon (See plates: 27, and especially 31 which show mucoid plaque in "loops" and "wormlike mucosal protrusions". Plate 46 shows mucoid plaque so thick that the duodenal folds are almost completely covered. Plates 63 and 66 of the colon **show obvious mucoid plaque that cannot be denied by anyone**.) These plates are reproduced at the end of this chapter for the reader's convenience.

---

[193] There is a difference between bile acid and acid bile. There are bile acids in alkaline bile. I believe that this form is normal and cannot cause harm. It is only after bile becomes too acid that bile acids can cause harm.

[194] Yamada, ed., pg. 1774 - 1776.

[195] Ibid., pg. 1776.

[196] Bernard Jensen, Ph.D., N.D., D.C., M.H., *Tissue Cleansing Through Bowel Management*, (Escondido, CA: Bernard Jensen Publications, 1981), page 28.

[197] Yamada, ed., pg. 1698 - 1699.

# Why Most Surgeons Are Unaware Of Mucoid Plaque

Surgeons and regular doctors *are not* trained in the subject of mucoid plaque and therefore remain unaware of this important bowel condition. The mucoid plaque is usually less than 1/4 of an inch in many areas of the bowel (except in heavy meat and dairy eaters). It usually develops from a semi-transparent liquid solution (mucin) and may look like it is part of the intestinal wall itself as it takes on the exact shapes, striations, and bulges of the intestinal wall. Until the mucoid plaque begins to mix with fecal matter, its color and texture may appear similar to healthy bowel mucosa. Unless one knows what they are looking for it may be difficult to identify, especially by sight. Therefore, to doctors using endoscopy and to surgeons, it is unnoticeable unless they are familiar with the many different appearances mucoid plaque may have.

When doctors are looking into the bowel, they are usually looking into an area of great disturbance. For example, when a surgeon is cutting out cancer, or a gastroenterologist is looking at colitis or other infections using endoscopy, they are looking at an extremely abnormal situation. Usually with serious bowel disturbances, the bowel chemistry is extremely over-acid. This *extreme* chemical solution may "burn away" the mucoid plaque. Under these conditions, the body may lack the sodium and other electrolyte reserves to create further mucoid plaque that would compensate for the acid conditions, therefore inflammation develops.[198]

## When Mucoid Plaque Fails

Doctors should consider that when the body is very depleted of organic sodium and the bile acid is strong and consistent for a long period of time, the acid may dissolve the mucoid plaque and create-colitis, Crohn's disease, ulcers or other bowel inflammation. If the body has the ability, it may fight back and form cyst-like formations or other harder fibric conditions such as those found in Crohn's disease, polyp formations, Carcinoid tumor, and most other severe gastrointestinal diseases. These plastic-like formations are much more resistant to acids than normal mucoid plaque; that may be why they are formed.

---

[198] Various types of bowel inflammation may also be perpetuated by diet and certain bacteria. This is also usually associated with the inability to digest certain foods. Some bacteria feed on undigested residues of carbohydrates, milk, soy products, etc., and their by-products can cause inflammation.

# Bowel Environment Alters Mucoid Plaque

When we think of mucoid plaque we often tend to visualize it as an unnatural, toxic, thick, firm, mucous-like substance, covering the mucosa of the intestinal wall. Indeed this is often the case, but it also may take various other forms. As the bowel environment changes, so does the mucoid plaque. For example:

♦ As the proportion of organic sodium drops in relation to calcium in the intestines, the mucoid plaque may become firmer.

♦ With the consistent use of table salt there is a tendency for the mucoid plaque to become hard, crystallized, and brittle. In this form it can be very difficult to remove.

♦ When taking aspirin, gastric mucosal pH drops quickly, and injury is sure and sometimes permanent. Mucus at this site may be very thick, or raw ulcers may form when there are not enough alkaline minerals[199] and the body is unable to form the healthy protective layer.

♦ When mucoid plaque is formed in response to extreme toxicity, the plaque may be a soft, thick mucus.[200]

♦ When mucoid plaque is formed because of acid bile, it may be soft, transparent, remain thin, or become thicker depending upon how strong the bile acid is and the composition of mucous secretion. The thickness depends upon the amount and strength of the acid in the bile and the compensational strength of the alkaline reserve.

♦ When the pH of the bowel drops below 4.5, mucoid plaque becomes firmer and forms a dense white precipitate.[201]

---

[199] Kauffman, Jr. and Ligumsky, "Role of Endogenous Prostaglandins in Gastric Mucosal Integrity," Found in: Allen, Bell and McQueen, "Mechanisms of Mucosal Protection of the Upper Gastrointestinal Tract," *Mucus and Mucosal Protection,*(Philadelphia, PA: Raven Press, 1984), pg. 317.

[200] Guyton, pg. 776.

[201] Forstner, pg. 707-708.

# Experienced Doctors on Mucoid Plaque

On page 23 of his book, *Tissue Cleansing Through Bowel Management*, Dr. Jensen describes mucoid plaque. "The heavy mucus coating in the colon thickens and becomes a host of putrefaction. The blood capillaries to the colon begin to pick up the toxins, poisons and noxious debris as they seep through the bowel wall. All tissues and organs of the body are now taking on toxic substances. Here is the beginning of true autointoxication on a physiological level." On page 27 he reveals his knowledge in this matter. "**One autopsy revealed a colon to be 9 inches in diameter with a passage through it no larger than a pencil. The rest was caked up layer upon layer of encrusted fecal material. This accumulation can have the consistency of truck tire rubber. It can be that hard and black.** Another autopsy **revealed a stagnant colon to weigh in at an incredible 40 pounds**. Imagine carrying around all that morbid accumulated waste." On page 42, Dr. Jensen talks about his old teacher Dr. John Harvey Kellogg at the Battle Creek Sanitarium, who "maintained that **that 90% of the diseases of civilization are due to improper functioning of the colon.**" Dr. Jensen explains that National College in Chicago performed over 300 autopsies. "According to the history of these persons, 285 had claimed they were not constipated and had normal movements and only 15 had admitted they were constipated. The autopsies showed the opposite to be the case, however, and only 15 were found not to have been constipated, while 285 were found to have been constipated. Some of the histories of these 285 persons stated they had had as many as 5 or 6 bowel movements daily, **yet autopsies revealed that in some of them the bowel was 12 inches in diameter**. The bowel walls were encrusted with material (in one case peanuts which had been lodged there for a very long time." Dr. Jensen explains: "As we work with **eliminating the encrusted mucus lining**, we must also consider nourishing the new cells below it.... **Bowel cleansing is an essential element in any lasting healing program. The toxic waste must be removed as quickly as possible to halt the downward spiral of failing health.** This is best done by **removing accumulated fecal material from the bowel.....**"

Another author, **Dr. Robert Gray**, has described the mucoid plaque in a manner similar to Dr. Jensen and myself when he talks about how constipation can be associated with "old, hardened feces" which stick to the walls of the colon and do not pass out with the regular bowel movements. He points out that fecal matter can become sticky and gluey and glues a coating of itself to the walls of the colon as it passes through. He claims that when "**layer after layer of gluey feces piles up in the colon, they often form into a tough, rubbery black substance.** Old feces may build up in pockets and they may coat the entire length of the colon and small intestines as well. They do not pass from the body with ordinary bowel movements but require special techniques to dissolve the glue which binds them in the body."[202] He also explains that parasites lodge themselves in the old matter that encrusts the walls of the intestinal tract. He believes that **without the mucoid plaque, intestinal parasites cannot maintain a foothold in the body and to remove the parasites, one must remove the "mucoid matter"**.[203] He further explains that malabsorption is related to the accumulation of mucoid plaque.[204]

Dr. Jensen and Dr. Gray had ideas different ideas than myself as to how the "mucoid plaque" is formed. Both of these authors felt that it was the acid-forming, mucus-forming, and highly processed foods that contributed towards the formation of mucoid plaque. I agree that they may contribute towards its composition, however, my studies indicate that excess intake of acid-forming foods drains electrolytes and *acidifies the bile* which then triggers mucin to coat the intestines. This is one reason why mucoid plaque seems to be smooth and fairly even in thickness throughout the gut.

**Dr. V.E. Irons**, a pioneer in colon cleansing theory and activity, and a staunch advocate against modern medicine wrote a booklet called: **"The Destruction of Your Own Natural Protective Mechanism."** In his booklet he made the following statements: "I challenge the world that you couldn't find in the USA, 1000 people who don't have a clogged colon. Just let me get them on the Colema Board and on the 7 Day Cleansing Program both at the same time we will show any challengers WHAT WE MEAN. We will let them see, feel and even hold in their hands exactly what has been thickening, hardening, and decaying in their colon for years, causing all types of disease. The condition of the colons in this entire country are FAR WORSE than either the doctors, the AMA, the Drug houses,.....or even the Natural Health industry have any conception..... *our theory* states that the **CAUSE OF MOST CONDITIONS OF ILL HEALTH IS AUTOINTOXICATION** and that 95% of their troubles start in the colon. We can prove that we can find hardened mucous with its foul smelling curd in the colons of 95% of the entire nation. HOW DO WE KNOW THIS? Because possibly 99% of all ages and sexes have violated two of the major Natural Laws from one to three times every day since they were 2 years old. What are the two laws? 1. The WRONG combination of foods. 2. The constant daily use of tremendous amounts of DEAD FOODS. The wrong application of both of these laws has caused the body's natural protective mechanism to secrete mucous into the colon

---

[202] Dr. Robert Gray, *The Colon Health Handbook*, (Reno, NV: Emerald Publishing, 1986), pg. 5-6.

[203] Ibid., pg. 8.

[204] Ibid., pg. 13.

to protect the body from absorbing the many poisons which those counterfeit foods create. **But we have simply OVERWORKED Nature's protective mechanism to the point that the mechanism instead of protecting us from poisons now itself poisons us.....** This protective mechanism was never designed to continue secreting mucous one layer on top of another layer for years with no time out or chance for its elimination. The result is that layer on top of layer is secreted until its accumulation thickens to 1/8" to 1/4" thick. Sometimes this layer or layers gets to 3/8" to 1/2" in thickness, becoming as hard and black as a piece of old hardened rubber you see on a highway from a truck tire. It cannot be cut with a knife but you can cut it with a razor blade. Usually it breaks into innumerable small pieces. But we have had specimens saved in alcohol from several inches to a few feet in length while the longest we have had was 27 ft. (In one piece). Sometimes it will come out as a pile weighing as much as 11 lbs... and continue to come out for several days to a week...before the old hardened accumulated mucous, so tightly imbedded in the colon for months or years, comes out. It has probably been slowly emitting poisons into your blood stream, causing all types of distorted symptoms. Once this hardened mucous starts to eliminate, it will be trapped in the colander so that you can wash it and examine it. Anyone who disagrees with any of the above - REMEMBER, you CAN PROVE it to your own satisfaction by what comes from your own body for the smallest conceivable investment. There is no substitute for experience, and we challenge everyone to experience this for themselves.....You (meaning the reader and 95% of the USA) DO HAVE THIS HARDENED MUCOUS IN YOUR COLON AND YOU WILL BE AMAZED AT WHAT COMES OUT OF YOU." **My experience has undoubtedly verified Dr. Irons descriptive explanations**.

A certain doctor from Mexico sent me a letter. I have not received permission to use his name publicly so I will only give you his credentials. **M.D., Ph.D., N.D., P.P. Gen. Adm.** Here is his testimony. "Dear Sirs: ... Many times when practicing autopsies on people who died from chronic illnesses, **I have always found a thick layer of organized mucus-like hardened material** all over from the tongue down to the stomach, small, large and recto-sigmoid colon. Usually **it is more common among milk drinkers and meat eaters**. If for some reason your products have the ability to detach this layer of morbus material, then a great deal of accomplishment will be achieved for these persons. This layer is composed of coagulated and racemized glycoproteins, which **really impair the GI tract function and also constitute a reservoir of bacteria and viruses that invade the lymph and the blood, causing a wearing down of the bodily defenses and a lot of burden on the liver detoxification function.** For that reason, Gerson, Kelly and Beard enfancied always on GI tract cleansing to obtain better results with their cancer treatments. **In the past we have even removed the entire colon to obtain an effective**

**relief from auto-intoxication,** especially with colon polyposis and diverticulosis and chronic ulcerative-colitis....."[205]

Unfortunately, there has been little interest on this subject by the medical profession and theories vary from one end of the spectrum to the other. Medical science basically avoids admitting any truth to the testimonies that many thousands of people, who first sought help from medical science, ended up finding help from the natural procedures that modern medicine resists and denies. As modern medicine once denied that Candidiasis was a cause to many illnesses for several decades after the alternative practitioners announced the problem, modern medicine has also denied the bowel problems associated with many diseases.[206] Could this tragedy be perpetuated because they have not found a way to capitalize upon this subject?

Many doctors have proven the effectiveness of cleansing the body, but this has been very well suppressed. We must dig out old clinical studies to find the work that has been done in the past. Why did this happen? **It is not because cleansing doesn't work. On the contrary, I believe it is because it works too well and doesn't bring in profits.** Restoring electrolyte minerals, cleansing the body, removing negative thoughts and feelings, using natural remedies that strengthen and build, along with a good alkaline diet of fresh food, are in my opinion, the most powerful and effective methods to restore health. Seldom will anyone need more than this, **but, doctors and hospitals cannot produce the massive profits to which they have grown accustomed, when using methods such as those described above.**

Medical science has also proven the power of the mind in its ability to heal the body even under the most severe conditions. Yet it fails to practice what it has learned. One of the most important functions of a doctor should be to establish in their patients the **hope** that they can get well. **Yet how can this be done when the doctor himself has no faith or hope in his own treatments?** I believe that it is second-degree murder, if a patient dies after a doctor sends him home telling him that he will die because there is no cure. **What the doctor should say is that he (the doctor) does not know what to do, therefore the patient should go to**

---

[205] This doctor was from Laboratorios Farmacobiologicos "IZUMAC".

[206] Examples of modern medicine's classic denials: 1) the need to wash hands before delivering babies; 2) that diet is important to health; 3) that eating of meat and dairy is responsible for heart disease and cancer epidemics; 4) that table salt will not work well as an electrolyte in the body; 5) that alternative medicine is superior in treating cancer, heart disease and most other diseases; 6) that gallstones can be easily removed with olive oil and lemon.

someone who does know. Or, the doctor could say, "Based upon what I know about your disease and what I know about my treatments, you will die in xx months, if you follow my program."!

# Tangible and Intangible Effects of Removing Mucoid Plaque

It appears that in average meat-eating persons, and vegetarians who eat too much grain and vegetarian meat substitutes, conditions such as described in the section before this one are rapidly developing. With my cleanse program, more than 90% of the people find large amounts of mucoid plaque coming out of their bowels. **It is not uncommon; in an average report the cleanser removes 35 to 45 feet of mucoid plaque in a seven day period.** During the first two or three cleanses, close to 90% of the cleansers find white or yellow pieces of polyps coming out of them. Many report tumors being released, various disease conditions improving or disappearing, as well as the release of other things that no one has been able to identify.

**When mucoid plaque is released by cleansers, many have also reported a corresponding release of old emotions and memories associated with those emotions.** After these releases, most people enjoy the disappearance of analogous disease conditions. Even when a specific past incident was not recalled by the cleansers, the passing of a piece of mucoid plaque often alleviated seemingly unrelated emotional stress. Many have theorized from this, that **emotional memories have the capacity to somehow attach themselves to mucoid plaque, where they continue to influence us in subtle, and sometimes, in quite significant ways until that plaque is removed.**

**Just as a piece of iron can be magnetized and then hold that magnetism, it seems that proteins and other molecular particles can hold on to the vibrational influence of thoughts and feelings.** Contained within this vibratory influence are memories. If this hypothesis has merit, it explains why it is so difficult to rid ourselves of grudges, angers, resentments, fears, guilt, etc. For these habits of consciousness are stuck in our cell tissues. I have found that through the right mental attitude and cleansing the body, we can make almost unbelievable advances in gaining control over our habits of thinking and feeling.

When using my program, this old mucoid plaque is usually eliminated in sections of one to two feet. One lady in Tucson had a piece that was 15 feet long ( the longest single piece known was 27 feet). She

# How to Identify Mucoid Plaque

said that after several feet came out, that she had to pull the last 10 feet out by hand! It is not uncommon for pieces to come out more than 2 to 4 feet long, but the average is 6-18 inches. Occasionally it is very stiff, something like an old piece of dried rawhide, but usually it is soft and flexible to the touch. It may also be in a more liquid state due to the action of the herbs, seeming gooey and mucus-like. Generally it holds together quite well (contrary to the cleanse shake substance which is clumping or jelly-like, and falls apart in water). In color, mucoid plaque can be gray, yellow, green or light green, or light brown to black, but usually is blackish green, which may indicate a relationship to bile. Strangely enough, for some people, the more we cleanse, the lighter the mucoid plaque becomes. The reason for this may be that new mucoid plaque is developing as fast as it is being removed. This could be a sign that something toxic is still in the bowel; perhaps pathogenic bacteria, parasites or yeast. Or possibly the bile is still too acid. However, that should not be the case if one has been eating the right foods, and drinking plenty of carrot juice.

Mucoid Plaque generally has a peculiar, distinctive odor that is not too bad, but with highly toxic people, it can have an unbelievable horribly foul odor, depending upon what is in it. Sometimes it will smell exactly like something we had eaten many years ago. I remember one time it smelled exactly like pork chops for about three days, something I had not eaten in over 20 years. Another time it smelled like roast beef, which I had not eaten in at least 14 years.

Some people eliminate worms as long as 30 feet (tape worms) with the cleanse. People have reported various sizes and colors of worms coming out. The red in some worms always indicates that they have been sucking blood. Some people report worm holes throughout their mucoid layers. They say, "It looks like they just go in and out."[207]

Often layered, the mucoid plaque can sometimes be so firm that it is difficult to cut with a knife. **Ron Sherr** of Tucson wrote: "Rich, the stuff that came out of me, well some of it was so tough that I couldn't cut it with a perforated knife, I had to use a hacksaw. It was at least 1 inch thick and over three feet long. Immediately after I passed it, my back problem was gone." Ron is a good friend of mine and I challenged him. I said, "Come on Ron, that is hard to believe; you must be exaggerating." He was a little perturbed that I doubted him, and he swore that this was not an exaggeration. In all the years I have known Ron, I have never found him to lie or exaggerate. He always prides himself on his honesty and integrity.

The mucoid plaque is usually, but not always, somewhat shiny, and often looks like thin or thick pieces of wet leather or rubber. Some pieces may look like rope. It may show striations, smoothness, overlaps, folds, or creases if it comes out in large enough pieces to see them. For mucoid plaque takes on the shape and texture of the portion of the intestine where it was formed.[208] Some intact sections of mucoid plaque may be sliced open, revealing the tube structure of the plaque layer, with the cleanse shake substance inside.

In the earlier stages of cleansing it is common to find popcorn-looking substance (polyps), or an amber or dark green jelly-like goop (lymph). Fun stuff! This is where cleansing becomes entertaining, scientific, and educational. You will soon consider yourself a qualified "intestinal discharge" examiner. It is a good idea to keep a pair of chopsticks in the bathroom during a Cleanse for examination and ease in measuring. If several family members or friends cleanse at the same time, it's fun to keep track of the number of feet and compare notes. Many times people who have read my book came to my house. Several of them came right out and asked me if they could see my bathroom. I asked them why? "I just wanted to see if you really have chopsticks near your toilet." So I let them see. Sure enough, there they were - nice, clean chopsticks.

---

[207] **See Chapter 6: Modern Digestion: A Distorted Picture, under "Parasites: A Widespread Problem."**

[208] **See Chapter 9: Facts About Dr. Anderson's Cleansing Program, under "Identifying the Origin of Mucoid Plaque."**

However, for what it is worth, I no longer have them, for I no longer have mucoid plaque coming out.

Looking into the toilet and seeing that mucoid substance, you will be filled with great joy. You'll want to go outside and shout it to the world. For you will be flushing away the cause of lack of energy, premature old age, failing eyesight, wrinkles, poor memory, liver and kidney weakness, gland dysfunction, and many other various diseases. Most of all you may have rid yourself of the toxic emotions that have become stuck in your - stuff! Then you will be pleased with yourself, because you had the wisdom, the courage, and the strength to do something really good for your life. Well, that is my opinion and it is the opinion of thousands of other people who have accomplished this program.

In addition to expelling the classic mucoid plaque, old toxic substances (possibly loaded with drugs, parasites, and dead tissue), may flow from any and all channels of elimination during a cleanse. These channels include: the kidneys, skin, lungs, mouth, nose, and ears. Please understand, that most people are likely to be extremely toxic and they should be careful when cleansing. Too much toxic release all at once can cause alarm and even harm. **Please read this book and cleansing instructions carefully.**

As you can see, mucoid plaque is an important consideration in the health of the digestive system and to the health and vitality of our bodies. However, as important as it is, there are many other factors that can cause disease in the bowel. Mucoid plaque is only one factor. Each and every factor is associated with living unnaturally according to the parameters of our species. As with every species of life on this earth, everything survives in a specific environment and also must have specific foods for health. Modern man has lost touch as to what is natural. Today, it is normal to not know what natural is. I believe that this disastrous lack of knowing is the primary cause of all the diseases and problems we face in today's society. I also believe that it was deliberately brought into play by those who wish to control, manipulate, and profit by mankind's weakness and disease. I refer to a group of men who are at the helm of world governments, education channels, news medias, the military, and medicine. Everyone on this planet is a victim and within a few years much of that which has been kept hidden will be revealed and the last major battle between the forces of good and the forces of evil will be over. In the meantime, I hope that this book will help people prepare themselves for the massive epidemics that are likely to occur within a few more years.

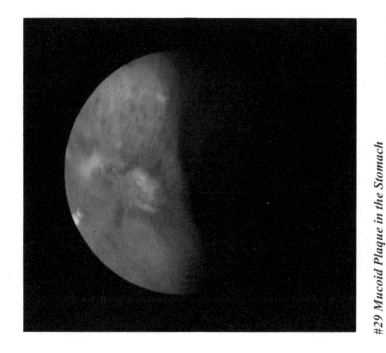

**#29 Mucoid Plaque in the Stomach**
*This ulcer, within the pyloric antrum, is surrounded by hard, brittle mucoid plaque with an abnormally large blood supply. The body has lost control over its natural mechanism and created a calcification-like mucin as a last-ditch effort to protect itself.*

**#27 Mucoid Plaque in the Stomach**
*The mottled appearance of the mucosa of the antrum (lower stomach) suggests chronic inflammation of the stomach. It could also be indicative of a patchy increase of mucin or mucoid plaque in response to continued inflammation of the antral (in the lower stomach) mucosa.*

**#46 Inflamed Duodenal Mucosa**
*In this section, there is a localized redness of the mucosa within the duodenum. The inflamed areas are raised suggesting an increase in the secretion of mucin in response to the inflamation.*

**#31 Mucoid Plaque in the Pyloric Area of the Stomach**
*Gastrojejunostomy (the surgical establishment of a direct passageway between the stomach and the jejunum to facilitate gastric drainage). The inlets to the jejunal loops moving toward the stomach and those moving away from the stomach are open, though it is hard to see amidst multiple layers of mucoid plaque. This picture presents one of the many different forms of mucoid plaque.*

**#63 Mucoid Plaque at the Opening to the Appendix**
*A mucosal whorl surrounding the opening to the appendix. Note the thickness of the mucin and the lack of any visible blood vessels. This is highly indicative of mucoid plaque. Compare this image to the previous one of a healthy colon.*

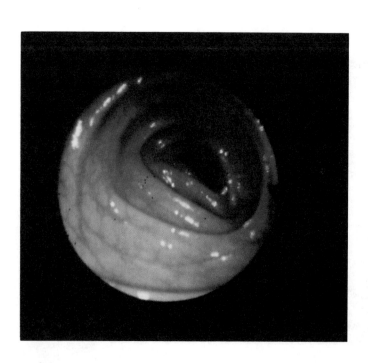

**#60 Normal Transverse Colon**
*The colonic folds are free of mucoid plaque and the network of blood vessels of the colon is readily visible. This is how a healthy colon looks.*

**#80 Chron's Iletis**
*The mucosa is thickened and ulcerated on the left side of the ileum (that portion of the small intestine just prior to the colon), while the right side is devoid of plaque.*

**#66 Severe Ulcerative-colitis**
*Notice the layers of mucoid plaque that form over the original wall of the colon. They appear to be brittle, with a continued secretion of mucin.*

**83 Acute Ischemic Colitis**
*With this condition, the blood supply is blocked. This appears to be the result of the thickened mucoid plaque that is actually breaking away in large pieces and blocking the lumen (passage way) of the colon.*

**#81 Acute Ischemic Colitis**
*Two things are readily apparent here. There is localized cell death in response to the pathology of the colon and an extreme thickening of the mucosa surrounding the diseased area. Notice the layering of the mucoid plaque.*

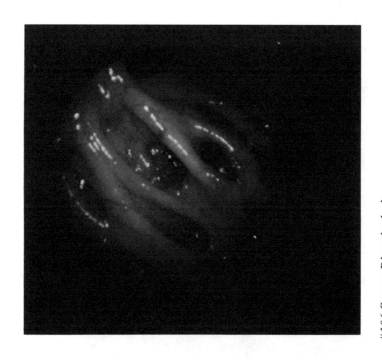

**#106 Severe Diverticulosis**
*The central diverticulum is oozing a small amount of bright red blood. The diverticulum beneath it is filled with fecal pellets.*

**#97 Polyp in the Sigmoid Colon**
*The long stalk of a sigmoid polyp (origination in the sigmoid colon) climbing over the mucosal fold. Polyps are another form of mucoid plaque.*

**#108 Severe Melanosis Coli**
*Characteristic of this condition are heavy deposits of dark pigment which impart a snake-like appearance to the mucosa of the ascending colon. The mucoid plaque can take various colors, as well as shapes and forms.*

# Chapter 4

# DOCTORS DISCUSS KEYS TO EXCEPTIONAL HEALTH IMPROVEMENT

*"As everything is impermanent, fluid and interdependent, how we act and think inevitably changes the future. There is no situation, however seemingly hopeless or terrible, such as a terminal disease, which we cannot use to evolve."*

## - Sogyal Rinpoche

**All physiological, chemical, and anatomical processes in every cell and all organs in our bodies are completely dependent upon the digestive system.** Yes, the brain, liver, heart, muscles, bones etc., all get their nourishment from that wonderful long tube, the digestive system. **Not only is it the source of nutrients, but it's also the main channel for elimination of body wastes.** It is sad to think that this is not taught in medical schools or even public schools, and that most doctors have failed to realize it on their own. A few doctors have had the wisdom to take care of this important mechanism.

## Doctors of Great Success

Doctor Bernard Jensen D.C., N.D., Ph.D., made the following statement: **"In the 50 years I've spent helping people to overcome illness, disability and disease, it has become crystal clear that poor bowel management lies at the root of most people's health problems.**[209] Dr. Bernard Jensen had studied with many very successful doctors throughout the United States and Europe. He then built his own sanitarium and practiced with an open mind for more than 50 years. His fame has traveled all over the world. He was even nominated for the Nobel

---

[209] Jensen, pg. 3.

Prize, but because he was not a "mainstream" doctor, his nomination was rejected.

Dr. Jensen [210] says: **"Every tissue is fed by the blood, which is supplied by the bowel. When the bowel is dirty, the blood is dirty, and so on to the organs and tissues....it is the bowel that invariably has to be cared for first before any effective healing can take place."** Dr. Jensen publicly stated that more than 90% of diseases in America can be traced to unhealthy conditions in the bowel. Privately, he told me that it's closer to 100%.

In his textbook on Iridology, Dr. Jensen explains: "Besides these world-renowned exponents of intestinal sanitation, other authorities have given recognition to the belief that cleanliness of the colon is necessary to good health. **It is believed that disorders such as appendicitis, infected tonsils, liver and gallbladder infections, dysfunction of the heart and blood vessels, sinusitis, arthritis, and rheumatism, etc., no doubt have their origin in a sluggish colon."**

My experience proves that he is absolutely correct, but I would add one thing - **it is not just the colon that must be cleansed; it's the entire intestinal tract, the stomach, duodenum, small intestine, and colon.**

Doctors who have achieved fame for their exceptional health improvement rates **always took care of the alimentary canal.** Dr. William Koch, Dr. Eugene Blass, Dr. John Kellogg of the Battle Creek Sanitarium, Sir Arbuthnot Lane, surgeon for the King of England, Dr. Bernard Jensen and Dr. J.H. Tilden are some of the exceptional individuals who used this knowledge.

In the early 1900's, **Dr. J.H. Tilden** of Denver, Colorado, specialized in healing pneumonia, which was at that time the number one killer. During that epidemic almost every doctor lost hundreds of their

---

[210] Dr. Bernard Jensen, Ph.D., N.D., D.C., M.H..is known as the father of Iridology. He has pioneered many new health concepts and improved many others. He has received many awards and honorary degrees from around the world, has even been knighted for his work, and received the Cross of the Order of St. John of Malta. He is the author of about 30 books and is recognized throughout the world for his work. He has been nominated for a Nobel prize but someone put a stop to the possibility of his receiving it. He has had one of the most successful careers in healing people in the 20th century. I believe he'll go down in history as one of the most effective pioneers in the health field. I am happy that he was one of my teachers.

patients to that deadly plague. Dr. Tilden had more pneumonia cases than any other doctor and he **never lost a patient. He used no drugs at all. He simply cleaned out the colon** (using enemas and colonics), used water therapy, and administered natural, live foods.[211] Even in those days, his success was considered miraculous because other doctors were relying on drugs and continually meeting with failure.

**Sir Arbuthnot Lane M.S., F.R.C.S., surgeon for the King of England,** made the following statement: "**There is but one disease and that is deficient drainage.**"[212] Dr. Lane spent many years specializing in bowel problems. He was an expert in removing sections of the bowel and stitching it back together. He taught this work to other doctors and gained an international reputation for his efficiency. During the years of this work, he began to notice a peculiar phenomenon. During the course of recovery from colonic surgery, **some of his patients experienced remarkable cures of diseases that had no apparent connection with his surgery.** For instance, a young boy who had had arthritis for many years, was in a wheelchair at the time of surgery. Six months later, this boy had recovered entirely from arthritis. Another case involved a woman with a goiter. **When a specific section of the bowel was removed in surgery, there ensued a definite remission of the goiter within six months.** These and similar experiences impressed him deeply, as he saw the relationship between the toxic bowel and the functioning of various organs in the body. After much thought about this relationship, he became very interested in changing the bowel through dietetic methods and spent the last 25 years of his life teaching people how to care for the bowel through cleansing and nutrition, and not surgery. **Sir Lane said, "All maladies are due to the lack of certain food principles, such as mineral salts or vitamins, or to the absence of the normal defenses of the body, such as the natural protective flora.** When this occurs, toxic bacteria invade the lower alimentary canal. **The poisons thus generated pollute the bloodstream, causing every tissue, gland, and organ of the body to gradually deteriorate and be destroyed.**[213] Lane made the statement that **arthritis could not develop in the absence of intestinal toxemia,** that there is clinical and x-ray evidence of stasis[214] in such patients, and that the

---

[211] If Dr. Tilden practiced today as he did in the 1900's, he would probably lose his license.

[212] Stan Malstrom, N.D., M.T., "Your Colon - Its Character, Care and Therapy," (Orem, Utah: BiWorld Pub. Inc., 1981), pg. 1.

[213] Dr. Bernard Jensen, D.C., N.D., Ph.D., *Iridology, The Science and Practice in the Healing Arts,* Volume II, (Escondido, CA: Bernard Jensen, Pub., 1982) pg. 408.

[214] Stasis: Stagnation, constipation, autointoxication of intestines. *Stedman's Medical Dictionary.*

symptoms disappear and patients recover sometimes with startling rapidity when the condition of stasis has been effectively dealt with. Sir Lane reports **a connection between intestinal toxemia and "several changes in the thyroid"** such as "adenomatous growths." He also made this statement to the staff of John Hopkins Hospital and Medical College, "Gentlemen, **I will never die of cancer. I am taking measures to prevent it. It is caused by poisons created in our bodies by the food we eat...."**

**Dr. Harvey Kellogg, M.D.** of the Kellogg Sanitarium said, **"Of the 22,000 operations that I have personally performed, I have never found a single normal colon, and of the 100,000 that were performed under my jurisdiction, not over 6% were normal."**[215] Dr. Kellogg said that he knew of many cases in which operations were prevented by cleansing and revitalizing the bowel. **He maintained that 90% of the diseases of civilization are due to improper functioning of the colon.**

**Dr. George C. Crile,** head of the Crile Clinic in Cleveland and one of the world's greatest surgeons, said: **"There is no natural death. All deaths that come from so-called natural causes are merely the end point of progressive acid saturation.** Many people go so far as to consider that sickness and disease are just a 'cross' or an element which God gave them to bear here on this earth. However, **if they would take care of their body and cleanse their colon and intestines, their problems would be pretty much eliminated** and they could eliminate their 'cross' by proper diet, proper exercise, and in general, proper living."[216] In other words, obey the laws of nature!

Many doctors have proven that the bowel was the key to health or disease and the most important part of our physical anatomy to take care of in order to achieve successful healing. The following cases were **obtained from medical journals.**

Dr. H. J. Bartle found in a study of 50 cases of intestinal toxemia that 72% of those cases had constipation. Dr. Satterlee found 84% of his patients had constipation when they had intestinal toxemia. This indicates that **serious bowel disease is associated with having constipation.** Dr. William Lintz, M.D., successfully treated 472 patients suffering from **allergies** by cleansing the bowel. Dr. Allan Eustis, M.D., Professor at Tulane University of Medicine in 1912, cured 121 cases of bronchial **asthma** by intestinal cleansing. Dr. D. Rochester, M.D., University of

---

[215] Jensen, D. C., N.D., Ph.D., *Iridology, The Science and Practice*, pg. 408.

[216] Malstrom, pg. 1.

Buffalo School of Medicine in 1906, made the statement that **after 23 years of years of observation, toxemia of gastrointestinal tract origin is the underlying cause of asthma.** Dr. Bassler reported that **by reducing intestinal toxemia, he had 100% success eliminating cardiac arrhythmia.**[217] Dr. Bainbridge, M.D. stated that intestinal toxemia is common among the causative factors of so-called functional **heart disease.** Dr. D. J. Barry stated, "There seems little doubt that substances having a deleterious action on the **heart musculature and nerves are formed both in the small and large intestine,** even under apparently normal circumstances." Dr. Hovel stated that "toxemia due to intestinal sepsis is a common cause of increased **blood pressure.**" Dr. J. A. Stucky, M.D.: "In several hundreds of cases of diseases of the nasal accessory **sinuses, middle and internal ear**... I have found unmistakable and marked evidence of toxemia of intestinal origin as evidenced by excessive indican in the urine, and when the condition causing this was removed, there was marked amelioration or entire relief of the disease." Dr. C. W. Hawley, M.D., treated many cases of **eye strain** and disease with success once again by relieving intestinal toxemia. In 1892, Dr. Herter, M.D. **linked intestinal putrefaction to epilepsy in 31 patients.**

I had one doctor take the Cleanse who had epilepsy. **During her cleanse she had her last seizure. Five years later she reported that she has never had a seizure since doing the cleanse and no other signs of epilepsy.** I have seen other epilepsy cases disappear while doing the cleanse. I used to wonder why the Cleanse was so effective against epilepsy. Now we have some important clues. Research involving autism has found that seizures are associated with certain toxic bacteria.[218] It appears that when these bacteria are present in certain individuals, seizures can occur. Digestive cleansing is obviously one of the most effective methods of reducing large amounts of pathogenic bacteria. This could be a problem when some people do a cleanse. If they have these bacteria, and they do a cleanse, they could stir up the little buggers and have a seizure

---

[217] Cardiac arrhythmia: Loss of normal rhythm of heartbeat. *Stedman's Medical Dictionary.*

[218] See Videotape Series: Tape 1, *Autism and Microorganisms*, William Shaw, Ph.D. Great Plains Laboratory, Overland Park, KS. Phone 913-341-8949. Dr. Shaw explains that bacteria and yeast produce certain specific compounds which are absorbed into the blood and eventually secreted into the urine. New sensitive equipment are now able to measure these compounds. It has been found that bowel toxins are far more prevalent than expected. Dr. Shaw relates bowel toxins to Rett's syndrome, seizures, adult & child psychosis, severe depression, attention deficit, hyperactivity, and hypoglycemia. A little more research and they may find much more than that.

during the cleanse. When people have epilepsy and do the cleanse, they sometimes have a seizure. As indicated above, this has happened, but fortunately, it may be the last one. It is impossible to know for sure. Doctors should really consider the importance of this. What is really happening when we do a cleanse? Is it removing massive amounts of toxin producing bacteria or something else? Maybe it is a combination of things; whatever it is, it is impressive!

Mental problems are another area where cleansing really can help. Drs. Satterlee and Eldridge reported their experience with 518 cases of **"mental symptoms"** including "mental sluggishness, dullness, and stupidity; loss of concentration and/or memory; mental incoordination, irritability, lack of confidence, excessive and useless worry, exaggerated introspection..." **Their success in eliminating these symptoms by surgically relieving intestinal toxemia is truly remarkable in the light of today's commonly-held beliefs.**

Dr. J.F. Burgess, Montreal General Hospital, reports the results of studying 109 cases of **eczema**. He states, "On the basis of clinical observations and sensitivity tests against various amino acids and ptomaine bases, **eczema is probably caused by intestinal toxemia.**"

It is my own opinion that all cancer, AIDS, liver disorders, kidney, brain, and heart disorders receive their toxic malformations from the intestines. And when it is not directly associated with the bowel, then it is because the liver, kidneys, or other organs have become weakened as a result of long term toxicity in the bowel. Other factors are nutrient deficient foods, negative thoughts, etc. **Sir W.A. Lane** tried to make it clear when he wrote that he was **"exceedingly impressed by the sequence of cancer and intestinal stasis."** We know that changes in the breast, caused by intestinal pollution, have been described by many doctors.

# A Positive Attitude is Essential

Evidence clearly shows that: no matter what the disease; **as long as a person has the right mental attitude, a strong desire to be healthy, the relentless determined drive to seek out the cure and cause, the willingness to do whatever is necessary to be well, and the willingness to forgive and Love those whom we feel hurt us; that person will bring into his or her world that which he/she desires, and will eventually find health.** If only health professionals would espouse this truth, the door would open to making (or allowing) it to happen. Too often, people lose hope because their doctor told them that there wasn't a cure. In many cases they were told that there was no hope for survival, that they were doomed to an early death; when in actuality, there was a method that would have brought them back to health. This is a common occurrence in the medical profession simply because the medical profession uses methods that are designed to modify symptoms rather than deal with causes.

When doctors tell a patient that there is no hope, that he or she is doomed to die, they place the death sentence upon someone who may be gullible enough to allow themselves to be so victimized. **What these doctors are really saying is: "Based upon what I know about your disease, if you follow my suggested treatment, you will die."** An intelligent patient will automatically reply: "Obviously you're the wrong doctor for me." **THERE IS NO SUCH THING AS AN INCURABLE DISEASE.** No matter what the disease, how terrible it is, or the stage of its development, someone has risen above it and found his or her cure. Even in the so-called latter stages, when there was "no hope", people have conquered illness.

**Did you know that we can cut out 25% of your liver and it will grow back again?** Not only that, but after it grows back we can cut out another 25% and then another 25% etc., and it keeps growing back again and again. Just as the body knows how to do that, it also knows how to heal and repair itself. We know that **each cell in the body has the intelligence to grow an entirely new body, and it doesn't matter whether the body is 2 years old or 120, the cells always know what to do**. The body has the intelligence to function perfectly 100% of the time, from an embryo to the very last breath. The main reason it appears to malfunction is because it has been abused.

**Disease is a natural result of an unnatural lifestyle.** It is an automatic consequence of a lack of Love and Joy, which is the source of energy, vitality, and life. Who has the wisdom to consider that we are responsible for our diseases and that they are due to our lifestyles, our attitudes, our diets, and our detrimental habits of thought and emotion? We tend to blame something besides ourselves - God, our parents, the husband or wife, even the weather. Come on, think. Think Cause! What caused this in the first place? Let's get to the cause and root it out - all of it. Get down to the deep roots, Cleanse & Purify; then we're free of it forever.

The most important step in healing ourselves is to realize that at some level we help create all our problems. One reason this is so vital is that only after we acknowledge our responsibility as a co-creator with the spiritual and natural forces of nature, can we open the door to the spiritual power within that can heal us. **Whenever people consider themselves victims (thinking: this is not my fault; it was imposed upon me!), then at the very moment they proclaim their belief, usually unconsciously, that they do not have the power to protect or heal.** It is the same as giving our power away and feeding the subconscious mind with the very programming that we would hope to avoid. And believe me, there are forces that do not want us to consciously use our creative powers. We all have made mistakes. That is one thing we all have in common. Let us admit that we made our mistakes, and through those mistakes we learned and grew; our mistakes have brought us to where we are and now we reclaim our power to change and recreate. The moment we do this, we take back our power and once again walk the road that leads to healing and success.

# Chapter 5

# THE INTENTIONAL DEVELOPMENT OF MODERN DISEASE

*"The message well I hear, but faith, alas is wanting.*
*Yes, the faith in a helper and savior is often put to a*
*hard test here.*
*The sick have been deceived so often and have buried*
*all hope. "*

- Adolf Just

*"Mopes Max von Pettenkofer, a German chemist, did not*
*contract the disease even though he deliberately swallowed*
*a cholera bacteria, a virulent culture. This was a source of*
*amazement for a century later. He also was one of the first*
*to state that hygiene was a matter of good health rather*
*than just good manners. "*

- Rudolph Hauschka, D. Sc.

## Forces Against Nature

If an angel came and gave a formula that would cure almost any disease, it would be against the law to claim its effectiveness. If the angel went about healing and curing people, the FDA would probably handcuff the angel at gun point and attempt to remove the angel from fulfilling his/her Divine Mission.[219] But explaining in simple, scientific terms how

---

[219] Contact the National Health Federation and ask about Jonathan Wright MD. The FDA broke his clinic door down five minutes before it was to open and walked in pointing guns. Dr. Wright wasn't guilty of anything nor was he charged with anything. Was he the only guiltless one that experienced the wrath of the gun pointing FDA? Certainly not. From Web Page about Jonathan Wright and the FDA: James DeMeo, Ph.D., Director of Research, "Anti-Constitutional Activities and Abuse of Police Power by the U.S. Food and Drug Administration and other

we destroy our own bodies and minds and how we may reverse that destruction, leaving out all claims, will hopefully not offend the AMA, FDA or the drug companies they support, will it? Though our freedom of choice in selecting the treatments we believe in to cure our bodies has largely been taken from us, we fortunately, live in a country that still guarantees freedom of speech, *to some degree*[220].

Unfortunately, people in this country are not well informed about a system of healing that has proven to be effective in curing and preventing chronic and degenerative diseases. In fact, they are terribly discouraged from using effective alternatives, sometimes by force. I believe the reason is that **effective treatments do not produce the massive profits that our modern medical system generates**. The health profession makes money on sick people, not healthy people. If doctors were to make everyone well with a system that works, they certainly wouldn't perpetuate their incomes. After all, there would be little use for this book or any other health book, nor the Cleanse Thyself Program, or even the entire health care system. How sincerely do we want to heal?

**Ignoring the intestinal tract, nutrition, and the power of the mind are among the greatest and most dangerous mistakes that medical doctors, other health professionals, and their patients can make.** It is the number one physiological reason for the failure to prevent and cure disease of any kind. Most Americans have serious problems in their intestinal tracts, whether they know it or not. And, almost all persons, even the majority of vegetarians, are deficient in minerals - especially electrolyte minerals.

## Conventional Medicine Suppresses Bowel Cleansing

It was very interesting to discover that almost no clinical studies have been written in medical journals about intestinal toxemia as the cause of disease since the late 1940's - about gastrointestinal diseases, yes, but not about toxic bowel conditions. Prior to the 40's, "intestinal toxemia" was a common term used by medical doctors. It was a term which

---

Federal Agencies," (Ashland, OR: Orgone Biophysical Research Lab, 1998).

[220] We receive many wonderful testimonies. The FDA will not allow us to print the testimonies unless we change them in ways that meet the FDA's guidelines. Therefore many of the testimonies you read in our literature have been significantly watered down.

indicated a major cause of disease. Understanding cause is **essential**, for until one knows the cause of disease, its treatment is a shot in the dark.

**Deny the cause and the cure remains a mystery**. The average American can understand this, so why do so many doctors resist this truth? Is it because the medical conspiracy is keeping it from reaching medical schools? If the medical world would treat the cause of disease with Nature's perfect way: good food, herbs,[221] cleansing and fasting; instead of relying on man-made harsh chemicals called drugs,[222] radiation, scalpels, saws, knives, and other dissection tools (treatments which always weaken rather than strengthen the body); their continual failures could become successes. Though this would not enhance the medical industry's pocketbooks and could even restructure the entire American economy, America would become a country of healthy people.[223] Perhaps it is necessary to ask whether people really want health, vitality, a clear mind and freedom. Or are they willing to sacrifice these blessings for a better house, a nicer car and toxic responsibility?

---

[221] "And the fruit thereof shall be for meat, and the leaf thereof for medicine." *The Holy Bible*, Ezekiel, 47:12.

[222] Eli Lilly, the pharmacutical magnate, himself said that a drug without toxic side effects is no drug at all. This is a good definition of a drug - "has toxic side effects." The FDA is attempting (with some success, unfortunately) to classify a drug as being *anything* used for medicinal purposes. This can include herbs, food and water. If the FDA achieves their goals, then they will have a law passed which will not allow medicinal herbs to be sold without a prescription from a medical doctor. This is one of the many diabolic ways of gaining greater control and maintaining high profits for the drug companies. Should this happen, herbs, all nutritional supplements, and super foods, will basically be outlawed. Unfortunately most doctors won't prescribe these things, but continue to support the drug companies because that is where the money comes from and because they do not know anything about the herbs and nutrition they may prescribe.

[223] A healthy America could shift the power of wealth, for approximately 13.6% of gross national product in the U.S. in 1995, consisted of dollars from the disease industry. This figure is projected to increase to 15% by the year 2000, representing a 7.2% growth rate in the industry over 5 years. Total expenditures on conventional medical treatment in the U.S. are projected to exceed 1.4 trillion dollars by that date. From: J. V. Vincenzio, "Trends in Medical Care Cost - Revisited," *Statistical Bulletin of Metropolitan Insurance Company*, 1997; July; Vol. 78, Issue (3), pg. 10-16. This does not include supermarkets, restaurants, meat, dairy, sugar, candy, chemical, and processed food industries which all support the disease industry. Yes, remove it all and allow our planet, to become a world of health, for if we have lost our health, all the riches in the world mean nothing.

Once I was talking about treating causes with a fellow who didn't see the point. He said, "When I get a flat tire, I just fix it. I don't worry about causes." I replied, "Would you try to fix the leaking hole in the tire while the nail was still in it?" He said, "Oh, I see what you mean." Then I said, "How about not getting the nail in the tire in the first place? That's preventive medicine."

Doctors do the very same thing as this mechanic when they cut cancer out, or remove a colon or breast and don't address diet, nutrition, pounds of toxicity, and emotions. They don't even touch the cause. They scarcely even consider it. It is like putting a patch over the nail in your tire. It may work until you pay your bill. Patients go home and pray that the cancer doesn't come back again. Seldom are they told to change their diets. [224] They are rarely given nutritional advice, even though they are terribly depleted of amino acids, minerals and vitamins. So patients of the Church of Modern Medicine[225] go on doing the exact same things that got them sick in the first place. What's really being said to them is: **"Go home and keep doing whatever it was that made you sick in the first place. Then we will see you again, and again, and again. And remember, as long as you have insurance or plenty of money, we are here to serve you."**

This habit that people and doctors have of **not** considering the cause is the result of super-brainwashing. We have been brainwashed into believing that meat is necessary for health, that dairy is good for our bones and teeth. Nothing could be further from the truth. **Yes, fresh human milk is good for human infants, and fresh raw cow milk is good for calves, but pasteurized cow milk is extremely harmful for both cows and people.**[226]

---

[224] When doctors do tell their patients to change their diets, it is usually unbelievably bad. When my mother was in the hospital for her operation, she said, "Even I know that their food is terrible." I saw the menu and wondered who designed it; certainly no one who knew anything about what is good for human bodies.

[225] "Church of Modern Medicine" is a term used by Dr. Robert Mendelsohn, M.D., formerly National Director of Project Head Start's Medical Consultation Service, Chairman of the Medical Licensing Commiting for the State of Illinois, etc. He is the excellent author of *Mal e Practice: How Doctors Manipulate Women; How to Raise a Healthy Child In Spite of Your Doctor;* and *Confessions of a Medical Heretic.* These three books have been widely available. Check your local health food store. Information on these books is listed in the Bibliography.

[226] Allen, et. al., "Protein-Induced Hypercalcuria: A Long Term Study," pg. 741-749. H. M. Linkswiler, M. B. Zemel, M. Hegsted, S. Schuette, "Protein-Induced Hypercalcuria," *Federal Proceedings*, 1981; 40: 2429.

There are many ways that the medical authorities squelch alternative treatments for disease. The medical community is still trying to say that no one recovers from AIDS. Their response to all the recovered AIDS patients is, "They probably didn't have AIDS". When they are confronted with the fact that their doctors said they did, they try to get out of it by saying, "The doctor may have made a mistake". What they are really saying is that if a hundred thousand AIDS patients take brand x and get well, it is not necessarily a proven cure. **They have to prove that it is scientifically a cure before they will accept it as such. That way they have all the time in the universe to not announce a cure.** For the standards on what is "scientific" may vary widely, and are easily manipulated for monetary reasons. This is one of the ways they maintain control. This rigid adherence to what is supposedly "scientific" is nothing but a business convenience in my opinion. It has nothing to do with science. They want to make sure the money keeps coming in for research and that they can keep selling drugs that are only partially effective. **If they sold drugs that worked, and everyone became healthy, then they would be out of business**. As bad as that sounds, that is exactly the way it is. [227]

During the years from 1880 to the late 1940's, incredible information had become available to support the theories that the cause of almost all diseases could be traced back to the gastrointestinal tract. **However, it was becoming obvious that if the disease industry was to ever expand and become the high-profit business which it is today, the knowledge of the causes and remedies of disease would have to be suppressed.** Before 1950 there was very little disease in America. It was the healthiest nation in the world. It was clear to many doctors and scientists that just cleansing the bowel and changing the diet would solve about 90% or better of all health problems. So the "disease industry",

---

Cow's milk is not only a negative source of calcium, but contributes towards inhibiting calcium from being absorbed and utilized from other food sources. No wonder vitamin D is added to cow's milk; they hope that it will help increase calcium absorption. Maybe it helps, but it is not enough. And, Dr. Ted Morter, *Your Health Choice*, (Hollywood, FL: Fell Publishers and Company, Inc., 1990), pg. 167.

[227] Many people wonder, if herbs work, why don't the drug companies and doctors use them. The reason is this: No one can patent herbs. Therefore, the drug companies cannot control the price, nor can they prevent their competition from using them and maintain control over the market. But, by making a specific drug, that no one else has, they can patent it, set whatever price on it they want, and never worry about competition. Take valium for example: In the very first year of sales in the early 1970's sales exceeded $750 million! (Peter Fuhrman, "No Need for Valium," *Forbes*, 1994; Jan. 31, pg. 84-85.) What would have been their profits if everyone used the herb valerian, which valium is made from?

which is comprised of the drug cartels, and all their supporting organizations, including food manufacturers, pharmacies, supermarkets, and the meat, dairy, sugar, candy, and processed food industries, made some important decisions. They clearly understood that **to produce massive profits and successfully achieve a medical monopoly,**[228] **it would be necessary to switch everyone's attention from cause to symptoms and stop teaching the importance of bowel cleansing and diet in medical schools. The success of their actions created the world's most profitable industry, and probably amazed the instigators themselves.** It was even more profitable, consistent, and deadly than the war industries. I realize this appears to be rather a rash statement, but the evidence is undeniable.

## The Germ Theory

The number one most effective scheme to increase disease and profits was to establish a concept called the "Germ Theory" or the "Theory of Infection". **This is a theory that implies that we are not responsible for disease; that disease is a condition imposed upon us from an outside source.** Based on Pasteur's original concepts, the idea is that disease is primarily caused by outside entities such as bacteria, viruses, fungus, etc. It is theorized that these "germs" attack our bodies, and there is little anyone can do to prevent this germ invasion. This is still the accepted theory of modern allopathic medicine. **We have all been programmed or brainwashed into believing in this "Germ Theory".**

After seeing disease overcome by countless people who have made changes in diet, lifestyle and thinking to cleanse their bodies, I have to conclude that: we create our own disease by our own life-styles and thought processes. Based on my own studies and observations with darkfield microscopy, while studying under Gaston Naessens, I believe that our bodies even have the ability to mutate microorganisms into various bacteria, yeast, and viruses and it is our own consciousness that regulates the species of microorganisms.

**All life on our planet depends upon a specific environment for survival.** You will not see penguins in Africa, or giraffes in the Arctic. You do not see flies in a clean garbage can, nor will you see pathogenic microorganisms having a field day in a truly clean and healthy person. Pathogenic germs must also have the specific environment they require. Germs are usually not the cause of disease, but are the result of disease. Germs are the smoke, not the fire. **It is what we do to ourselves that produces the internal chemistry that is necessary for germs to survive.**

---

[228] Instigated by John D. Rockefeller, see Griffin, pg. 359-368.

When this is fully realized in our society, disease will be on the endangered species list. **Truly, it is the unnatural things we do that force the body into one situation after another until it loses its ability to maintain natural balance.** Because of what we do, we change the internal chemistry (inner environment) of the body - especially in the bowels, then the blood, etc..

In contrast to the Germ Theory, **the "Theory of Toxicity"** is a concept which asserts that **disease is primarily caused by toxic internal environment which causes congestion and malfunction. It proclaims that we are indeed responsible for our health.** This theory suggests that **it is what we do to ourselves (diet, emotions, etc.) that provides specific internal environments in which disease and germs can thrive.**

*The primary problem with the Germ Theory, is not whether or not a bacteria or virus causes a disease. The main problem is that the **Germ Theory does not address the physiological and psychological factors which allow the germ or disease to develop. It subtly denies the power within ourselves which allows each of us to control our lives.***

# Three Reasons Why the Germ Theory is Devastating

## 1. Suggests Diet and Lifestyle are Unimportant

**First:** **It encourages harmful habits by suggesting that it doesn't matter what we do or eat.** Supposedly, diseases are caused by germs or carcinogens attacking us, and there is nothing we can do to avoid them except to use vaccines and get regular check-ups. **This theory perpetuates extremely harmful and unnatural dietary and other lifestyle habits which flood our bodies with toxic acids, mucus, and many other poisonous substances.** These acids and toxins activate a disease cycle which is a pleomorphic [229] process that causes mutation of normal life forms within our bodies. From this gradual mutation process, disease develops, and if the cause is not abated, various diseases are allowed to advance into chronic and degenerative states. Adherents of the Germ

---

[229] Pleomorphic: Polymorphic; Multiform. Occurring in more than one morphologic form. Polymorphism: existence in the same species or other natural group of more than one morphologic type. *Stedman's Medical Dictionary.* In plain English, it means: life form species respond to the chemical environment they live in, and are capable of mutating into other forms which may appear to be unrelated to the original type.

Theory intentionally believe that it doesn't matter what we eat - that eating has nothing to do with health or disease - yet even most children know better than that. It has only been in the last few years that the trend has begun to change. More and more medical doctors are realizing that their college professors did not have all the answers, and that there is a great need for doctors to think for themselves.

## 2. Deadly Treatments Suppress Symptoms and Stop Healthy Toxin Elimination

**Second: The germ theory encourages medical doctors to use costly, ineffective, often harmful, and sometimes deadly methods of treatment** - treatments that often cause serious future diseases. Medical practices, with the blessings of the AMA and the FDA, bombard our bodies with even more toxic contaminants by using treatments (drugs and radiation) which seldom produce the desired effect, or do so only on a short term basis, while causing many complications, further weakness and disease.[230] Antibiotics are only one example and compared to other drugs, a mild example.[231, 232] However, there is probably more disease caused by

---

[230] Chemotherapy drugs are toxic. They suppress the immune system, leaving the body vulnerable to infections. They also have many terrible side effects as does radiation. They both can cause nausea, diarrhea, extreme fatigue. David Larson, M.D., Editor-in-chief, *Mayo Clinic Family Health Book*, ( New York, NY: William Morrow and Co., 1990), pg. 1245. **See Appendix: Chemotherapy.**

[231] Antibiotics that kill off part of the intestinal flora can upset its balance and may open the door to infection or pathological overgrowth. Overgrowth of Clostridium difficile, initiated by antibiotics, produces severe inflammation of the colon with diarrhea (pseudo membranous colitis). Samuel Baron, *Medical Microbiology*, 3rd Edition, (New York, NY: Addison-Wesley Publishing, 1981), pg. 1172.

Various antibiotic drugs can cause infections which include brain abscess, aspiration pneumonia, thoracic emphysema, intra-abdominal infections, postoperative wound infection, infections related to gynecologic disease or surgery, etc.. The exotoxins of Clostridium tetani and C. botulinum are among the most potent poisons known to man (estimated to be one million times as potent as rattlesnake poison). Heavy fungal growth is often stimulated by commonly employed antibiotics and may be associated with fungal infections often complicating therapy. Mattman, pg. 243-247.

[232] Antimicrobial drugs have spread new varieties of microorganisms (mutated species) that are resistant to antibiotics. Gerard J.Tortora, Berdell R. Funke, Christine L. Case, *Microbiology, An Introduction*, 3rd

antibiotics than any other thing in this world, except diet, and negative thinking. For antibiotics upset the feeding system of our bodies. The fundamental core of our being, which every system, every organ, tissues, fluids, and chemistry depends. It is ironic how clearly antibiotics have saved the lives of thousands of people, but promoted massive suffering and death to millions. But it occurred so gradually, that it has taken decades to finally realize what they have done. Should we really blame antibiotics? I don't think so, **for the truth is, each of us had to make the decision to go against what is natural**. Not only that, but our minds, through the habits of thinking and feeling, pull us into the situations we experience. Chemotherapy drugs and other drugs often poison healthy cells and suppress the body's elimination processes, driving disease deeper into the tissues, which may bring temporary relief, but only postpones the body ridding itself of the potential deadly conditions that caused the disease in the first place.

Drugs can force the body to stop the process of eliminating the toxicity and other conditions which have already caused the internal environment to alter. **Most drugs merely postpone disease eruptions, which are very likely to occur** repeatedly **in the future.** It is far better for a patient to deal with a disease at the earliest possible moment and eliminate the filthy sludge that germs thrive upon, rather than when the body may be older, weaker, more toxic, and unable to deal with the future eruptions. **Even medical statistics reveal that medical practice contributes towards the tenth highest fatality rate in the U.S., which is doctor-caused disease or death.** Statisticians even have a name for it, "iatrogenic."[233] However, a little further research in statistics reveals that they left out important figures and failed to include deaths caused by medical drugs and infections contracted in hospitals. Medical drugs were the third leading cause of death, and hospital contracted infections was fifth! Out of a total of 392,556 deaths tabulated under leading causes of death in 1996, 17.74% were caused by the practice of conventional medicine.[234]

---

Edition, (New York, NY: The Benjamin/Cummings Publisher, 1989), pg. 12-13.

*Ask yourself this: Why is it that doctors **do not** tell us these things?

[233] Iatrogenic - Denoting an unfavorable response to medical or surgical treatment, induced by the treatment itself. *Stedman's Medical Dictionary.*

[234] Web Page of Earl Mindell, Ph.D.; *Time Magazine*; *Journal of Community Health*, 1980; Spring; Vol.5, No. 3., pg. 149-158. All other figures from the National Center for Health Statistics through the U.S. Dept. of Health and Human Services, Centers for Disease Control.

## 3. Teaches Denial of Inward Healing Power

Third: **The germ theory subtlely, thoroughly, and very effectively, causes the believer to deny his/her own trust and faith in the Innate Intelligence (Infinite Intelligence, God) which actually does the healing.** It is this intelligence that is the basic intelligence in our DNA. Just as a surgeon's scalpel accurately and effectively cuts away specific tissues, so **the germ theory destroys the faith and often the hope of our own beings by subtly and unconsciously persuading the patient to reject their trust in Divine influence and the natural laws of nature.**

The germ theory is the basic belief of the world's most profitable and powerful religious organization (modern medicine), which is wise enough to not call itself a religion. Yet it is. And **it takes away the natural faith of gullible victims, causing them to trust in man-made intelligence, man-made inventions, man-made cleverness, and decisions.** This religion takes away the faith that health can be restored, the hope of perfect health, and the possibility of future health.

The use of vaccines, which is based on the Germ Theory, is destroying our children and their minds, and genetically engineering future generations.[235] See the end of this Chapter for more information. These substances do not cleanse or strengthen the body, they contaminate it. The scalpel, drugs, and radiation do absolutely nothing to eliminate the cause of disease. On the contrary, **the belief in these things prevents people from seeking out the more basic cause, which is always a result of habitual thoughts and feelings which are soul based.**

## Summary: Basic Causes Must be Addressed to Recover Good Health

Drugs (especially vaccines and antibiotics), chlorinated and fluorinated water and air pollution, acid-forming foods, processed foods, mineral deficient foods, unnatural chemicals and hormones in foods, and harmful emotions, are not the way to good health. We need to understand what these things do to our bodies, what we can do to prevent them, how to correct the harm already done, and then develop the inner strength to live a healthy lifestyle. For it does take a unique strength to live healthfully. Indeed, there are many things that may present obstacles: social pressure,

---

[235] Read some of the books listed in the back of this book, about vaccines.

difficulties in obtaining pure and wholesome foods, higher prices, bad habits and the effort it takes to develop new ones.

And yet, after all I have pointed out, I want to say that there may be rare times when a drug may be the only thing that can solve a problem. The difficulty is knowing when it should be used.

# Why Medical Science Chose the Germ Theory

Even though Pasteur's work triggered development of the "Germ Theory," also known as the "Theory of Infection," Pasteur himself later rejected the theory.[236] Medical science, however, adopted it. Here was the beginning of the downfall of the healthiest nation in the world. In only 80 years America would drop from the healthiest to become the sickest nation in the world.[237] During this time the medical industry grew exponentially. **It is mainly because of adherence to the Germ Theory, that even today, most medical doctors do not believe that it matters what we eat.** Medical science does not even teach nutrition to medical doctors.[238] Further, they want us to believe that all the filthy, slimy, moving garbage we see in a sick person's blood is sterile.[239] They want to give us all sorts

---

[236] Later Pasteur changed his viewpoint and agreed with Beauchamp that disease is a result of "terrain" (internal environment). Neil Z. Miller, *Vaccines: Are They Really Safe and Effective?*, (Santa Fe, NM: New Atlantean Press, 1993), pg. 66-67.

[237] Out of 100 nations coordinating with the U.S. Dept. of Health, America was the healthiest nation in 1920. By 1987, America was on the bottom of the list. We can't get any lower, but we can get even sicker. Irons, pg. 2-3.

[238] Only 30 medical schools in the U.S. have any required courses in nutrition. A Senate investigation revealed that the average physician in the United States received less than 3 hours of training in nutrition during 4 years of medical schools. Robbins, pg. 150.

[239] Contrary to medical belief that the blood is sterile, the blood is not sterile, but it contains microorganisms and filth capable of causing disease when the internal environment of our bodies has produced the suitable condition. It is easy to see under a microscope, all sorts of pathogenic microorganisms swimming, vibrating, and wiggling in the blood. Many of them are unnatural, harmful, and definitely not sterile. Would you think that the blood is sterile when you can see various bacterial and parasite forms swimming in the blood? How about yeasts and other weird indescribable forms wiggling and growing in the blood?

of vaccines, shots, tests, radiation, drugs, operations, etc., because they want us to believe that we need to attack and kill these entities which have invaded our bodies, rather than clean the environment that makes their propagation possible.[240]

Why are medical doctors taught this? How much money will drug companies and doctors make if they send their patients home and tell them to change their diet, cleanse their bodies using herbs, fasting, and enemas, or simply use natural means to help improve the body's elimination? What will be their future profits if disease is eradicated?

How much money will drug companies and doctors make if they tell their patients that they need more tests to discover what germ is at fault, where it is located, how severe it has become and then take even more tests - that they need to spend more time at the hospital, that they need to take more drugs or get operated on. Of course, if the solution has not presented itself by then, they instruct that you repeat the process all over again. What will be their future profits if disease is increased?

---

The few medical doctors who use microscopy in their work, usually use only phase contrast. They are also trained to put dyes into the blood, which kills the microbes. Therefore, they can never view what is really going on in the living blood because they kill it before they view it. The somatids, their forms, and most of the pollution that can be seen, are easily viewed with darkfield microscopy, not phase contrast. I have many blood atlases with thousands of pictures, and not one picture using darkfield. There is so much more that can be seen using darkfield. Why don't more medical doctors use it? Maybe they don't want to know that the blood is indeed, polluted! Because if they knew it was polluted - what do you think the logical treatment would be? Get rid of the pollution! Right? Will drugs remove pollution? No! Drugs cause pollution. So what would they do? Those who study natural medicine, the naturopathic doctors, the natural medical doctors, and others, should know exactly what to do.

[240] Indeed we live in a murderous society. They want to kill microbes in our bodies. We have been trained from childhood to kill bugs in our orchards, gardens, and farms, rather than go to the trouble of using organically grown farming methods that strengthen plants to resist the bugs. Our society is full of hunters who want to kill deer and anything else that fly's, crawls, or walks. The majority of our society feeds on innocent animals that are killed unnecessarily for our food. We are programmed from childhood to kill or fight. Think about all the killing and fighting we see in movies and on TV. And if you still have doubts, just watch your TV on Saturday mornings and observe what children get to see.

# Other Ways Medical Science Has Increased Disease

## High Protein Diets

**Next to the Germ Theory, the most treacherous scheme to increase disease has been to encourage high-protein diets.**

High-protein diets, long touted as essential to health, lack fiber, and are very acid-producing. In reality, the high protein diet:
1. Causes excessive acids and toxins
2. Depletes minerals
3. Reduces oxygen potential
4. Reduces peristalsis
5. Causes the body to create excessive mucus and congestion
6. Damages the digestive tract
7. Weakens the liver and other organs

Auto-intoxication is a result of intestinal toxemia which is primarily a result of a high-protein diet, mineral deficient food, an excess of processed food, and too much cooked food.

Success in promoting the high protein diet was achieved through many educational techniques, some of which included changing the 12 Basic Food Groups which contained more alkaline-forming foods, to the standard 4 Basic Food Groups which contain more acid-forming foods. The meat, dairy industries, and medical industry, of course, loved the increased profits of their disease-causing products, as did the cereal companies; for it was well-known that harmful bacteria in the bowels was a major cause of disease, and that high-protein diets changed the helpful, friendly bacteria into harmful, putrefactive bacteria. Now the 4 Basic Food Groups have been revised again and fortunately it was an improvement this time.[241]

People who have been indoctrinated into belief in a high protein diet have asked me, "Where do you get your protein?" I tell them, "From watermelon, and my wife gets hers from lettuce." It is almost impossible to not get enough protein. Protein is in all foods except oils.[242] Where do cows get their protein? From grass. Where should people get their

---

[241] New Food Pyramid developed by U.S.D.A.
http:\\www.knoxnews.com\health\weightmanagement\pyramid.html

[242] Keith Akers, *A Vegetarian Sourcebook*, (New York: Putnam, 1983), pg. 24.

protein? From fruits and vegetables and a few nuts, grains and legumes. The only way anyone can not get enough protein is: 1) they don't eat enough of the above foods, or 2) their digestive system has failed, or is functioning so poorly that they cannot digest or assimilate the food they eat. Don't buy into the protein scare - it is a lie that is designed to make money!

### Bad Bacteria, Toxins and Candida

**Ammonium, clostridium, indole, skatole, urea, and guanidine are some of the toxins produced by the bad bacteria which thrive on high-protein diets.** Many of these toxins affect the central nervous system. It was found by 11 independent labs that schizophrenics have 5 times more indole and skatole in their urine than what is normal. The liver cannot protect us from all harmful toxicity produced by the putrefactive bacteria, even when we have strong, healthy livers, and it has been estimated that a high percentage of people have weak livers.

There is strong evidence to support the fact that all cancer, AIDS, liver disorders, kidney, brain, and heart disorders receive their toxic malformations from toxic intestines. Note especially Sir Arbuthnot Lane's comments in Chapter 4. He was convinced that intestinal stasis was a forerunner to cancer.

Candidiasis is a terrible yeast infection that can create overwhelming levels of toxicity, and is associated with the onset of many serious diseases. It was only discovered in the 1970's and in a high percentage of all cases, can be attributed to the use of antibiotics. It was known by 1988 that one-third of the American people have Candidiasis, and it can affect all body systems. After the discovery that Candida albicans was a serious cause of so many illnesses, a few natural practitioners were able to successfully treat the problem. However, the AMA and the medical world at large, denied its existence for about 15 years. Either due to the pressure of successful holistic medicine, or because a profitable drug was made to treat the disease, the AMA finally put their tails between their legs and admitted that the "quacks" were once again right.

# Making Things Complicated

Medical science loves to make things extremely complicated. It keeps people, including doctors, confused. That is another way of producing a monopoly. Every profiteer loves a monopoly; that is, *if* they are in control of it. Imagine the oil industry's reaction if someone found out how to power our cars with water. People have been killed to stop such inventions. Do you think the medical religion would want to admit that by using certain herbs and by changing the diet, most health problems would be solved?

Now if by some chance you find people that still don't believe that there is a serious problem in our society with conventional medicine, learn what Dr. Robert Mendelsohn, M.D. has to say about it. But first let me ask: are you impressed by credentials? See this footnote.[243] This is what he has said about the medicine that is currently practiced (that's a great term - the practice of medicine. I guess that means they haven't gotten it right yet! They need more practice.): "The greatest danger to your health is the doctor who practices Modern Medicine....I believe that Modern Medicine's treatments for disease are seldom effective, and that they're *often more dangerous than the disease they're designed to treat*....I believe that more than 90% of Modern Medicine could disappear from the face of the earth - doctors, hospitals, drugs, and equipment-and the effect on our health would be immediate and beneficial.....Every drug stresses and hurts your body in some way." He went on to say that the most dangerous place in the world is in a hospital and the second is in a medical doctor's office.

The modern medical system, officially known as allopathic medicine, is the most dangerous system in terms of the survival of the human race. In number of casualties, it has outranked war[244] by many times. Yet, the vast majority of people in the Western World adhere to it like glue, support it like it was their friend, trust in it like it was God, and like cattle walking to the slaughterhouse, become weaker, maimed and often, dead—long before their time.

Like Dr. Jensen, I have been keeping an eye on each new generation of people. Through the iris of the eyes, we can observe the strengths and weaknesses of people. It is frightening to see each new generation becoming weaker and weaker. **OUR ENTIRE SOCIETY HAS DEVOLVED TO SUPPORT THE DETERIORATION OF PEOPLE, NOT THEIR WELL-BEING!**

---

[243] Dr. Robert Mendelsohn, M.D., was the National Medical Director of Project Head Start, Chairman of the Medical Licensing Committee for the State of Illinois, associate professor at the University of Illinois Medical School, director of Chicago's Michael Reese Hospital, and the excellent author of *Male Practice: How Doctors Manipulate Women*; *How to Raise a Healthy Child In spite of Your Doctor*; and *Confessions of a Medical Heretic*.

[244] Total U.S. casualties during all four years of W.W.II equal 234,874, as compared to 392,556 medical casualties in 1996 alone.

# Change is Possible

At this point in time the medical industry has several advantages. People have been so conditioned by our fast-paced society to expect quick fixes and instant gratification, that it is difficult to change habits and diet. The food industry has been catering to the ever changing faster and faster pace with quick meals that are proving to be unhealthy. It takes an effort to eat a properly prepared diet. Any person who has the guts to break away from the destructive lifestyles of the Western World is labeled as weird. It is possible, however, to change. And someday this will be turned around and these people will be looked upon as enlightened - those who had the intelligence to dare to turn away from the destructive tide of man's pathetic weakness.

Those of us who are doing so are to be commended. We are also finding ourselves rewarded with greater vitality, awareness and fitness. We are awakening and advancing mentally, spiritually and emotionally. We are remembering to think of cause and effect. As we remember, we will find the strength to change our habits and release unhealthy desires. On the other side of those mind-dulling and body-desensitizing habits and foods is a world of alertness, intelligence, joy, inner peace, harmony, greater awareness, and best of all, love - love for everything.

# Politics of Illness

## Freedom to Choose?

**How can anyone respect a country that forces it's people to use deforming and deadly treatments, such as chemotherapy, radiation, surgery and other potentially deadly drugs to attempt to cure diseases such as cancer?** After such severe treatments, the whole body's immune system is essentially destroyed. The body is then so weak, how could it possibly go about healing itself? Such treatments are not the part of wisdom. There may be times when these man-made radical treatments will work, (that is usually when the patient's belief in the treatment is incredibly strong) but usually they leave the victims terribly weakened. I believe that whenever they have worked, the healing would have worked better using natural methods. However, I believe that surgery is occasionally a good approach, but only when the infected mass is so huge that it is better to remove it than for the body to absorb it. But the surgeon should then instruct the patients to cleanse, rebuild, improve diet, remove negative emotions, etc. In other words, they should encourage the patient to put an end to the cause.

## Amazing Cleanse Results - An Unwanted Challenge to Drugs?

Tens of thousands of people have experienced some very impressive results with my cleansing program. But few people have seen it from my point of view. For I was hearing from hundreds, even thousands of people who have experienced amazing results both during and after the cleanse. In other words, I have had the wonderful opportunity to witness the benefits of so many people as a result of cleansing that I can't help but get excited. From this point of view, I've realized that there is nothing else that is responsible for such amazing miracles. After the first year of seeing these results, I knew that we probably had the greatest health program the world had yet to see. And now after 11 years, I am fully convinced of it. Because of the efficacy of my cleanse, I initially refused to advertise because I didn't want the FDA or the AMA to find out about it. After all, herbs work, and without any of the death or disease-causing side-effects which drugs are known to have. And, as I saw it, my cleansing program has been so remarkably effective that it could have the potential of reducing drug sales. There have been incidents where it has appeared that they have gone out of their way to make herbs and natural healing look bad. And that's putting it mildly - very mildly. When the following incident took place, I had to ask myself if my fears had manifested.

One of my products was mysteriously contaminated, and many people got sick, including myself, because I use my own products. We immediately recalled the affected batches. We sent samples of the batches to one lab after another to try and find out what the problem was. We checked everything we could imagine that could possibly cause the symptoms our people were having, including: lead, other heavy metals, bacteria, parasites, toxic chemicals, etc. Finally, a toxicologist in Massachusetts detected digoxin in the blood of one of the victims, and from that the FDA was able to determine the cause: a low grade digitalis (*of the quality that would have been rejected by pharmaceutical companies in their process of making the heart medicine, digitalis*). Digitalis is derived from the weed commonly known as Woolly Foxglove, and can be very toxic. This situation prompted us to initiate a major recall, and the timing was perfect if it was designed to put us out of business. It almost did, but we hung in there. Yet it was truly a nightmare for us and for the many customers who were affected.

This unlikely contamination, which was previously never known to occur in plantain, was a major shock, not only to us, but also to over 100 other companies which the FDA discovered had purchased these same plantain supplies. Another shock was when the FDA discovered that the affected batches came from Germany! We had been told by our supplier, who was a personal friend, that it was grown in America and wildcrafted. We paid extra for that, too!

When the FDA announced to the entire world that one of our favorite formulas was potentially deadly, they omitted that the problem was confined to certain batches. Now here is a good question for you. Why is it that the FDA announced through several worldwide media channels that this product was potentially deadly and demanded that people stop using it immediately, but they do not do this with drugs, even with drugs that KILLLLLL!!!! However, look at how many people have died from FDA approved drugs recently and the FDA doesn't bother to tell the public! Look how many people died at the hands of AMA approved procedures. I think that something is deadly wrong!

♦ More than 2,556 deaths a year are caused by the use of *over-the-counter drugs!*[245]

♦ In the last 10 years, more than **18 million Americans** suffered serious, toxic side-effects from medical drugs and had to be hospitalized. That number now averages over 2 million Americans a year![246]

♦ In 1980, **150,000 patients in hospitals died as a result of an infection that they did not have prior to entering the hospital.** More recent figures are not being released.

♦ American deaths from the adverse effects of prescribed drugs in 1995 was over 160,000![247]

♦ **Total conventional medicine-caused deaths is *392,556 = 17.74%* of all the leading causes of deaths in America.**

♦ That figure (from only one year - 1996) is **nearly double the *total American causalities during all four years of W.W.II!*[248]** Are Americans at war with medical doctors and/or drug companies? Imagine a war where one side doesn't have enough sense to know that they are being killed by their enemies. And if that isn't bad enough, imagine that the side that is loosing is financially and socially supporting their enemies in their own self destruction and encouraging their friends, families, and even their children to do the same! Has our society gone totally insane!

♦ At the 1996 level of medical doctor-related deaths (and it is always increasing), **in less than 3 years, medical doctors would be responsible for more deaths than ALL THE WARS AMERICA HAS EVER HAD!**[249]

---

[245] The Web Page of Earl Mindell, Ph.D.

[246] U.S. News and World Report quoted in "Health Realities," by Queen and Company.

[247] Source: The Web Page of Earl Mindell, Ph.D.

[248] Total U.S. casualties in W.W. II = 234,874. From: http:\\www.army.mil\cmh-pg\war.htm.

♦ About 90% of the patients who visit doctors have conditions that will either improve on their own or that are out of reach of modern medicine's ability to solve.[250]

# Is There a Medical Conspiracy?

In my opinion, anyone who does not believe that there is a medical conspiracy should easily qualify to become an ostrich in their next life! Do you have any idea how many doctors have lost their licenses[251] because they treated people with alternative methods? Many have even been severely harassed, professionally ruined,[252] and killed.[253] The results? Americans have become slaves to systems that do not work, and medical doctors and other professionals are afraid to speak up. But it happened so gradually, so cleverly, that 'we the people' got sucked into it. We trusted in credentials instead of common sense. We trusted a science led by

---

[249] Average annual American WWII deaths 58,000. All the American wars together equal 1,089,200. Source: http:/www.va.gov/pressrel/amwars,97.htm

[250] T.A. Brennan, L.L. Leap, N.M. Liard, L. Herbert, A.R. Localio, A.G. Lawthers, J.P. Newhouse, P.C. Weiler, H.H. Hiatt, "Incidence of Adverse Event and Negligence in Hospitalized Patients. Results of the Harvard Medical Practice Study," *New England Journal of Medicine*, 1991; Feb. 7; pg. 370-376.

[251] Barry Lynes, *The Healing of Cancer - The Cures, the Cover-ups and the Solution Now.* (Queensville, Ontario, CAN: Marcus Books, 1989), pg. 32.

[252] This is only one example of many I have heard. Andrew Ivy, Vice President and professor of physiology at the University of Illinois was former chairman of the National Cancer Institute's National Adversary Council on Cancer. He was an internationally recognized scholar and prolific author of scientific papers. He made the mistake of supporting a cancer-curing serum called Krebiozen - which over 20,000 cancer patients had supposedly benefited from. One U.S. Senate Committee lawyer personally assessed 530 cases and concluded that Krebiozen was effective. Another supporter was Major General Wallace Graham, Physician to the President of the U.S., who announced that he had seen "unusually good results with Krebiozen". The FDA spent multi-million dollars in prosecuting Dr. Ivy, ruining him publically and professionally, and illegally and without facts, destroyed the credibility of Krebiozen. Source: Ibid., pg. 58-59.

[253] Barry Lynes, *The Healing of Cancer, The Cures - the Cover-ups and the Solution Now!*, (Queenville, Ontario, CAN: Marcus Books, 1989), pg. 31, 161.

in credentials instead of common sense. We trusted a science led by conspirators instead of nature and God. Now we are beginning to see that we have become victims of almost unbelievable treachery. People suffer and die by the millions and we never stop to think why.

**Leading causes of death in US in 1996**[254]

|     |                          |             |
| --- | ------------------------ | ----------- |
|     | All causes               | 2,262,903   |
| 1.  | Heart disease            | 733,834     |
| 2.  | Cancer                   | 544,278     |
| 3.  | **Medical drugs**        | **162,556**[255] |
| 4.  | Stroke                   | 160,431     |
| 5.  | **Infections in hospitals** | **150,000**[256] |
| 6.  | Lung disease             | 106,140     |
| 7.  | Accidents                | 93,874      |
| 8.  | Pneumonia/Influenza      | 82,579      |
| 9.  | **Iatrogenic disease**   | **80,000**[257] |
| 10. | Diabetes                 | 61,559      |
| 11. | HIV/AIDS                 | 32,655      |
| 12. | Suicide                  | 30,862      |
| 13. | Liver disease            | 25,135[258] |

Am I the only one that cares? Is there something wrong with me that I care so much? Anyone else out there who cares? Yes, but darn few.

Even worse than promoting death and disease-causing treatments while outlawing effective and safe treatments, is the forcing of innocent

---

[254] **Even more current information which confirms the conclusion that medical drugs are extremely dangerous is reflected in further statistics** that have come to my attention, just as this book is going to print! See an article from *The Washington Post*, **Wednesday, April 15, 1998 on page A-1, titled: "Correctly Prescribed Drugs Take Heavy Toll,"** by Rick Weiss, Washington Post Staff Writer.

[255] Web Page of Earl Mindell, Ph.D.

[256] *Journal of Community Health*, 1980; Spring; Vol. 5, No. 3, pg. 149-158. (You can be certain that this statistic is far worse today than in 1980.)

[257] Source: American Iatrogenic Association's Home Page - aia.iatrogenic.org (They cite this statistic as coming from Time Magazine). American Iatrogenic Association, 2513 S. Gessner #232, Houston, TX 77063.

[258] All other figures came from the National Center for Health Statistics through US Dept. of health & Human Services Centers for Disease Control.

children to be stabbed with poison containing needles (vaccines) when no one knows what the long term effects will be. Especially when there is a history[259] of disease, deformity, and death associated with vaccines.

In spite of my convictions about using the most natural treatments, I believe that the best therapy a patient can have is usually that which the patient believes in the most, for the belief of a patient is the most important factor of all in getting well. If chemotherapy - then I say go-for-it. If radiation is what they believe in, I would say do it. That is how powerful I believe the mind can be. **But, to neglect nutrition and diet is often a form of suicide or murder, and to neglect cleansing and psychological change is simply ignorance.** I believe that we should all have the choice to choose. **We all should have the right to choose whatever treatment we believe in, but we don't have that right; it has been taken from us. If information or availability of a treatment that works is kept from us then we cannot exercise our right to choose.**

## Misinformation

I think that in this world of extreme deception and almost constant programming through the news media, television, and uneducated educational systems, people's minds are constantly being manipulated into denying the facts and truth about their health and today's medical industry. The vast majority of people live lifestyles that are downright destructive and the really sad part of it is that most of them have no idea that they are creating a tremendous amount of disease in themselves and their family.

For an example: If you take an average American family with four children, and they eat the standard American diet (SAD), go to the standard American doctors (another SAD), and basically live the lifestyle of the standard American, here are the statistics of their four children: One will die of cancer and another will have cancer and the other two are likely to die of heart disease although there is a better than 70% chance that one will die at the hands of conventional medicine.[260] If by some remote chance they all lived to be 90 (which they wouldn't), they *all* would have diverticulitis as well as many, many other diseases.[261]

---

[259] Read the books about vaccines under: Suggested Reading in the back of this book.

[260] I figured out these projections based upon average leading causes of death over the past 20 years.

[261] *Merck Manual of Diagnosis and Therapy*, 15th Edition, (Rahway, NJ: Merck Sharp and Dohme Research Laboratories, Division of Merck and Company, 1987), pg. 813-815. See Colorectal Diverticular Disease in Index.

**Due to restrictions on the flow of health related information, and due to the outlawing of some alternative treatments, in many situations it appears that there is no choice.** I have had to turn away many people who wanted me to treat them for cancer. But the law prevents me. I can only say, "Change the law, and I will be there for you."

### Effective Anti-cancer Formulas 'Lost' and Suppressed - Three Doctors Killed

Dr. Koch had developed one of the most successful cancer treatments ever recorded. With cases of advanced cancer, he had a 46% cure rate. When patients were not in a terminal stage, the cure rate averaged 72%.[262] His formula saved many lives and was especially effective for leukemia. Dr. Koch had about 4,000 doctors using his "Glyoxylide" before the FDA and AMA found out about it. *Then he was arrested and a six month trial ensued.* **During the trial, one doctor who was testifying in Koch's behalf, was poisoned to death, and another was run down and killed by a car. Dr. Koch survived 13 assassination attempts.** He won the case and fled the United States. The Brazilian government offered him the highest position in the Brazilian medical services. He accepted the position, but reportedly did not survive the next attempt on his life; he was poisoned. The Glyoxylide formula was apparently lost forever.[263] Was this an unusual situation? Unusual in the sense that it is rare for someone to come up with an effective cancer cure, but certainly not rare for the FDA and AMA to stop it.[264]

Linus Pauling said that "Everyone should know that the 'war on cancer' is largely a fraud, and that the National Cancer Society and the American Cancer Society are derelict in their duties to the people who support them."[265] Robert C. Atkins, M.D. stated specifically, "There is not one, but many cures for cancer available. But they are all being

---

[262] William F. Koch, Ph.D., MD., *The Survival Factor in Neoplastic and Viral Diseases*, (Detroit, MI: The Vanderkloot Press, Inc., 1958), pg. 210.

[263] Barry Lynes, *The Healing of Cancer, The Cures - the Cover-Ups and the Solution Now!*, (Queenville, Ontario CAN: Marcus Books, 1989), pg. 31, 161.

[264] Ibid., See Chapter 2: The FDA, and Chapter 3: The AMA.

[265] From: the back cover of *"The Cancer Industry,"* by Ralph W. Moss, Ph.D.

systematically suppressed."[266] The distinguished medical journal Lancet reported, in 1975, a study which compared chemotherapy and no treatment at all. The report concluded that no treatment proved a significantly better policy for patients survival and for quality of remaining life.[267]

# Vaccines, Are They Good or Bad?

In 1918, the US Army forced the vaccination of 3,285,376 natives in the Philippines when no epidemic was brewing, only the sporadic cases of the usual mild nature. Of the vaccinated persons, 47,369 came down with small-pox, and of these 16,477 died. In 1919 the experiment was doubled. 7,670,252 natives were vaccinated. Of these 65,180 victims came down with small-pox, and 44,408 died. In the first experiment, one-third died, and in the second, two-thirds of the infected ones died. **Here was the beginning of the great vaccine experiment, and it continues today - experimentation.**[268] I obtained this from Dr. William Koch's book, *The Survival Factor in Neoplastic and Viral Diseases.*

Dr. Koch, by the way, has been considered by many people as the greatest doctor who ever lived. About vaccines and other drugs, he said this: **"The injection of any serum, vaccine, or even penicillin has shown a very marked increase in the incidence of polio - at least 400 percent. Statistics on this are so conclusive, no one can deny it."**[269]

The Federal Centers for Disease Control admitted between 1973 and 1983, **87% of all cases of polio in the US were caused by the polio vaccine, and from 1980 through 1989, it was 100%.** Not only that but some people outside of the US who "caught" polio, had previously been vaccinated against the disease. Lot of good the vaccine did, right?[270]

About **50% of all people who contract diphtheria, have been fully vaccinated and 33% of the fatal cases had been fully vaccinated.**[271] Lot of good the vaccine did, right?

---

[266] Lynes, pg. 7.

[267] Lynes, pg. 9.

[268] Koch, Ph.D., MD., pg. 19.

[269] Irons, pg. 2-3.

[270] Neil Z. Miller, *Vaccines: Are They Really Safe And Effective? A Parent's Guide To Childhood Shots*, (Santa Fe, New Mexico: New Atlantan Press, 1992), pg. 22.

Eight years before the first measles vaccine was injected into a human body, the death rate of **the epidemic had declined 97.7% and was still dropping**. Yet the drug companies took the credit for eliminating the disease. This is a typical propaganda technique in the vaccine brain washing experiment.[272]

According to the World Health Organization (WHO), **those who have been vaccinated for measles have a 14 times greater chance of getting the disease.** Lot of good the vaccine does, right?[273]

In 1976 more than 500 people who received their **flu shots** were paralyzed with Guillain-Barré syndrome. **30 died.** That same year, **this disease was at least 50% greater among the vaccinated US Army personnel than unvaccinated civilians.**[274]

DPT. If ever there was a diabolical sinister activity directed against children it is DPT vaccination. **Nothing to my knowledge has caused such horrible and unnecessary suffering and death to children other than DPT.** Thousands of children, after going through unbelievable agony and long screaming fits, experienced the following: permanent blindness, continuous seizures, inability to speak, permanent dyslexia, shock, hallucinations, permanent disablement, permanent brain damage, convulsions, and death. Studies have shown that approximately 1 out of 200 children have suffered severe reactions. Other studies have shown that **children who received the DPT shot have an 8 times greater chance of dying in childhood than normal.** Dr. Viera Scheibnerova, the author of one of the studies announced that **"vaccination is the single most prevalent and most preventable cause of infant deaths".** Another study of 103 children who died of SIDS, found that two-thirds had been vaccinated with DPT prior to dying.[275] And they force this on our children by law. Not my children. No way![276] Based upon information available in 1985, I have figured that **approximately 4,000 children die each year from DPT vaccine.**

---

[271] Ibid., pg. 24.

[272] Ibid., pg. 24.

[273] Ibid., pg. 22, 25.

[274] Ibid., pg. 44.

[275] Ibid., pg. 36

[276] Ibid., pg. 22. Also, Harris L. Coulter and Barbara Loe Fisher, *A Shot In The Dark*, (Garden City Park, New York: Avery Publishing Group Inc., 1991). Also read other books about vaccines listed in the back of this book.

I agree with Dr. Hodge: **"Compulsory vaccination ranks with human slavery and religious persecution, as one of the most flagrant outrages upon the rights of the human race."**[277]

Excerpts from a letter from Eleanor McBean, Ph.D. to Governor Edmund G. Brown of California, October 1964: "......I have uncovered some shocking data, showing that **our government, medical and military authorities know that vaccination has killed and crippled thousands of innocent people; but the facts have been suppressed.** The vaccine business has continued to thrive **in spite of its disastrous failure, for the mere reason that it nets millions of dollars for the promoters, and this buys power with governments and propaganda control over the masses who don't know how to think for themselves."**[278]

Let me give you an example of some the substances they put into vaccines. Here is a list: substances from the skin of calves inoculated with seed virus, inactivated virus from infected cattle tongue epithelium, live virus attenuated by embryonate egg or mouse passage and propagated in tissue culture, virus strains prepared in chick embryo cell culture, rabies from duck embryo origin. Other vaccines contain live virus prepared from duck embryo or human diploid cell culture, calf lymph, a formaldehyde-inactivated suspension of *Rickettsia prowazekii* grown in embryonate eggs, a suspension of dried mouse brain infected with French neurotropic strain of yellow fever virus.[279] Further vaccine ingredients may include: rotten horse blood (for diphtheria toxin and antitoxin), macerated cancerous breasts, sweepings from vacuum cleaners (for asthma and hay fever), pus from sores on diseased animals, metallic poisons, powdered insects, mucus from the throats of children with colds and whooping cough, decomposed fecal matter from typhoid patients, sewage, urine, fecal matter, and cow sore pus.[280] Do you believe in witchcraft? Some people actually believe that witchcraft, or something like Satanism, is the intelligence behind the medical conspiracy. But do you really believe that even witches would use the ingredients just described?

**Many doctors believe that the massive epidemics today of cancer, heart disease, chronic fatigue syndrome and more are related to vaccines.** I agree. Many of us believe that it is only a matter of time

---

[277] Hannah Allen, *Don't Get Stuck! The Case Against Vaccinations and Injections*, (Tampa, Florida: American Natural Hygiene Society, 1985), pg. 115.

[278] Ibid., pg. 130.

[279] *Stedman's Medical Dictionary*, pg. 1680-1681.

[280] Hannah Allen, pg. 22-23.

now, that our modern disease epidemics[281] will turn into massive death epidemics. Mankind is well prepared. We've been drugged beyond logic, programmed to eat unnatural and toxic foods, forced to drink polluted water and breathe toxic air. Our daily lives are full of stress and fear, and now, we even experience serious electronic pollution on a daily basis. Indeed, we have been well prepared for major disasters. For the last 70 years or so, each generation has been well prepared by our medical system, news media, schools, etc. Each generation produces a weaker generation. It is very illuminating to examine a whole family. I have studied the irises of a grandmother, then the mother, then the children. The iris reveals the constitutional strengths and weaknesses of the person. When I've compared the children with the grandmother, I wonder how the children are even alive. No way will they live like their grandmother to be 90. And so it is. Children are becoming weaker and weaker, and you may have noticed, fatter and fatter, like hogs being prepared for slaughter. Disease is becoming more and more prevalent, and no government agency is doing anything about it. There is a reason why they vaccinated the Filipinos. Do you know what the reason is? It is the same reason they vaccinate everywhere else in the world where people are gullible enough to allow it. It is the same reason they want to do it to our children. There are not many doctors who know the reason, because: 1.) It is beyond their imagination and 2.) They have been well programmed in believing that it is doing people some good. Nothing could be further from the truth.

**The reason for vaccination is that there is nothing more effective in weakening the bodies, minds, wills, imagination, sensitivity, awareness, and spiritual awareness of any person than putting highly toxic, foreign DNA, and poisonous substance into the body and disabling the immune system.** For our immune systems were never meant to function in the way that vaccines necessitate. Our society is a highly programmed society. I believe it is highly controlled by forces that most people know nothing about. These forces have gone to great lengths to keep this kind of information out of the hands of the people. They have deliberately and successfully programmed society to not believe that these forces even exist.

So now, most people are so conditioned that they cannot believe the truth when it is presented. Evidence indicates that when cattle are walking down the chute to be slaughtered, they know something is terribly wrong; they act as if they are filled with fear. Are cattle more aware than humans? Indeed, the masses of mankind have no idea how they are being controlled and manipulated into sheep-like consciousness. Is it too late to turn the tide? I believe it may well be too late very soon.

---

[281] Cancer, heart disease, chronic fatigue, bowel problems, and etc.

In summary, I quote Dr. J.M. Peebles, MD., "**Vaccination is the most outrageous insult that can be offered to any pure-minded man or woman. It is the boldest and most impious attempt to mar the work of God that has been attempted for ages. ...It is time that free American citizens arise in their might and blot out the whole blood-poisoning business.**"[282] I strongly suggest that you read the books about vaccines which are listed in the back of this book. You may learn that the massive increase in cancer, heart disease, AIDS, Candida albicans, and many other diseases may be associated with vaccines. Yet because vaccines have this delayed time-bomb effect, it may be difficult to trace diseases back to vaccines.

**Wake up America and the world! It is almost too late! For many it is too late. For those who still have a chance, cleanse and purify thyselves, get rid of the deadly programming and poisons within you, and pray daily for the protection of your loved ones and the rest of the world. Eat the foods intended by the creator, fresh fruits, vegetables, nuts, seeds, and sprouted grains. Cleanse and rebuild. Eliminate all that is unnatural.**

---

[282] Hannah Allen, pg. 173.

# Chapter 6

# IMPAIRED DIGESTION AND ITS OUTCOMES

## The Creation of Toxicity

When the intestines have *any* mucoid plaque there is always an interference with the digestive process. Even when a person has just a thin lining of mucoid plaque in the intestinal tract, they could have sluggish peristaltic action, inhibited assimilation, and the beginning of toxic accumulations. This usually occurs first in the upper alimentary canal and then throughout the rest of the bowel. At this point, some degree of disease begins to manifest as symptoms.

Mucoid plaque build-up represents the potential for putrefaction (rotting), depletion of oxygen, reduced circulation and abnormal bowel function. This condition offers the perfect environment for a wide variety of pathogenic microorganisms such as bacteria, yeast, parasites, and possibly things we've never heard of before.

## An Overview of Functional Problems Caused by Intestinal Mucoid Plaque

### Poor Circulation: Key to Disease

One of the main problems with this plaque is that it inhibits the in- and outflow of the gastric and intestinal fluids and seems to inhibit nerve function as well. The inflow is critical; it allows assimilation of nutrients necessary for health. The outflow, just as essential, permits the cellular and metabolic waste products from the lymph and intestinal fluids to be released into the bowel and then eliminated from the body. When this flow is blocked, or decreased, the natural chemical balance is altered, causing a wide range of negative chain reactions.

This is a necessary scenario before most of the bowel diseases can manifest, including cancer. When we study intestinal biopsies, we wonder why epithelium so persistently secretes mucin. Seemingly, from deep within the mucosa, the mucosa is attempting to rid itself of toxins, and release toxins contained in the lymph. But, if it cannot do so because of a lack of circulation, toxin accumulation is imminent. The body has to have circulation or it begins to die at the point of congestion. Just as when you leave your hands in water for too long and your skin begins to crinkle or if you leave a bandage on a sore and the skin cannot get oxygen, the skin begins to die. This is a sign of a lack of circulation - the inability to bring oxygen or other nutriments necessary for cell life. It only takes a few minutes of total lack of circulation before decay sets in. With most bowel diseases, circulation has been decreased, but not totally. Therefore, only partial decay sets in and it takes years before problems develop into chronic or degenerative states.

**Following is the most important missing link in today's health. It has been lost, forgotten, or ignored by almost every doctor on this planet, even naturopaths.** There is a great deal of discussion about diet, nutrition, and hundreds of treatments and supplements, but almost nothing about cleansing and rebuilding the core of the body's ability to circulate life sustaining nutrients to the cells - the digestive system. Only a tiny percentage of doctors have realized the importance of this essential life-support system. Indeed, as Go and Summerskill pointed out; **"Digestion is the great secret of life."**[283]   I believe that the digestive system is indeed one of the secrets of health and disease. With few exceptions, every disease begins first in the mind and feelings, and then the digestive system. The digestive system is the first and most important part of our body that must be addressed with all diseases, if good health is to be achieved and maintained.

## Impacts of a Disabled Digestive System

* When the acid/alkaline balance in the alimentary canal is upset as it is when mucoid plaque forms, it opens the door for other strains of undesired bacteria and may severely weaken the friendly bacteria required for proper digestion. This directly results in failure to assimilate proteins, vitamins, minerals(especially calcium), fats, and other needed substances. From this alone, the body loses control of cholesterol, and the blood pressure may be affected. Even more importantly, the ability to *manufacture* certain amino acids, B vitamins(especially B-12), vitamin K, natural antibiotics, enzymes and other things may be reduced.

---

[283] V.L.W. Go and W.H.J. Summerskill. "Digestion, Maldigestion, and the Gastrointestinal Hormones," *American Journal of Clinical Nutrition*, 1971; 24, pg. 160-167.

\* The nerve and electrical reflex points in the bowel wall short-circuit wherever the plaque accumulates. This alone can precipitate disease throughout the body.[284]

\* Some cleansers have reported feeling a sensation in lymph gland areas which they believed was lymph drainage, when certain sections of the intestines were freed of mucoid plaque[285]. Subsequently they also reported reduced or no congestion remaining in lymph glands, along with improved immune function. This has prompted me to theorize that there may be lymph drainage sites in the intestines which become blocked by mucoid plaque and toxic, causing lymphatic back-up. It follows that this may result in lymphatic disease, obesity, malnutrition, excessive toxicity, and thickening of the bowel wall.

\* The peristalsis slows[286] with the buildup of mucoid plaque. This can cause another chain reaction of negative events. As the time it takes for food to move through the alimentary canal increases, fecal matter becomes drier and then begins to contribute to the mucoid plaque. The birth of serious bowel pockets and diverticula begins. At this point people may develop excessive thickening and ballooning of the bowel.

---

[284] **See the Diagram on colon reflex points in Chapter 8: How to Determine If You Need A Cleansing Program.**

[285] The idea of lymph draining into the intestines contradicts the popularly held medical theory that lymph drains into the blood. However, there seems to be a significant level of experience among cleansers which would indicate that somehow the removal of mucoid plaque from certain areas of the intestines does facilitate the lymph draining, sometimes very dramatically and quickly. Hence an overweight person may lose 50 pounds or so in one week while cleansing, when certain areas of the intestines are freed of mucoid plaque. The weight is lost both in large amounts of mucoid plaque being expelled, and in copious quantities of urine. I believe this is because the lymph is finally able to release stored toxins and the excess liquid required to store them.

[286] Daily bowel movements: If you eat three meals daily, you should have four bowel movements daily. One first thing in the morning, and the other 15 to 45 minutes after each meal. Anything less than this is moving toward constipation. Anytime a person has less than two bowel movements daily, and they eat 3 meals, they are constipated and are moving towards disease. If they only go once a day, disease has already developed and is becoming serious. -Dr. Richard Anderson, N.D., N.M.D.

## Mucoid Plaque in the Small Intestine

Most nourishment is assimilated in the small intestine (which is composed of the duodenum, jejunum, and ileum), although some nourishment may be absorbed through the stomach and colon. The small intestine is called small, although it is actually six times longer than the large intestine, or colon. The small intestine is more than 22 feet long and is of greater importance when considering digestion, assimilation, and malnutrition, because mucoid plaque in the small intestines may block assimilation of nutrients as well as interfering with reflex points.[287] If mucoid plaque from the jejunum and ileum is eliminated[288], we know that the body's ability to assimilate food properly may have been impaired. We could have been eating the most perfect, organic foods, using digestive enzymes and chewing our food well, and still not have had good absorption.

# Pathogenic Bacteria

Along with the presence of the mucoid layers, there is generally an imbalance of intestinal flora (with the presence of various pathogenic bacteria which thrive in the mucoid plaque environment). These "bad" bacteria further impair digestive ability as they overrun the friendly bacteria needed to produce and assimilate various nutrients, as noted under "Impacts of an Impaired Digestive System." It is estimated that these toxic, undesirable bacteria are predominant in the greater part of the population of the United States. This is obvious when we realize that disease is so epidemic despite almost everyone in the Western World having taken antibiotics. This is because antibiotics devastate friendly bacteria as well as the troublesome bacteria targeted, and leave the body susceptible to anything that comes along. I am convinced that anybody who has disease has already lost his or her ideal bacterial profile. Pathogenic bacteria are known to cause the following:

### How Pathogenic Bacteria May Affect the Human Body

1. Interfere with digestion especially with carbohydrates and proteins.
2. Prevent absorption of B vitamins, amino acids, and especially vitamin B-12.
3. Cause pre-mature cell breakdown.

---

[287] **See the Chart on Reflex Points under "Colon Reflex Points" in Chapter 8: How to Determine if You Need a Cleansing Program.**

[288] **See Chapter 9: Facts About an Optimal Cleansing Program, under "Identifying the Origin of Mucoid Plaque."**

4. Weaken the liver and other organs.
5. Create free radicals which are a major cause of what is called old age.
6. Produce bizarre reactions.
7. Cause gas.
8. Contribute to the breakdown of our immune system.
9. Drain a person's energy.
10. Intensify pH imbalances which pave the way for further bowel disorders.

Some *E. coli* bacteria have been known to cause cancer in laboratory animals. Most people who have cancer never find out why. It is interesting to note that cancer among meat-eaters is more than 90% higher than among life-long vegetarians, and the primary sustenance of the bacillus coli is meat.

Other contributing factors to pathogenic bacteria overgrowth are overcooked foods and undigested proteins. Meat substitutes are high on the list of the primary detrimental foods for vegetarians. Vegetarians should beware of highly processed soy, rice and bean concoctions, which are often used as meat and dairy substitutes.

After cleansing away the causes of imbalances in intestinal flora, **it is imperative to replace the harmful bacteria with "friendly bacteria."**[289]  Once the entire gastrointestinal tract is cleansed of the mucoid matter, friendly flora is established and we are consistently eating foods that maintain that purity, we will begin to reap the benefits. Actually, just getting a little out has helped thousands of people enormously. We should always remember; the closer we stay to nature, the healthier we will be. Everything that is processed by man is unnatural to our bodies and will trigger imbalances in our bodies and minds.

---

[289] **See Chapter 9 under, "Friendly Bacteria Essential," and Chapter 14 under "Friendly Bacteria."**

# Toxicity in the Colon

When mucoid plaque becomes a chronic condition, stagnant pockets of over-acid toxic debris may settle and cause "bowel pockets", the perfect environment to nurture overgrowths of pathogenic bacteria, yeasts, parasites, etc. These bowel pockets are the thickened areas that some doctors describe in association with bowel cancer and diverticula.[290] Bowel pockets are also the pre-cursor to diverticulitis, a condition where the diverticula become infected and inflamed. Bowel pockets can accumulate to such a degree that the colon's circumference may expand to four or more times its normal size causing a ballooned bowel. This unnatural stretching of the bowel wall is one of the causes of "leaky bowel syndrome."

Toxins, poisons, and free radicals from the plaque itself, and from pathogenic bacteria and parasites living in and under the plaque, constantly seep into the bloodstream and lymph, settling in the weaker areas of the body, especially the liver, kidneys, and spleen. Once these eliminative organs become over-loaded with toxins, they become sluggish and are unable to perform their proper functions. Then the toxins overflow and can go into any weak area of the body. **This is why with any disease, especially chronic disease, the bowel needs to be cleansed and renewed.** Then the liver and kidneys should be cleansed and rejuvenated. For if these organs give way to the toxic overloads, disease develops. As Dr. Jensen has said many times, "The name of a disease depends upon where the poisons settle." Thus, from the same base cause, various diseases evolve.

**Even if one succeeds in strengthening the weak area or suppressing the symptom, the toxic flow from the bowel will find another area to settle.** This is what many drugs do. Some drugs merely deaden the sensitive nerves and some push toxins out of one area as they move to another area. In the meantime the doctor looks like a hero for the symptoms quickly disappeared. Not only that, but his practice is guaranteed another visit, for it will only be a matter of time and his patient will have some other symptom as soon as those toxins accumulate in another area. Now the patient not only has his original toxins to contend with, but the added the toxins from the drug also. As these areas of toxic settlement become more and more congested, the oxygen supply is gradually reduced, waste from the cells backs up and accumulates, nutrients have difficulty entering the cells, and the sodium/potassium ratios inside and outside the cell can reverse. Then cells become more acidic until finally they reach a chronic degenerative state and may mutate into cancer or other serious diseases.

---

[290] Whitehead, pg. 85, 432.

# Development of Bowel Disorders

Some people believe that most bowel diseases have similar causes, yet there are so many names for bowel diseases that it is totally amazing. There are about 33 different names for just polyps listed in Stedman's Medical Dictionary. Polyps are commonly eliminated by people who do the cleanse. They look like small pieces of popcorn kernels, they are usually off-white or yellow. After a few cleanses, they are no longer seen. As described earlier in various medical terms, a polyp is a general descriptive term used with reference to any mass of tissue that bulges or projects outward from the normal surface level. Polyps, often considered a precursor of adenocarcinoma, develop on an average at age 25 years and become symptomatic at age 33 years.[291] On an average, adenocarcinoma are usually present for about ten years before symptoms of rectal bleeding, diarrhea, mucus discharge and abdominal pain develop. The average age of diagnoses is 39 and **the mean survival time after diagnosis is three years.[292] The three years probably applies to those who are treated by M.D.'s. According to Dr. Jones of the University of Southern California at Berkeley, their survival time would probably have been about 12 years had they not been treated by conventional medicine.** However, had they been treated with proper diet, deep cleansing, effective antioxidants and other alternative procedures, I believe most of these people could get well.

## Early Signs

An early sign that bowel disease is developing is alternating constipation and diarrhea. Diarrhea is often constipation in disguise. Constipation is almost always associated with pathogenic microorganisms, and with mucoid plaque according to my research. When the growth of these unfriendly microorganisms reaches a level where they are attacking the epithelium, these cells respond by secreting massive amounts of mucus and liquids and this causes diarrhea.

Constipation is the slowing down of peristalsis. As peristalsis becomes more and more inhibited, the transit time of food through the alimentary canal becomes slower and slower. As it slows, food begins to rot and ferment, which often creates gas[293] before it can exit. (Lack of

---

[291] Whitehead, pg. 893.

[292] Ibid.

[293] Yamada, ed., pg. 1525.

sufficient enzymes can also cause gas.) If one fails to drink enough water, the stool loses moisture, causing it to become dry and sticky. The fecal matter then has a tendency to stick to the walls of the intestines, blending or amalgamating with the mucoid plaque and bowel pockets. This creates an even greater thickening of the mucoid plaque. When peristalsis slows it takes greater and greater pressure to move fecal matter through the system. When fecal matter backs up, the pressure may become so great that it causes bulges and other protrusions in the gut wall which are called diverticuli. Here the muscle wall is stretched into pockets, which are often filled with stagnate fecal matter containing pathogenic bacteria, etc. Diverticulitis is the condition that occurs when the diverticuli become inflamed.

# Development of a Diverticula
## Cross Section of Intestines

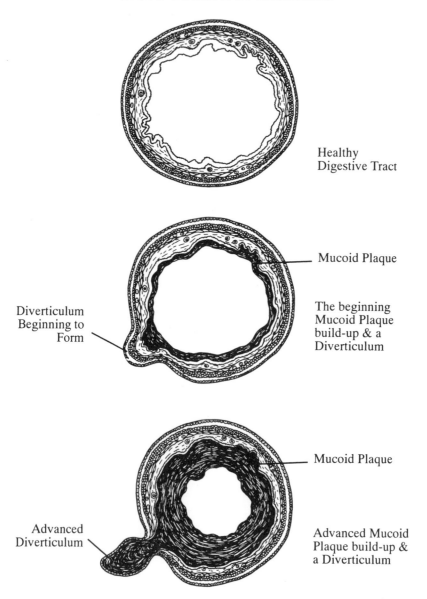

Healthy
Digestive Tract

Mucoid Plaque

Diverticulum
Beginning to
Form

The beginning
Mucoid Plaque
build-up & a
Diverticulum

Mucoid Plaque

Advanced
Diverticulum

Advanced Mucoid
Plaque build-up &
a Diverticulum

# Diverticulitis

Diverticulitis is becoming more common every day, because people's diets have become worse. It is estimated from autopsy studies that 30% of adults have diverticular disease and over 50% of those over 40.[294],[295] Diverticulitis is associated with a meat eaters diet and processed food. Before the 1920's, this disease was almost unknown. It is a twentieth century disease, as is heart disease, cancer, and most of the diseases people create. Dr. Bernard Jensen had a patient who had 113 diverticula.[296] The most common symptom of intestinal diverticulitis is a cramping pain usually in the lower left side of the abdomen, associated with nausea and fever. If ever one of these pockets should break, surgery may be necessary. Here is one situation where we can appreciate a surgeon.

It takes many years of bad habits to weaken the bowel enough to form diverticula. It is rare in parts of the world where dietary fiber intake is high (vegetarian). Science is still trying to determine the reason why vegetarians do not get diverticula. They like to think it is because of the high fiber in their diets, but admit that it could simply be because meat diets produce bowel disease.[297] Perhaps it's animal revenge. Diets low in fiber (such as meat and dairy diets, and diets high in processed foods) result in small stools that require high intra-colonic pressures for their propulsion in the colon. This high pressure leads to protrusion of the mucous membrane through the weak and toxic points in the colon's musculature at the sites where blood vessels enter the colon wall.[298] Diverticula [299] are common in the small intestine as well as the colon. Jejunal (upper small intestine) diverticula are usually asymptomatic, yet this may lead to malabsorption of vitamin B-12.[300] Often these diverticula protrusions are

---

[294] Whitehead, pg. 431.

[295] Berkow, pg. 813. (the Merck Manual)

[296] Jensen, *Iridology, The Science and Practice in the Healing Arts*, Volume 2, (Escondido, CA: Bernard Jensen, 1982), pg. 234.

[297] Whitehead, pg. 431.

[298] R. E. Pounder, M. C. Allison, A . P. Dhillon, *Color Atlas of the Digestive Tract*, (Chicago, IL: Year Book Medical Publisher, Inc., 1989), pg. 427.

[299] B. C. Morson, *Color Atlas of Gastrointestinal Pathology*,(London, England: Harvey Miller Publishers/W.B. Saunders Co., 1988), See pictures of diverticula from both the inside and outside, pg. 214.

[300] Pounder, Allison, and Dhillon, pg. 304.

at the entryway of blood vessels which means, of course, that toxic waste will more easily spill into the bloodstream.

As explained in the previous section on "Toxicity in the Colon," these conditions, as well as further bowel problems are a result of mucoid plaque, an acid bowel, electrolyte deficiencies, and other nutritional deficiencies. Use of antibiotics and vaccinations may also contribute. The combination creates the perfect environment for worms, parasites, and various types of destructive bacteria and yeast.[301]

# Candida - "Yeast"

It has been estimated that one third of the American people[302] now have Candidiasis. Candidiasis is common in all the Western industrialized countries, as well as every other country that has diet and medicines similar to those in America. It is very rare for anyone with Candidiasis to not have had antibiotics or vaccinations.[303] Even people with extremely over-acid

---

[301] Yeast problems are not usually caused by mucoid plaque. Yeast diseases usually occur after the use of antibiotics, which then alters the internal chemistry of the bowel. We can also create yeast by allowing filth to develop in the bowel.

[302] John Parks Trowbridge, M.D. and Morton Walker, D.P.M., *The Yeast Syndrome*, (Toronto, CAN: Bantam Books, 1988), pg. XVI.

[303] Vaccinations: In my opinion, there may be rare situations in which vaccines may have a place, such as in tetanus or snake bites, but even that I doubt. To vaccinate mass populations as they are doing is, in my opinion, total insanity. I believe that this is a direct action initiated by individuals who do not have any good intentions for the masses of mankind. Those behind this insidious affair are, in my opinion, connected to the dark forces, the sinister forces that cause so much pain and suffering in this world. If ever anyone doubted that a medical conspiracy against the Western populations exists, they should look into vaccines. It is the most treacherous method of perpetuating the disease industry. Forced vaccinations of innocent babies and children is one of the most vicious schemes the sinister forces have yet devised. Vaccines are nothing but experiments. Many thousands of children have died and many more thousands have been severely damaged for life because of vaccines. Who is to know what the long-term effect will be upon future generations? These experiments are often deadly. See Allen, *Don't Get Stuck!* and *The Case Against Vaccinations and Injections*, (a quote from William Koch, Ph.D., M.D.) pg. 148.
　　As I said before, things are covered up. Hundreds of thousands of innocent people have been murdered and many more have been needlessly crippled and deformed by vaccines. Not only is this

conditions usually do not get Candidiasis unless they have had antibiotics at some time.

The reason that antibiotics cause Candida, is simply that antibiotics destroy most of the friendly bacteria in the bowels. When we lose the friendly bacteria in our intestines, then Candida can flourish. First it begins in the bowel, then if leaky bowel syndrome is present, it can travel into other parts of the body that are not strong enough to resist its infiltration. Candida is basically a living, fungal parasite that releases very toxic waste which can get into the bloodstream and cause various symptoms. The most common are fatigue, depression, brain fog, and poor memory. **It also helps further drain our electrolytes**. Other common symptoms are yeast vaginitis, oral thrush, diaper-rash, other rashes, menstrual cramps, chronic diarrhea, all types of infections, asthma, headaches, bloating, impotence, prostatitis, bad breath, burning eyes or failing vision, pain in the ears, etc. etc. The list is endless.

The really bad part of this disease is that it gradually weakens the whole body, especially the immune system. It then opens the way for all sorts of other diseases. Candidiasis is one of the main conditions that is strongly associated with AIDS development.[304] Though antibiotics are the primary trigger, successful Candida overgrowth requires weakened digestive and immune systems, a toxic body, and usually emotional suppression. It seems to be associated with unconscious feelings of rejection and unresolved relationships; feelings that are based upon an underlying destructive point of view.

### Causes of Candidiasis and Other Microflora Imbalances

| Doctor-Caused (Iatrogenic) | Self-Caused |
| --- | --- |
| Antibiotics | Poor diet |
| Steroids | Electrolyte deficiency |
| Vaccines | Long-term depression |
| Oral contraceptives | Mercury amalgam "silver" |
| Gastric operations | fillings |
| X-rays, irradiation of abdomen | |

Many, many pathogenic bacteria, yeasts, fungi, and other rather nasty critters live in our bodies all the time. As long as all systems,

---

concealed from the public, but those in power do not even inform their own doctors. It is kept quiet.

[304] Anthony James Degidio, D.O., M.D., *Everything You Need to Know About AIDS*, (Burlingame, CA: New Additions Publishing, 1994), pg. 11 and 29.

especially our digestive and immune systems, are functioning properly, these pathogens are kept in check, but when our internal environment becomes more and more polluted, the liver, digestive system, immune system, and other organs and glands lose their efficiency. Then toxins build up and these microorganisms begin to proliferate. A good example of what happens is how Candida albicans grows into Candidiasis. If you have developed Candida, you may want to consider using supplements of friendly bacteria which can aid in overcoming Candida.[305]

Candida albicans is a yeast, but as our internal environment changes, this yeast biologically transmutes into a fungus. In this form, it produces long, root-like structures that penetrate the mucosa lining of the intestinal wall. This penetration can weaken the epithelium creating "leaky bowel syndrome".[306]

# Leaky Bowel Syndrome

Some doctors believe that the "Leaky Gut Syndrome" is almost always associated with auto-immune disease and that repairing the gut lining is essential in order to reverse auto-immune disorders.[307] When undigested protein molecules are assimilated into the bloodstream, the immune system produces antibodies against these protein molecules, for it views them as foreign particles. When this happens people become sensitive to the foods and drinks they consume. In this process, the body begins to attack these foreign invaders. The sensitivity problem occurs because the antigenic sites of these foods and other protein substances are similar to our own physiological tissues. This means that in some people, the body's own antigens fail to recognize the difference and attack the body itself, as well as the particles that pass through the leaky gut.

The entry of these incomplete proteins and other undigested foods, various bacteria, parasites, particles etc. into the bloodstream causes a severe overload of the immune system as well as intense toxicity. These people will experience feeling good one minute and in a few moments feel poorly. In particular, those who feel bad after eating may have leaky bowel syndrome. (Remember, I said that most people with AIDS have Candida

---

[305] See Chapter 9: Facts About An Optimal Cleansing Program, under "Cleansing and Candida," and Chapter 12: Rebuilding Vital Organs, under "Using the Two Probiotic Formulas to Fight Candida and Pathogenic Organisms."

[306] Yamada, pg.1525.

[307] From the web page of Dr. Zoltan P. Rona M.D., M.Sc.

albicans first.) As these conditions advance, all sorts of problems can occur in various combinations and intensities. Common ones are various types of allergies, digestive problems, muscle weakness, skin problems, memory loss, chest pains, joint pains, fingernail problems, depression, mood swings, and feeling spacey and unable to concentrate.

## Causes of Leaky Bowel Syndrome

| | |
|---|---|
| Alcohol | Bile acids |
| Changes in bowel caused by antibiotics | Constipation |
| Dairy products | Eating foods we are allergic to |
| Fried foods and other acids in bowel | Parasites |
| Pathogenic bacteria | Processed foods |

Too much consumption of acid-forming foods, meat, wheat products Safflower, corn, and sunflower oil.[308] These oils cause irritation to the intestinal wall, which in time weakens the villi and microvilli.

## Common Conditions Associated with Leaky Bowel Syndrome

| | | |
|---|---|---|
| Brain fog | Candida albicans | Chronic fatigue |
| Extreme energy shifts | Environmental sensitivity | General toxicity |
| Hay-fever | Headaches | Indigestion |
| Irritable bowel syndrome | Memory problems | Mood changes |
| Pains throughout the body | Sensitivity to foods | |

## Other Diseases Associated with Leaky Bowel Syndrome:

| | | |
|---|---|---|
| Acute gastroenteritis | After use of antibiotics | Allergies |
| Alopecia areata | Any bowel diseases | Atopy |
| Back pains | Bacterial infections | Blood in stool |
| Bowel Cancer | Calcium problems | Chest pains |
| Chronic fatigue syndrome | Colitis | Concentration problems |
| Consistent heartburn | Crohn's disease | Cystic fibrosis |
| Depression | Diabetes | Diarrhea |
| Digestive problems | Exocrine pancreatic defects | Fibromyalgia |
| Fingernail problems | Food sensitivities | Gastroenteritis |
| Joint pains | Iron deficiency | Kidney trouble |
| Liver problems | Lupus Erythmatosis | Memory loss |
| Mood swings | Multiple sclerosis | Muscle weakness |

---

[308] Yamada, pg. 1895.

| Pain in eyes | Pancreatic problems | Polymyalgia rheumatica |
| Raynaud's disease | Rheumatoid arthritis | Sjogren's syndrome |
| Skin problems | Spleen problems | Thyroiditis |
| Unusual gas | Urticaria (hives) | Vasculitis |
| Vitiligo | | |

These are just a few of the many symptoms. It gets more serious when we realize that in this process, the immune system is getting weaker, and other organs such as the liver, spleen, kidneys, brain, heart, and glands are becoming weaker, by the minute. It is no wonder that Candidiasis, especially with leaky gut syndrome, is considered a forerunner of many diseases. Directly, it is associated with bronchitis, asthma, chronic infections, depression, gastritis, colitis, allergies,[309] and AIDS.[310]

Those with leaky bowel syndrome will need to embrace a program to rebuild the bowel wall.[311]

## Parasites: A Widespread Problem

It is an illusion to think that Americans are free of parasites. *Foundations Of Parasitology* (1989) a medical textbook, reported that **more than 55 million American children are infected with worms and that this is a gross underestimation if one includes parasites such as pinworms.** This textbook reported that a doctor in Amherst, Massachusetts, claimed that over the years of his practice, he had treated virtually every major parasitic disease of humans. That would include foreign or tropical parasites. More than one quarter of all the annual deaths in the world, are children who suffered from parasites which caused malnutrition and intestinal infection. On a world-wide basis, worms outrank cancer as man's deadliest enemy. In fact, the World Health Organization has named parasitic disease among the six most harmful infectious diseases in humans.

Some common worms such as *Ascaris* roundworms lay more than 200,000 eggs a day. *Ascaris* can perforate the bowel wall and cause intestinal obstruction if present in large enough numbers. They are fairly common in the Western World and can dramatically compete with the host's nutritional needs. In some malnourished children, *Ascaris* were

---

[309] Trowbridge, M.D., Walker, D.P.M., pg. XVII and page 12.

[310] Degidio, pg. 11 and 29.

[311] **See Chapter 12: Rebuilding Vital Organs under "The Bowel."**

present in such large numbers that they reached as much as 10% of the child's body weight. They can also invade other organs.[312]

In Brazil one parasite disease called *American Trypanosomiasis* causes 30% of adult deaths. Relative to other countries, it was thought that North Americans suffered little from parasite diseases because of our "good health," "good nutrition," climate, and sanitation. Climate, yes. Sanitation, yes. But the fact that we are one of the sickest nations in the world reflects poor nutrition. Increasingly poor eating habits are beginning to catch up with each new generation. Parasite diseases in America have increased significantly just in the last two decades. Parasite epidemics have occurred in New York, Colorado, Washington, and New Hampshire, with serious outbreaks in other states.

By definition, a parasite is an organism that injures its host to some degree. The common definition of a parasite is **an organism that lives on or in another, draws its nourishment therefrom and often injures its host** Some parasites can coat the inside lining of the small intestine and prevent the lining from absorbing nutrients in food. They can also cause severe constipation by blocking or plugging the alimentary canal. Some parasites, such as *F. Buski,* produce severe damage to the intestinal wall by their powerful suckers. As noted, *Ascaris* attacks and may block the bowel, causing malnutrition in the host; it may also invade the bile duct, appendix, and other organs. Many parasites damage their host by devouring essential substances that the host needs. The hookworm for an example, sucks blood and deprives the host of more iron than is replaced by diet. This causes anemia. Hookworms lay 5,000 - 10,000 eggs a day and can live for about fourteen years. The broad fish tapeworm selectively removes vitamin B-12 from the alimentary tract and produces megaloblastic anemia. *E. Histolytica* erodes the intestinal wall by excreting a proteolytic enzyme. This is a very common method of internal destruction by parasites.

There is good evidence that parasites and worms thrive in mucoid layers. They may even feed on it. **Parasites protect themselves from most vermifuges (de-worming measures) by burying themselves inside or underneath the impacted mucoid layers.** There they remain, happily nestled in their perfect habitat, until the mucoid fecal layers are removed once and for all, the bowel pH returned to normal, the intestinal mucosa normalized, and the correct bacteria rule the intestinal lumen.[313] The diet

---

[312] D.B. Jelliffe, "Ascaris Lubricoides and Malnutrition in Young Children," *Documenta de Medicina Geographica et Tropica,* 1953; 5, pg. 314.

[313] Lumen - the hollow part of an organ. *Stedman's Medical Dictionary.*

must be cleaned up, for **parasites thrive upon undigested proteins, carbohydrates and processed foods.**

## Experiences with Parasites

Years ago I suspected that I might have a tapeworm and who knows what else. After much cleansing of my intestinal tract I tried several herbal formulas to kill and extract the little buggers, including black walnut, an herbal formula, garlic, and pumpkin seeds. I went on several weeks, off two weeks, and back on again to get the eggs. It didn't do a thing. Later, Dr. Jensen told us that the only truly effective means he knew of to kill worms was to eat nothing but raw onions and garlic for three days and take a strong herbal laxative (overdose) the last night. The next morning, when it was time for a bowel movement, we were to sit in warm milk. As strange as this sounds, worms *love* warm milk. The theory is that the weakened worms will end up in the colon after fleeing from the raw onion and garlic, but scurry back up when feeling the cold air at the anus. If they sense the warm milk instead, they will go for it.

Since I never recommended anything I hadn't tried, a friend and I took off to the mountains. We went through three days of agony, eating nothing but raw onions and garlic, and on the last day, even sat in the warm milk at the crucial moment. The last part was the most hilarious moment of my life-but that shall remain confidential. The only thing that came out was a one-inch hookworm. Although this procedure is an effective method for treating some parasitic infections, I have definitely found a better way to do it. Anyone who suspects they may have parasites may call my office for information on the herbal products I have available to overcome parasites.

Several years ago, I was in Tucson. A friend, my wife (at that time), and I were all on the Cleanse but experimenting with what became the phase of cleansing that involves taking one meal a day with herbs and shakes. At this time I felt I was about 90% cleaned out. About the only part of my digestive system that was not completely free of mucoid matter was the stomach and maybe a few other spots here and there (where I had stuck emotions). I was certain of this because I still had an apparent hydrochloric acid deficiency and a spot of mucus still remained on my tongue. We were on our fourth day of cleansing. I had just finished taking a psyllium shake. I suddenly gulped for air. I doubled over and grabbed by stomach. For about 20 minutes I had to hold my stomach and found that I couldn't stand up straight. I felt like something was trying to turn my stomach inside-out. It wasn't really painful, but was a very weird feeling. Then just as suddenly as it had come, it disappeared and never returned. The next morning I passed a tapeworm about four feet long. And the morning after that, I passed either another one or a piece of the previous one that was about a foot long. Once we start cleansing seriously, we need to be aware that such an experience may happen. We should be thankful if it does.

Junk foods overwork the stomach, pancreas, kidneys, liver, heart, thyroid, and more. They severely strain the body's immune system. By junk foods, I mean foods made with white flour, sugar, salted foods, processed cereals and all other "foods", that are unnatural to a truly healthy body. These so-called foods produce the ideal breeding ground for parasites.

Several years ago, two doctors came to see me. One was very thin and sickly. He told me his story about how a few years ago, he was a vibrant healthy person and had a good medical practice. He went out of the country on vacation and about three weeks after his return his health began to decline. A year or so later, he had to quit working and concentrate on taking care of himself. He ended up going all over the U.S. trying to get help from various doctors. Several times he almost died. After almost an hour of telling me all this problems, I began to say to myself; "It sounds like *Entamoeba histolytica*." Finally, I asked; "Were you ever checked for parasites?" He replied; "I can't tell you how many times I asked the doctors to check me for parasites, but they all said that it can't be parasites. Then, about a week ago, I went to a parasite specialist in Phoenix. He found that I had *Entamoeba histolytica*. This is not an unusual situation. Many people have died from parasites, and their doctors never even thought to look into it.

## Where Parasites Live

Parasites can live anywhere in the body; be it intestines, lungs, liver, lymph glands, heart, prostate, bile ducts, skin, appendix, muscles, brain, or any organ. One autopsy revealed five tapeworms in a woman's head. I know of a doctor who was examining a patient's eye with a microscope and saw a tiny worm crawl from one part of the eye to the other side and disappear under the eyelid. **Parasites may be microscopic in size or as long as 30 feet (or longer). Parasite disease symptoms mimic many other diseases, thereby avoiding easy diagnosis.** Most parasites are not deadly, but they can cause a lot of trouble. If they cause damage to the nerves in the head or spine, symptoms can occur anywhere in the body - from one end to the other. Similarly, if worms are in the intestinal tract, they can, by their toxic secretions or by reflex disturbance, cause problems in the heart, liver, kidneys, brain, etc.

## Conventional Medicine on Parasites

Similar to their long-held position on Candida (that it did not exist and those who treated it naturally were quacks!) practitioners of conventional medicine do not recognize the abundance of parasites in the American people and they have not thoroughly investigated what parasite invasion can do throughout the body. Most doctors do not effectively test for parasites. **Current stool or blood tests are not effective.** These tests work only by chance. For, as noted previously, parasites can hide beneath mucoid plaque. **In order to accurately test for parasites in the bowel, it is essential to take a sample from inside the rectum, by gently scraping the plaque, which the doctor will think is normal mucosa, and testing that sample.** This method of testing should reveal any parasites and eggs that are present. Conventional medical treatments sometimes work very well, and other times not at all. They are often dangerous, and can have horrendous side effects.

## A Partial List of Parasite Disease Symptoms

| | | |
|---|---|---|
| Abdominal pain | Abscess near lymphatics | Acute muscle inflammation |
| Acute, chronic constipation | Anemia | Anorexia |
| Appendicitis | Ascites | Asthma, bronchial attacks |
| B-12 deficiency | Bleeding rectum | Blindness |
| Blood in feces | Bloody spit | Blurry vision |
| Burning urination | Burping | Calabar swellings |
| Central nervous system impairment | Cerebral calcifications | Chagoma on head, neck, abdomen |
| Chest pains | Chills | Chyluria |
| Colitis | Coma | Conjunctivitis |
| Constipation | Convulsions | Coughing |
| Dermatitis | Diarrhea | Digestive disturbance |
| Disfigurement | Dizziness | Dysentery |
| Edema | Elephantiasis | Eosinophilia |
| Epididymitis | Fevers | Funiculitis |
| Headaches | Hematuria | Hemoglobinuria |
| Hepatitis | Hepatomegaly | Hives |
| Hyperpigmentation | Intestinal obstruction | Irritability |
| Itching | Jaundice | Joint pain |
| Leukocytosis | Leukopenia | Loss of sleep |
| Lung/ bronchial congestion | Lymphangitis | Lymphocytosis |
| Malaria-like chills/ fevers | Malnutrition | Melena |
| Muscle pain/spasms | Myocarditis | Myositis |
| Nausea | Neurologic symptoms | Night sweating |
| Nodules | Peritonitis | Pica |
| Pneumonitis | Proteinuria | Pruritus ani |
| Pulmonary symptoms | Rashes | Rectal prolapse |
| Retinochoroiditis | Shock | Shortness of breath |
| Skin ulcers | Steatorrhea (fat in stools) | Sweating |
| Swelling of eyes, face, etc. | Tachycardia (fast pulse) | |

| Typhoid fever symptoms | Ulcers, cutaneous | Urethritis |
| Vomiting | Weak immunity | Weakness |
| Weight gain | Weight loss | |

Vaginitis - vaginal inflammation with yellow, frothy foul-smelling discharges

Enlargement and malfunction of organs such as liver, spleen, lymph nodes, heart, gall bladder, etc.

You may be asking **how clean-living persons could possibly become infested with parasites**. They can't really. They have to first have weakened themselves to a significant degree, or they would be immune to any kind of infection from an outside source. So, for the typical average person, the most common source in America **is eating** insufficiently-cooked pork, beef, fish or any other creatures that have eyeballs, legs, fins, or pinchers (yes, that includes crab, lobster and all other shellfish). For the **eggs of parasites are extremely tough and can resist a great deal of heat and freezing. In addition, touching infected dogs, cats, and other animals** is a very common method of picking up parasite eggs or sometimes parasites themselves.

## Common Methods of Parasite Infection

- Drinking infected water
- Being bitten by flies, mosquitoes, and animals (usually in the tropics)
- Contacting filthy environments or infected animals by breathing or touching (remember, just like cockroaches, parasites thrive in a filthy environment)
- Eating foods grown in infected soil, especially soil which has been fertilized with animal dung (pig dung is particularly contagious)
- Eating unclean, raw vegetation, grown with infected animal fertilizer
- Walking barefoot on infected soil
- The body develops them through the pleomorphic process of somatid mutation

Once parasites are in the body, the only sure way to get them out is to get rid of their environment of filth, for that is where they live and that is their food - filth. Have you ever seen flies in a clean garbage can? Take away their environment and take away their food, and they will go away with the help of herbal vermifuges. Remember the promise and take heart: "Cleanse and purify thyself and I will exalt thee to the throne of power!" What do you think the throne of power is? The porcelain throne in the bathroom, of course! That's how you get your power - sitting on the throne; you poop enough of the right stuff, and you'll be powerful![314] In most cases, cleansing is the first step that should be

---

[314] **See Chapter 12: Rebuilding Vital Organs: Essential Cleanse Follow-Up, under "Eliminate Parasites."**

taken to remove parasites. This should be followed with parasite specific remedies. However, in some cases of severe infestation, cleansing may cause such rapid parasite die-off that the cleanser becomes too ill from the resulting flood of toxins to proceed. In these situations, a qualified practitioner, familiar with an ideal cleanse program, should be enlisted for guidance and support, and parasite specific remedies may need to be used before the cleanse can be accomplished.

## Advanced Bowel Disorders

Unfriendly bacteria, fungus and parasites, all produce highly toxic acids as waste products. These then compound the over-acidity due to poor diet and stress, and weaken the intestinal wall severely. In some persons, the body may become so compromised that it may even become unable to continue forming the protective mucoid plaque barrier. This extreme acidity may then begin to eat away portions of the plaque itself, as well as underlying tissues. This may lead to such severe conditions as IBS, ulcerative-colitis, and perhaps may even trigger the further development of extremely tough plastic-like polyps, cysts, growths and even tumors, as a distorted, last-ditch attempt to protect those areas where the plaque has failed.[315]

However in many cases the plaque simply continues to build up. And as the mucoid plaque [316] becomes jammed with fecal matter, its thickness is further increased. One autopsy revealed an extreme case; **a colon twelve inches in diameter was packed with layer upon layer of encrusted mucoid fecal material, leaving a tiny one-fourth inch opening.**[317] What's your waistline? If it's larger than you know it should be, keep reading. Another autopsy exposed a colon so packed with mucoid substance that it weighed 40 pounds! A healthy colon should weigh four to six pounds. **Increased weight of the transverse colon weakens its structure and causes prolapsus, which in turn puts pressure upon the lower organs and weakens them.** This can create problems in the

---

[315] **See Chapter 3: Mucoid Plaque, under "When Mucoid Plaque Fails," as well as, "Mucoid Plaque and Cancer," and "Mucoid Plaque Mutates!"**

[316] Pounder, Allison, and Dhillon, plate #439. Their comment, "a particularly bizarre stool, from a young woman with irritable bowel syndrome". This picture is similar to many specimens expelled by those who are cleansing.

[317] Jensen, *Tissue Cleansing Through Bowel Management*, pg. 43.

ovaries, uterus, and other female problems, as well as prostate and bladder problems.

Colitis, diverticulitis, cancer of the bowel and candida are becoming as common as Coca Cola. If toxicity is not removed from the bowel, the body fights a losing battle with these and other diseases. The other organs meant to eliminate toxins, the liver, kidneys, lungs and skin then become clogged and sluggish, and eventually the immune system will become extremely challenged; the enzymes will become ineffective, and the body will begin to deteriorate at an ever-accelerating rate. As the years go by, these conditions only get worse, unless something is done about it.

Removing mucoid plaque while providing the alkalizing minerals the body needs to eliminate over-acidity and toxins is likely to be beneficial to any body that has developed bowel disease. Anyone with bowel disease is encouraged to first read this book, then begin the most gentle phase of an ideal cleanse program, *following the instructions carefully*. An attending, qualified health practitioner who is familiar with your condition and with cleansing, and preferably this program, should work with you to monitor your condition and progress as you cleanse, and to assist you with any problems that could arise. It is very important to take the program slowly until your body is strong enough to handle faster and deeper cleansing.[318]

---

[318] **See Chapter 12 under "The Bowel."**

# Chapter 7

# WHY CLEANSE?
# THE GOAL AND BENEFITS

**LOVE**
is the happiest and most fun thing in the universe.

**LOVE**
flows naturally when we have removed the resistance to it.

**JOY AND HAPPINESS**
are the natural by-products of Love.

## Cultivate Love and Joy for Healing

Love and joy, can be cultivated to such a degree that not only can they heal our own bodies, but they also can heal those with whom we come in contact. Those who Love enough never want for anything. It does not matter whether you are a saint, a devil, or in between! **To cultivate the power of Love is the wisest venture anyone can ever initiate. For nothing, absolutely nothing in all the universe will bring greater benefits and happiness.**

Happiness is a form of Love. People seek relationships because of the feelings of happiness they desire. People seek better jobs, homes, wealth, power, etc., because they think that these "things" will make them happier. In fact, the primary purpose of every effort people make is based upon trying to be happier. **And there is nothing wrong in trying to be happier, it seems to be an innate urge within all of us. But, there is a secret to being happy and about 99% of us have missed it.**

A little logic will make this clear. **The feeling of happiness everyone enjoys now and then, comes from within and never from without.** If you acquire something that you have longed for, for a long time you will feel happy in acquiring it. But this feeling is nothing but a point of view based entirely upon the programming you created for yourself. Let's say that you created a point of view that once you have that car you feel you need and desire, then you will be happy. You achieve the goal and you are happy. It was a programming that allowed our mental sentinel, our point of view, permission to be happy when the goal was achieved. We can create another point of view to make us just as happy and even more so by another programming. **If we are wise, we will develop a point of view that allows us to be happy for no reason at all.** Simply because we want to be.

**The advantage to this is we are never dependent upon other people, places, conditions, or things to make us happy, for none of these "things" are permanent.** Not only that, but we have little control over "things". Things break, wear out, die, change, or are not available. **To place the condition of our happiness on "things" is foolish, unwise, unhealthy, and actually childish.** Especially when we realize that there is only one thing that will always bring us happiness and that is our choice to be that way. It is nothing more than developing the right point of view. In the words of Maxwell Maltz, M.D., author of Psychocybernetics: **"Men are disturbed, not by the things that happen, but by their opinion of the things that happen."**

Many doctors have realized that almost all disease is based upon negative thinking and the stress negative thinking creates. All these stresses were activated by disappointment, fear, anger, resentments, etc., etc. **Of these emotions, every single one is entirely dependent upon certain points of view.** And every one of these situations were based upon, sorry to say, a childish point of view; we didn't get what we wanted or reacted negatively because of what happened to us.

**We cannot always control the events in our lives, but we have full freedom to control how we will respond, or feel about what happens to us.** I look back in my life and see what caused the suffering I experienced and I can say that all of it was based upon my childish points of view. When I was pushed around and beaten, criticized, yelled at, had things taken from me, no food to eat, was cold, wet, hungry, etc., oh how I wish that I had had the point of view that would have allowed me to remain calm and happy inside in spite of the abuse I was experiencing. Had I been able to accomplish that back then, I would not have suffered the heart, liver, kidney, eye pain, head and ear problems, financial difficulties, etc., that I have had to handle. **When I look back, I am tempted to stand up and kick myself in the butt for the foolish mistakes I've made. But, instead I rejoice that I have finally learned that I can be happy no matter what the circumstances.** Yes, it is a challenge - the greatest challenge I have ever had. But I have made progress. I have allowed the past momentum of my negative energy to work its way out and I am finally beginning to feel the freedom I've craved.

**When we realize that "things" do not bring us happiness and that happiness is nothing but a point of view which is a result of our programming, we take an important step in gaining control over our lives, and that includes our health.** With a little thought we can easily conclude that: 1.) Happiness is based upon a certain point of view - always!, and 2.) To achieve the highest happiness is to cultivate the wisest point of view that opens us up to unconditional love for everyone and everything. **Why be satisfied with anything else?** All the negativity we have ever created was really based upon a distorted point of view that interfered with our opportunity to feel love. **Negative feelings are points of view that are tainted with the acid of selfishness.** Instead of settling for a distorted alloy, why not go for the uncontaminated gold itself - love! **The goal therefore, is to achieve unconditional Love for everybody and everything and then, to amplify it continuously.**

Imagine a most precious and valuable jewel sought after by everyone in the Universe. It is capable of healing our bodies, greatly increasing our wisdom and intelligence, solving all our problems, and giving us unending happiness and joy. Wouldn't you do everything in your power to obtain such a jewel? The truth is, the kind of love that I have been talking about will accomplish all the above. It is something that is within the reach of everybody. **There is a way to activate it, nourish it, and help it grow.** As I said in the first chapter, love is the cohesive power of the universe and it is everywhere. **The great key is to open and allow it to flow through us. It is not something that we have to create. It is already created.** All we need to do is become the vessel for its flow. **One of the other keys in achieving this goal is to remove all the interference that would block it.** Yes, the poison of negative thoughts and feelings, long suppressed, must be released, and replaced with love. Our attitudes and beliefs that interfere with the natural flow of Love, joy, happiness, health, and abundance, must be released. This release brings us into incredible potential for assisting the well-being of our own selves as well as others, and assisting others is fun and infinitely rewarding.

The resistance to Love, health, prosperity, and achieving our goals is the momentum of our own negative feelings, as well as those we accept from others. **Our negative feelings are the kinks that produce every undesirable experience that we have ever had or ever will have in our lives. Indeed, we reap what we sow.** There are very few exceptions to this. Therefore, the following four steps will benefit each of us tremendously:

1. If you do want this kind of love, ask the highest part of yourself - ask that which you know as God to help you achieve it.
2. Stop creating negative thoughts and feelings, and do not feel guilty when you slip up.
3. Do not deny negative feelings that arise, but ask God to help you release forever the cause and the effects. Cleanse the guts.
4. Practice Love for everybody and everything in every situation.
5. Practice being non-judgmental.

If we truly want abiding happiness, these things should be considered the most important work in our lives.

Though achieving these goals is extremely difficult and requires tremendous effort and determination, it is worth every effort. Only in this way are we assured of perfect health, perfect wealth, and unending happiness. Isn't that what we all want? Happiness? All the struggle and pain that everyone goes through is nothing more than each person's way of striving for happiness. Unfortunately, most people's efforts are distorted, bringing pain rather than joy. I know a man who sincerely made the following statement. "I'm my happiest when I'm my unhappiest." I was stunned when I heard him speak those words because I intuitively knew that it was true for him. This man was so numbed out from this previous programming that the only feelings he could feel were extreme negativity, and that gave him some kind of sensation. The problem is that most people do not understand the laws of the Universe and of Nature and therefore are like a man who doesn't understand the law of gravity and is standing on top of Yosemite Falls. Two thousand feet down and he stands on the edge looking down and has no concept of what will happen if he steps over the edge. **People need to understand the laws and use them wisely**. We all use them, but unwisely. **The creation of negative thinking through distorted judgment is utilizing the laws of our being unwisely**.

Negative feelings sooner or later seep into our energy fields that sustain physical function. **The more negative energy, the more interference with cell function**. When qualified by our misguided thinking and the resulting negative emotions, this energy is **capable of distorting DNA, and attracts toxicity or malformations**. This is why emotions can produce such profound physiological changes so rapidly. Negative consciousness actually becomes part of our cells. Many times when we are going through emotional stress, those feelings have already become stuck within our cell structure. We can go through all the psychological maneuvers that therapists have to offer and never fully rid ourselves of these "stuck emotions" because they have become part of the physical body. However, **by cleansing the body and mentally holding on to the new patterns we desire, we can eventually remove these toxic emotions - forever**.

It is imperative to do both - cleanse the body and practice maintaining a positive mental pattern, along with positive feeling. Cells are replaced fairly rapidly. Through cleansing and fasting, we can release unneeded cells extremely rapidly. But here is a very important point missed by most therapists. **Even though we can replace old cells rapidly, negative consciousness from the old cells can become attached to the new cells and take on the same qualities**. Therefore, it is essential to steadily hold the new pattern of what we want to be.

It is this concept which gives us the key to overcoming the aging process. Some scientists have questioned: 'Can we make the cell immortal?' But why bother? Our bodies make new cells every few weeks, days and even hours. So the question among scientists is: 'How is it that the slow deterioration of old age occurs with almost everyone?' **For more than 90% of the human body is completely renewed in less than a year.**

The answer is, **our new cells take on the negative consciousness which was attached to the old cells,** and then take on even more negativity through our increasingly distorted judgments. In this way, we literally suffocate in our own negativity.

I spent more than 10 years doing a research project to determine if physical immortality was a fact or fiction. I concluded it to be a fact. The forces that control society do everything they can to prevent people from knowing this. **Even the Christian churches worship One who taught this and yet the churches deny its possibility.** Indeed, following are the words of Jesus Christ, **"Verily, verily, I say unto you, if a man keep my saying, he shall never see death."**[319] And Paul's statement confirms; **"The last enemy to overcome is death."** These were not idle words, but words of encouragement for those who had the wisdom of understanding, the desire, determination, and persistence to know the truth.

## The Secret of Removing Negative Consciousness

The point is: **there are ways to release negative consciousness by removing the old cells which contain the negativity.** We do this by **maintaining the positive consciousness during the cleansing process and allowing the old negative consciousness to be released without judgment.**[320] **For it is the judgment that binds it to the new cells.**

There are many methods that help people get in control of their emotions and thought patterns. Anything that will help us do this is good. However, there is a problem with most of the psychological methods available today. The methods that are successful are usually successful because they help create new patterns. There is nothing wrong with that except that just creating new patterns does nothing to rid us of the old negative ones. To sweep dirt under the rug may hide it from view, but it is still capable of fermenting and breeding all sorts of undesirable results.

---

[319] The Holy Bible, John 8:51, 1 Corinthians 15: 26

[320] There is much that needs to be said here, but it goes beyond the scope of this book.

If we want to be free of all the self-created pain and undesirable experiences in life, we must cleanse and purify every aspect of our bodies and minds and fill our beings with pure Love, Joy, and Harmony. Jesus' story about not putting new wine into old wineskins is an excellent truth. We must clean out by the roots and not just cover up and suppress things with something better. Cleansing the entire body at every level is essential; and beginning with the guts is one of the most powerful tools for accomplishing this that has ever been created. Yet it is only a tool; there is much more that can be done. Chapter 10: Optimize Your Cleanse covers this in more detail. I only bring this subject up because those who do a full program are going to experience these things in a real manner. Cleansers will find emotions surfacing and they will feel them, they also will find some old feelings disappearing forever.

Cleansing the entire digestive tract, when done properly, can have benefits that go far beyond the physical level. This is why the second most common testimony we receive from those who do this program is, "I feel closer to God". The reason they do is because they have removed so much toxicity from their beings and to a degree, purified their emotions. This allows the essence of the Universe to flow more. With no effort on their part, except to have cleansed, they feel significantly more Love. Even then, it is only a small portion of the great potential which awaits. (The first most common testimony we receive is that people have more energy.)

# The Mystery of Aging

## Science and Religion
## Two views: A Shared Reality

We live in a very materialistic society. Basically, there are two influencing extremes in our society: gross materialism and gross religiosity. The first blindly cancels out the possibility of the spiritual side of life and accepts only that which can be seen, touched, or measured as truth. The other blindly accepts the spiritual side, without examination or experience, and bases all recognition of truth upon certain opinions and writings. Both view the other as extremist.

To me, both sides have much to offer. Leaving out the spiritual aspect of science, inhibits accurate investigation and blocks truth. And conversely, leaving out logical, careful examination and facts, the religious side becomes lost in superstition, tradition, and dogma. Each side is constantly trying to prove things that cannot be proved without the whole. It is like trying to build a boat with only one substance. Just try and build a boat with only wood and no screws, glue, paint, etc. Certainly wouldn't be a boat that I would trust.

Throughout the ages, there have always been a few people who functioned in balance - between the two extremes. They were able to verify the reality of both sides and they accomplished many things that neither side alone was able to accomplish. They learned to know, to do, and for their own protection, to remain silent.

One evening I was having dinner with an electrical engineer who was up to date on the latest scientific research in physics. He was explaining a remarkable event that began in 1895. Annie Besant and Charles W. Leadbeater had developed extraordinary abilities in clairvoyant research. In 1895 they conducted research into chemical elements which included the structure of the atom. My friend explained that the book these two people published in 1919,[321] **revealed various aspects of the atom that have only recently been discovered by science**. I draw several conclusions from this: 1) At least some human beings have extraordinary untapped potential that can be developed. 2) There are far better methods to study science than by killing millions of innocent animals through experimentation. 3) There are those who know more about some scientific concepts than scientists.

## DNA (Deoxyribonucleic acid) and Aging

DNA may be a major link in the scientific discovery of man's greater potential. It is amazing how much science has discovered about DNA. Yet, I believe that it is only a very small portion of what can be known. We have all been taught in school that DNA is the material from which the chromosomes of a cell's nucleus are formed, and which governs cell growth and inheritance. It forms the genetic code inside each cell and regulates most of the activities that take place in our cells throughout a lifetime. This implies intelligence. The great question is: where does that intelligence come from? To me, DNA is a link from a greater intelligence to cellular intelligence. Can DNA intelligence change? Science knows that it can, but does not know how to change it. **We know that DNA changes or we would not age. If we knew how to keep our DNA from altering to an old age profile, our bodies would not age! Aging therefore, is a mental concept that our DNA accepts.** I believe that I understand the process of modifying the DNA in such a way as to prevent aging and

---

[321] Annie Besant, P.T.S. and Charles W. Leadbeater, *Occult Chemistry - Clairvoyant Observations on the Chemical Elements*, (London, England: Theosophical Publishing House, 1919).

disease. However, knowing and doing are not the same. But, if we at least know, then we have the opportunity to begin working to transform the situation.

As I implied above, one of the great mysteries of science is the cause of aging. Science knows that within one year, almost all the cells of our bodies have been replaced with new ones. So how do we age? Science now knows that in the process of digestion, after the food particles have been broken down into a form in which the blood and lymph can pick them up, there is a process that takes place in the intestinal wall that attaches a DNA to the food substance. From there it is sent to the specific spot in the body where it is most needed. **What do you suppose happens when that food particle is attached to a DNA that is impure or contaminated by associated negative consciousness?** Having now a DNA, that food particle will become a part of the cell tissue, contaminating and weakening the tissue at that point. This process happens at a very slow rate, so we are hardly aware of it. I am convinced that another thing that happens with all of us is that **we contaminate our DNA through our habitual negative thoughts and feelings**.

I am suggesting that our feelings and belief systems are capable of altering our DNA, and that habitual feelings of love can alter the DNA favorably. Dr. Deepak Chopra, M.D., said; **"We are the only creatures on earth who can change our biology by what we think and feel."** If we believe that we will age like most people, our DNA will accommodate our expectations. Indeed, according to our faith it is done unto us. The same thing applies to fear. I knew of a man who feared getting a very rare disease. After many years of expecting it - it developed. Did the disease kill him or did his expectations?

# Unexpected Potential with Cleansing

Cleansing the intestines and the stomach opens hidden doors of incredible potential. **The digestive system is the hub of the entire body**. It is one of the great secrets of life. As it becomes more and more cleansed, other parts of the body begin to also eliminate their toxic overloads. **The more pure our cells and organs become, the more efficient they become. There comes a point when the channels of energy are unblocked and energy begins to flow such as few have experienced before**. I am not talking about just getting our energy back to normal. I am talking about something that is incredibly more potent than most people have ever experienced. Yet, energy stimulates. Too much energy in an unprepared vehicle can cause trouble. But in a strong prepared vehicle, it brings strength.

Each year thousands of people make the climb to the top of Mt. Shasta, a 14,164 foot mountain. The average person in good shape will do the climb, starting at the 8,000-foot level, in about 8 hours. Those who can make it in around 5 hours are known to be in outstanding shape. Anyone who can do it in less than 3 hours is considered almost super human. A friend of mind, Robert Webb, broke a 50-year world's record in climbing Mt. Shasta. From the 8,000 foot level, he began his ascent to 14,164 feet. **It took him 1 hour and 39 minutes.**[322] **The next closest record was 2 hours and 24 minutes.** Robert reported to the newspaper that when he is in the mountains, **he has the ability to access a source of energy that gives him his strength and endurance.** Everyone who climbs with him will agree. He flies by everyone with little effort. Even the most outstanding athletes are left in the dust by Robert.

Robert also happens to be a cleansing enthusiast. As I write this, Robert is on my cleanse program, for he is planning to set two new world records this summer. This is one of the ways he prepares - he considers it 'reducing resistance.' I am also helping him with nutrition to build maximum strength and endurance.

Anyone who ever made the climb will tell you that by the time s/he got back to the 8,000 foot level, s/he was beat. And to walk the last mile back to the car is almost unbearable to most people. For most, it will take days to recover. But Robert set another World's Record in 1997. **He climbed Mt. Shasta 5 times in 24 hours, setting the World's Record for elevation gain in a 24-hour period.** He climbed more than 30,000 feet in elevation in 24 hours, and all of it was above 8,000 feet in elevation! Not only that, but his average climbs that day were less than 3 hours. Will this record ever be broken? Probably, but only by a vegetarian![323]

Many people have heard of Tibetan lamas who **are able to sit on snow and ice in 40 degree below zero weather, with almost no clothing on, for as long as they like**. I have heard that some have contests to see who can burrow a hole in the snow the deepest with nothing but their body heat. **My research has verified these stories and many more wonderful stories of those who tapped the greater potential within**. Yet it is one thing to read or hear about stories like this, and another thing to embody these abilities. We should not assume that because one human body can do something like this, that all can, without proper preparation. And it is more than just a matter of the will. Those who have not sufficiently

---

[322] This was officially recorded by members of the Sierra Club.

[323] **See the sections related to eating meat in Chapter 13: Eating for Good Health.**

cleansed and purified themselves *on **all** levels of their beings*, should not place themselves in danger by attempting something like this.

An interesting event occurred in April of 1986. I was camping with two friends along the upper Skagit River in Washington state. This time of the year **the rivers of the North Cascades are icy cold**. Snow still lingered on the ridges just above our camp. Just before sunset we all decided to take a bath in the icy Skagit river. I was also experimenting with cold water therapy, therefore, I stayed in the water longer than normal and received quit a chill. Finally, I climbed out of the river and about then the sun had set and we all crawled into our freezing cold sleeping bags. I began to shiver as I watched the stars coming out. I thought about how I have always had below normal body heat and how long it takes for me to warm up. "Burr", I thought. "This could be a cold night. Maybe I should get out of my sleeping bag and run for a mile or so." I made a comment to my friends implying that I was freezing cold and there was not any warmth in my body to heat up my sleeping bag. One of them half joking and half serious replied, **"Declare the temperature you want to experience** like the yogis." We all laughed and then discussed it a bit. After all, we had heard many stories of how yogi's could sit on ice, completely naked in sub zero temperatures for days, and remain comfortable. "That's for me." I thought. So I decided to give it a try. I laid there and asked the Infinite to show me what to do. I proceeded to visualize myself being engulfed with hot roaring golden flames. I purposely formed a barrier in my mind that prevented me from feeling doubt. **After about two minutes, and to my absolute amazement, a sudden and unexpected rush of heat flowed through my entire body. Within a few seconds I had to unzip my sleeping bag, for I was beginning to sweat**.

What is this energy? Is it something anyone can tap into? Can it be used for healing? Can it be used to prolong our life if we wish it? Can it stimulate and strengthen our minds to a much higher level? Yes to every question. However, the body must be made very strong and stable, almost to perfection, before we dare tap into this awesome energy.

# Body Reflects Consciousness Perfectly

When our bodies were formed, did we or our mothers make decisions concerning the growth of our bodily processes? How is it that one of our arms didn't end up as a nose, or an ear didn't get put on the elbow? I am saying that **an intelligence beyond the usual conscious awareness controls our bodies' processes all the way from the first cell to the last breath**. This intelligence is called by science, "Innate Intelligence." You can call it God-Intelligence if you like and be just as correct. Every cell in your body has this intelligence. **Each cell always knows exactly what to do under every circumstance. It is impossible for your body to make a single mistake; it always responds perfectly according to the conditions imposed upon it** (again hereditary, genetic, mental and emotional patterns, plus food, environment, etc.).

Just as the intelligence which directs the body knows exactly how to make the body, **it also knows exactly how to heal and perfect it,** as long as we do not get in the way; all the body requires is its natural food, water and harmony. You may wonder: if the body knows exactly what to do at all times, then how can people become sick? **Every disease and illness the body can ever have, is a situation in which the body is forced to function in an unnatural way.** It may be because it was poisoned by the wrong foods, or too much food which caused toxic overload, or the food didn't contain needed nutrients, or perhaps the body is responding to hereditary, genetic, or emotional/thought patterns. The main point is that the body is designed to function perfectly: it automatically keeps itself alive. After all, keeping the body alive is the first priority, even if it has to drain itself of needed minerals to do so.

**The good thing about this is that when we finally do everything necessary to improve our health, such as cleansing, purifying, and giving the body the natural elements it so desperately needs, then it is quick to respond and rebuild itself.** Alkalizing the body and using an ideal cleansing program are the first two steps in this process of cleansing and purifying.

One day I dropped my calculator into a mop bucket full of dirty water, and it totally short-circuited. This would not have happened if it had been distilled water, as it is pure. Regular tap water is contaminated with inorganic minerals and will short-circuit electrical currents. The same thing is true of our bodies. If we put impure food, drink, or thoughts into ourselves, we short-circuit from toxicity. When we cleanse those substances from our bodies, incredible things begin to happen.

# Releasing Thought Patterns Stuck In Mucoid Plaque

My personal belief is that if we purify enough, that not only can we overcome all disease, but we can possibly conquer the "last enemy, death". I know that sounds very far-fetched to many. Scientifically, it is very possible. Spiritually, it is indicated. My research shows that many have accomplished it, so why can't we?[324] The problem is that most people have never heard of such a thing. In both the East and the West, there are numerous legends and stories of those incredible individuals who sought truth, purified themselves, became younger even at older ages, and went on living for hundreds of years until finally they just disappeared from the world. **Some believe these things, but many do not because of their "conditioning".** I personally have met several of these individuals and have become quite convinced of this reality. The key is to eliminate the cause, effect, record and memory of all negativity within us.

Many persons who have purified themselves, using the cleanse, have reported recalling long forgotten incidents and related intense emotions when releasing mucoid plaque. It is as if the emotions we felt while eating under stress were somehow recorded by our bodies in the food substance itself, and subsequently in the resulting mucoid plaque. This makes it quite evident why we should refrain from eating, and especially from "pigging out" when we are upset. The very feelings we may seek to avoid by stuffing food into our mouths under stress, ironically stay with us in the resulting mucoid plaque for years to come, and unless we cleanse and purify, for a lifetime. People who have had this sort of experience upon releasing mucoid plaque report that initially they will find some old emotional state arising, seemingly without cause. Then usually within a few hours they will release a section of mucoid plaque. **At that point the emotions disappear, as if by magic, and often a diseased physical condition disappears at the same time.**

*"Depression and worry were a way of life for me. In the week and one-half that I've been on the Gentle Phase,* **depression and worry have vanished - replaced by realistic assessment and joy**. *My stomach has reduced in size, and I have had no need to visit the chiropractor for help with a heart condition and diabetes." - Sherry Stanley, Alexandria, VA*

---

[324] The *Dead Sea Scrolls* contain records of some of the Essene members. These explain that Jesus was not the only one who conquered death during those times. His mother Mary, her husband Joesph, and the one known as John the Divine all reached this high level of attainment. Paramhansa Yogananda gives several examples in his impressive book; *Autobiography of a Yogi*. Theosophical literature also includes various individuals who accomplished this great level. Even the French archives include a very famous person known throughout history as the "Wonderman of Europe", the Count Saint Germain, whom many authorities have claimed was Sir Francis Bacon who faked his death, went to Tibet for about 75 years and returned as the Count, and then worked in Europe for over 100 years. Streets, rivers and towns are named after him. Many people claim to be in touch with him even today.

> "During the cleanse with partial fasting, (after releasing feet of accumulated 'dark green rubber') **I became aware of mistreatments to the SELF - emotional eating**, eating of improper or "dead" foods, habitual eating, abusive eating. **I became aware of toxic thoughts, toxic emotions and began to release everything**..."
> - Genevieve Gowman, San Francisco, CA

From these testimonies and many others like them, I developed a theory that **emotional stress had the capacity to bind to cellular tissue, and especially mucoid plaque.**[325] I believe a major amount of negative consciousness is stored in the mucoid plaque in the stomach, small intestine, and the colon. **Compared to toxins stored in the rest of the body, the mucoid plaque is the easiest to extract. After we have cleansed out the plaque from the bowel, it then becomes possible to cleanse cellular tissue in other organs and parts of the body.** Then the potential for freedom from old mental/emotional/physical patterns can become a reality.

I am convinced that **as heat radiates from fire, or as magnetic energy radiates from a magnet, so does toxic accumulation in mucoid plaque radiate death into the mental, emotional, and physical bodies,** further perpetuating negative feelings, thoughts, habits, and disease. This may reveal why the great spiritual geniuses of antiquity always fasted - often for 40 days or so - before they achieved their exalted consciousness.

# Testimonies

The following are true reports from individuals who have used my cleansing program:

### The Cleanse Removes Negative Thoughts and Deep Emotional Stress

Avona L'Carttier of Seattle stated, "Over the past 14 or 15 months I have done the full cleanse with fasting three times and the cleanse with two meals each day for five weeks on and off since my first full cleanse. Since that time, in addition to many physical benefits, such as having more energy, needing less sleep, and the loss of a lot of cellulite, my mind is clearer than I can ever remember. I have always had a good memory and quick mind (I majored in mathematics in college), but I noticed a

---

[325] There is a great need for scientific research to explore more fully the relationship of consciousness to the physical structure of our bodies. It is obvious, as many doctors will testify, that our bodies are an extension of our consciousness - but to what degree?

significant difference. It's great. I feel that part of this is due to **the release of a build-up of denied emotions I've held since my childhood. I truly believe the physical cleansing triggered deeper emotional cleansing than I had been able to achieve before.** Over the past summer, which I started with a full cleanse in late spring, I did a cleanse with one meal per day, taking mostly juices for lunch and dinner, off and on all summer. **I was motivated to continually dig deeper and deeper into the emotional traumas of my childhood and release them.** With each cleanse, I find that I am also driven to clean my house very thoroughly. I have given away bags and boxes of possessions, too. **The emotional releases, however, are most profound because I am now affected so little by others' issues. I find I respond lovingly and understandingly instead of having my own 'buttons' pushed.** The way others describe it to me is that I am not judgmental, very tolerant. It's great. My ability to see clairvoyantly continues to expand and I finally find myself moving from a place of deep inner joy, instead of simply deciding to just be happy."

### Transcendental Bliss, Energy, and Love, in Place of Chronic Fatigue and Stress

S. B. of Port Angeles, Washington wrote, "I'm a 26-year-old male attorney who works very long hours, endures a lot of stress and confronts a lot of unhappiness in both my clients and the court room. I used a 10-day cleanse and released approximately 18 ft. of hard stale smelling fecal matter. Some of my stuff was even black!! I reached a point during the program where **I actually felt transcendental - my spirit was freed!!! The 'terrible problems' I faced on a daily basis weren't so terrible; my chronic fatigue disappeared**; the bags under my eyes vanished along with the tiny crow's feet around my eyes; my handwriting even changed!!! **I felt incredible feelings of Love for family and friends. I entered a state of bliss that I had never experienced <u>and</u> have not since experienced. I actually felt close to God.** Tears come to my eyes as I describe this to you. You must all know that [your cleansing program] is a godsend - its effects are real and revealing."

### Recovered from the Deadly Effect of Medical Radiation

One health practitioner, Catherine of Tucson, Arizona, wrote about one of her clients, "...who had bladder cancer three or so years ago, and **they over-radiated her and she had no control over her bowels.** They said it would be that way for the rest of her life. **After one week [of cleansing on your program] her bowels are moving on their own** in the morning and no uncontrollable diarrhea."

### Bone Cancer Pain Reduced

A man was sent to me with bone cancer. He was in terrible pain. After his first cleanse he reported, "Rich, **at least 75% of the pain just disappeared.**"

## Critical High Blood Pressure Back to Normal

**Every person I know who had critical high blood pressure reported that it was normal before they completed my cleanse program.** There was only one exception to this, and that person's high blood pressure dropped halfway to normal, but there was a good reason for it. He was in and out of the hospital while taking the cleanse, and he had to sneak in the ingredients. L. James in California told me after she did the cleanse, "I had very dangerous high blood pressure for over a year. Nothing the doctors did ever helped my condition, but, on the sixth day of using your cleanse, I went back to the doctor for a checkup. He was shocked to discover my blood pressure was normal."

## Skin Problems Improved or Gone

One person reported that she had a serious skin problem, a rash from head to toe, bloody and with sores in many places, which made it difficult to sit or lay down. After the usual going from doctor to doctor routine, and after trying anything and everything, she finally did my cleanse program, and almost all of the rash was gone within 7 days.

A registered nurse who **had a rash for 30 years found it shrank to a tiny spot by the end of her first cleanse.**

## End of That Most Deadly Disease - Constipation

Marie Smith in Missouri reported that doing [my cleanse] probably saved her life several times. She says she hasn't had to go to the hospital for a long time now, as she used to do. Her big problem was extreme constipation. Constipation is perhaps the most deadly forerunner of most diseases. Most medical doctors need to be educated in this area, and I have heard that they have many times told their patients that having bowel movements once every two or three days was normal. It may be average, but it is not normal for a healthy body.

## A Doctor's Epilepsy Disappears

A doctor in Seattle reported that during her Cleanse, **she had her last epileptic seizure. That was five years ago.**

## Eyes Turn Color - From Brown to Sparkling Green

Jonni Sue of Mt. Shasta wrote: "Thank you, Rich (and your Teacher), for bringing us this uplifting method of purification. I have done the [your full cleanse program] six times so far, plus a few [cleanses with one meal per day] in between. **My eyes have always been a light brown color**. My mother was surprised when she saw **how GREEN they are now,** as my body is getting cleaner and more aware. People say my eyes sparkle, too. I feel safe to do longer water fasts now, and to start purifying on the deep cellular level. Also, I think I'm finally scraping the bottom of the barrel. On my first three cleanses, I got rid of tons of mucoid plaque from the colon. However, my fourth cleanse had lots of gristly mucoid plaque from the small intestines and only a little colon mucoid plaque. My fifth and sixth cleanses had almost no colon plaque at all, but still some from the small intestines. The sixth cleanse removed several large pieces of duodenum plaque which really lifted my spirits. When it's all gone and I can stick to a fruit diet, plus eliminate all judgments, maybe my eyes will turn blue!"

### Stomach Pains and Lumps Gone

Mildred, of Rosemead, California, wrote a letter and said, "God Bless You. I Love you and I thank you for [your cleanse program]. Several years ago, the doctors thought I had a tumor and I had to have several ultrasounds. There wasn't one. They sure did not know what was the matter. I had a large, hard stomach and suffered pain a lot. I told one doctor, 'If you can't help me, find someone who can!' While using your cleanse my stomach started to disappear. I was amazed. The hard lumps were getting smaller. I also was constipated, had sensitivity to plants and foods, had floaters, anemia, and edema. Noise pollution had me shaking. I had a flaky rash between my eyebrows and on my forehead in two spots. The rash on my forehead and brow went away just taking the herbs and my face felt softer within a few days. I used to think that going to the rest room once a day was great, but I realized I was wrong. I started to have 3 to 5 bowel movements a day with the herbs alone. During a 7-day cleanse, I got 50-3/4 feet out. **All my symptoms and pain were gone."**

### Gained Control Over Food

There was a wide variety of testimonies in this category. One lady wrote and said, "I thank God for sending you to us with this wonderful revelation of how to return to life as He meant us to live in these bodies. If I never gained one more thing from this program and were to die tomorrow - from any cause - I would die ecstatically happy - because I have overcome a major karmic hurdle - since reading your book, **I have for the first time, gained control over food."**

### Bowels Function Normally Again

Joseph Schechter, 39 years young wrote: "I am impressed with the effectiveness of your products and I'm very happy with the results of their use. I've taken the cleanse numerous times and it has changed me for the better. I feel more energetic, alert, and alive. **My digestive system is now working properly. The natural urge to eliminate within 30 minutes after a meal is fully restored**. I used to suffer badly from airborne allergens. The cleanse and change in my diet have resulted in a **great reduction of allergy symptoms**. My eyes clearly reflect my vastly improved health in all my bodily functions. I feel this is just the beginning of a life-long journey towards supreme health and fitness."

### What Goes In Doesn't Always Come Out Until You Cleanse

A lady in Idaho reported that ever since she could remember she had a hard lump in her abdomen, then about halfway through her first cleanse she had a very strange sensation just below her stomach. She drove home as fast as she could and soon **passed a hard piece of material about 6 or 7 inches long and about two inches thick.** She cleaned it off and when her husband looked at it, he clanked it on the toilet and it sounded almost like metal. Then he hit it hard and broke it. Inside were multi-colors. When she saw that, **she instantly knew that it was from all the color crayons that she had eaten when she was about five years old.** The lump was gone and she was so impressed that she told perhaps 50 or more people about [this cleanse program].

### Cancer Pain Gone - Plus Happy Side Benefits

Tony Miles from San Francisco had Lymphoma cancer under his right arm. Talk about pain! After using my cleanse program, **the pain was completely gone.** He was so happy that he became very serious about cleansing. He went on the cleanse nine times and **lost about 75 pounds of unnecessary weight.** His overall **energy increased two to three times, and he eliminated an enormous amount of "emotional stuff, day-to-day worries, and other basic fears".** His self-esteem greatly increased and he is confident that he can now find the happiness he seeks.

### Deep Cleansing Gets Results

Warren Brown, age 54, from Venice, California, wrote that the pains in his intestines, months-old accumulation of phlegm in his lungs, shortness of breath, and **15 pounds of unneeded weight disappeared after 10 days on Dr. Anderson's cleanse** and eating one raw vegetable meal each day. He said that he was looking at a clear way to avoid a bucketful of medical bills and extend his life expectancy far into the future.

### A Crippled Lady Walks Normally Again

Another time that I was in California studying with Dr. Jensen, I met Marie Mauger. She walked painfully, even using a cane. I told her about intestinal cleansing and she replied that she had used several colon cleanses, but they never helped her situation. **I explained that our program is not the same as the other colon cleanses.** Soon she was reading my book and then was on the cleanse. Here is an example of a person who was determined to be healed. It had to happen and it did.

This is her story: "For the last seven years, I have been dealing with a steadily increasing amount of pain in my right hip. For the last six months, the pain had become so great that I was using a cane regularly outside of the house. X-rays showed that the cartilage had worn off the head of the femur. An infection had also developed. The nerves at the head of the femur were telling my brain to immobilize the right leg. In spite of many different types of therapy to reverse the steady downward spiral, nothing seemed to turn the gradual decline around.

The different therapies I tried included and still do include chiropractic treatments, therapeutic massage, nutrition, exercise, emotional and mental awareness, spiritual practices, homeopathy, yoga, as well as colon cleansing using Dr. Jensen's program. Things I tried that I no longer do, included acupuncture, mega-vitamin therapy, body electronics, Biotron and Enterro treatments.

Approximately ten weeks ago, I started using Dr. Anderson's herbal products in preparation for a one-week intestinal cleanse. I took his herbs for six weeks before beginning the cleanse. For the cleanse, I did everything he suggested in the book, *Cleanse & Purify Thyself.* **On the second day of the cleanse, approximately 50% of the pain left my body and I stopped using the cane at that time.** On the third day of the cleanse, I did a little yoga with my yoga students for the first time in over a year. They were watching me with their mouths dropped open because their most recent experience of me was seeing a person move with great agony and pain.

In the five weeks since the cleanse, I have primarily been eating all fresh and raw foods with one to three pints of fresh vegetable juice daily. I haven't used the cane except on one occasion where I knew there was going to be a lot of walking. In general, the pain level has remained much less than prior to cleansing. For the first time in seven years, I'm seeing the reversal of the down spiral."

After a few more cleanses she was normal again, began teaching others how to do this kind of cleansing, and then became a world traveler.

**Serious Back Problems Gone**
A man named Gabriel Diamond had tried everything and finally found this cleansing program. "Dear Rich, this is the third cleanse that I am going on and have experienced dramatic increases in my overall energy and health. **Your program has been the most effective method for improving my health where all others have failed or have only provided temporary relief.** On only the second day of this cleanse I have had one of my more dramatic experiences while purifying my body.

I have had lower back and left leg problems for about five years. The most notable being sciatica, sometimes being so bad it's hard for me to walk. On the morning of the second day I felt pretty bad and I knew, because of my other cleansing that toxic material was moving about. During my enema I discharged a piece of mucoid from my colon about six inches long and over three inches in diameter. **After this piece passed I noticed that the pain and discomfort in my leg had decreased about**

**75%.** This convinced me even more about the importance of cleaning the alimentary canal. Little do people realize the true cause of their problems; mucoid and toxic buildup, and how easy it is to remove this toxic load and experience levels of well-being they have totally forgotten. I have improved after each cleanse. I'm going to see how good it is possible to feel."

Many people have commented on how their back problems disappeared after the Cleanse. One man, Ron Sherr in Arizona, told me that now he can go back to lifting weights again, because **his back improved after each Cleanse.** After his third Cleanse his pain was finally completely gone. I explained to him that had he improved his diet after the first Cleanse, his pain would have vanished more quickly.

### Cancer, Irritable Bowel Syndrome, Depression

"In Testimony to Rich Anderson's cleansing program, I received the following benefits: The GID (Gastrointestinal disorder) I had suffered from for years, GONE. The **IBS (Irritable Bowel Syndrome) and toxemia that developed, GONE.** An Esophageal Reflex condition that was increasing in intensity the past year, GONE. Toxemia of the body, I had developed from above, GONE. Brought to my awareness the mental depression I was in. Changed my eating, lifestyle, and food preparation; **lost 30 pounds of unneeded weight. Slowed (reduced by 23%) the progress of Prostate Cancer.**[326] Made me develop a personal CHOICE in

---

[326] This man did the full cleanse with fasting about five to seven times in a three-month period. His daughter told me that he had a great deal of pressure from his family who were very orthodox in their medical thinking. His brother was an M.D., his wife and son were dentists, and he was a pharmacist. He had to resist them every time he turned around. During this time, his niece who also had cancer, was giving him the worst time of all. She kept calling him on the phone and telling him that he had gone off his rocker, and was killing himself by doing this "insane" cleanse. This is typical thinking of those who have been severely brainwashed. She had been following the advice of allopathic M.D.'s, and her hair had fallen out, she had been sick for over a month, she had no energy, her skin had a grayish tint to it, and she was either depressed or angry. One day after her uncle had been on the program for about two months, she dropped in to see him. With great effort she crawled out of the car and dragged herself into his house. He had lost about 25 pounds of useless blubber and looked about 10 years younger than when she saw him last. As she stared at his bright eyes, glowing complexion, vibrant energy, and upgraded attitude, her mouth dropped open in dis-belief, and she immediately stopped preaching to him. It was clear as glass that he was getting better and she was getting worse. He also told me that he had suffered from depression for many years and that too went away. I was really proud of this man coming from such orthodox conditions and going through such incredible cleansing. His daughter, Rachel, was the force behind his success. It was as though he stepped out of hell and into

how I wanted to live my life; physically, emotionally, mentally, and spiritually. I would recommend this program to anyone who has similar conditions."

### Children Benefit Too
A mother wrote to me: "**My six-year-old**, after four weeks of cleansing with two meals per day and mostly raw foods, passed a six-inch chunk of old, blackish-brown, dried mucoid matter with striations that looked like finger prints. Proof that, **'Yup! he did need it too.'** We're both more excited now that we're seeing results. We'll be back in touch post-cleanse with the rest of our 'poop scoop'. Glad you're there. Thanks, Pamela."

Many children have benefited from this program, all the way from two years old and up. I only wish my parents had me do this when I was that age. What a difference that could have made!

### It's Almost Unbelievable
The Stuff That's Eliminated! - Sandra from Tucson wrote: "Greetings from a cleaner and more pure Sandy Ward. I came off the Cleanse today and I am SO IMPRESSED! I could not believe the filth and slime that came out! And so MUCH of it! Where does it all come from? AMAZING!"

### The Solution to a Life-Long Problem
Joy LaMarr, of Tucson, Arizona, shared her story: "Due to a bowel injury as a toddler, I've had a chronic problem with constipation my entire life. I lost count long ago of the number of doctors I've consulted and tests that have been conducted on me regarding this single problem. During the past 50 years, I've used countless varieties of stool softeners, laxatives, etc. Finally about three years ago, I resorted to using mineral oil (which worked, somewhat, but was still unsatisfactory). But I'm happy to report that in March, 1990, I began taking some of the herbs every night before going to bed, and have no problem with constipation anymore. Not once, in 4 months. It gives me a very warm feeling to know that my final, long-lasting remedy is safe, all natural ingredients." She also would have even greater success if she would do a cleanse, at least the one with two meals per day, and then get the proper bacteria in there.

### Dr. Anderson's Herbal Combination - Effective and Easy on Our Bodies
According to Nancy Peters, of Venice California, "Your herbal formulas are the first formulas of herbs or vitamins for glandular organs that

---

heaven. That is the way it can be with those suffering from a serious disease. It is a great opportunity to change into a new being.

I have been able to easily take consistently for the past 6 months. My body has said, 'no' to everything else, even with extensive Applied Kinesiology and Clinical Kinesiology work. I had great results with your products. On the second day of the cleanse some movement in my tail bone and corresponding movement in my jaw has allowed my back to shift into a position that allows energy to move through my body and shifted the position of my teeth so that they are better aligned! This is significant because after an auto accident 3 years ago and thousands of dollars for medical and alternative people, I have had a block in my energy that has presented me with consistent fatigue and pain for the first time in my life. As a result of [using your cleanse], I can place my body into a sitting position comfortably, my joints are 20% more flexible, the creaks in my neck every time I moved it are GONE! I feel my organs getting energy and beginning to work efficiently. I exist on very little food and have energy! My cellular texture of **my skin is more supple and alive, spots on my eyes that hadn't changed since my photos 10 years ago are gone. I have more laughter!** It's been easier to experience a bigger context in my life. I see the fields of belief that people are living from more clearly, and I have clearer intuition."

### A Man in His Eighties

Alfred Israel from Phoenix, Arizona was ecstatic: "I was on the cleanse for the full seven days. **Forty-five feet of beautiful Mucoid Sheaths were expelled.** What should I do with It? It is laying on the bathroom floor on aluminum wrap - the answer? I'll take pictures of it. I feel so much better and have more energy to continue my art work. This was a great birthday gift. I plan to continue experimenting with this. I think that possibly the cataract might be corrected in time."

### A Mother Wrote Concerning Her Daughter

Ramona of Los Angeles was convinced: "I am writing you about your wonderful *Cleanse & Purify Thyself* book and **how much you helped my daughter. She was in PAIN for years**. It was so bad that sometimes she couldn't speak! **She went to doctor after doctor and hospital after hospital** and they tested her in all their ways, but we couldn't find the reason for the pain. Until she went on your cleansing program. Thank you for writing such a brilliant book and helping my daughter lose all that prehistoric fecal matter. She is a new girl. I am going on the program myself."

### Good-bye Hay Fever and Pain, Hello New Lustrous Skin

"This note is to thank you - for your Love, compassion, caring, hard work, and research. Your cleanse was unbelievable! The best thing I've done for myself! 35 feet of 'filthy stuff' came out of me! So many positive and amazing things happened to me! The first real noticeable thing is **my skin. It's clearer and has a luster I don't remember it ever having before**. Others have commented on it too! I've been seeing an acupuncturist for 5 months - trying to open channels enough to release excessive amounts of toxins from my body. **I've had a large lump in my knee and it's been very painful. But...now... after my 1st cleanse the toxins are all cleared. My knee is great!** In fact all my energy is flowing so perfectly now that I don't need to go back to see him for a long while! Yah! (He was very amazed too!) And my hay fever? During the cleanse with two meals it started to lessen and during the full cleanse with fasting, **I had NO hay fever at all**. It's now been a week since the 8th day and the sneezing is starting again. I know after a few more cleanses it will be gone for good. I have no words to adequately describe how I feel right now. It's a 'clean' and a 'lightness' I don't remember having. Every time I released more 'stuff' I felt such a relief and Love for myself. I guess for me that's the most wonderful thing...a new discovery of Love for myself. So...I say please keep working and sharing. I send you all my Love and aloha and strength. Much Love, Jennett."

### A Lady from Canada

Mrs. Dallas Urgwhart had a graphic description! "I tried it. On the second day I could not believe how good I felt and the stuff that came out of me looked like the gunk when an alien starts disintegrating."

### Diabetes

"Dear Dr. Anderson, when my doctor told me I had diabetes I was really frightened. I had gone to see him because I had no energy. I was always tired and had to stay in bed most of the time. I'm 71 years old and always had a lot of energy and stamina, so when all of a sudden I had to stay in bed and could hardly get through the day when I worked, I was really scared.

"My late husband and sister had diabetes and other health problems, and I saw what the insulin and other drugs did to them. It was horrible. My husband and sister had high blood pressure and so did I. My daughter saw you on television and bought your book and had gone on your detox program. She said she couldn't believe how nice her skin looked. She had a terrible acne problem at 48 because of prescription drugs she had been taking. I had prayed and asked God to show me a way out of taking drugs for my health problems. When my daughter told me about your program, I didn't hesitate starting right away. The first week I started on the program I felt an immediate difference. I felt wonderful for the first time in months. I had no symptoms and my energy returned within the first two weeks. My tongue did turn very black about the third week. White Crow said not to worry, my body was just releasing toxins. My tongue turned its normal color after a few days and I have not taken anything my doctor prescribed since I started on your program. Thank you very much, you were the answer to my prayer. Sincerely, Clara Perea, Tucson."

### Worms, Parasites And Crawly Things Being Removed

Many people report worms being eliminated, all different sizes and shapes, from microscopic to over 30 feet. Barney Davis of Tucson said, "I'm gaining more and more energy, vitality, and have a new-found energy. **The total length of worms that came out of me in 7 days equaled 335.4 inches.**" (27.9 feet).

### Diabetes - She Reduced the Insulin

One lady was sure that her diabetes had brought her near the point of death. She could not function normally and was unable to hold a job. She would often just blank out and was in several auto accidents. She had to take up to 30 units of insulin twice a day. After she took the first Cleanse she was able to drop her insulin down to 10 units once a day. Her energy level increased enormously. She could then work and function as a mother once again. She continued to cleanse and work on her diet. She kept getting better and better. Not all her problems were with diabetes, of course, and she would occasionally have severe fatigue problems. One day she called to tell me that she could barely walk or talk. I asked her to come over and let me check her out. She had to take a bus because she didn't trust her driving. I began to test her for various things and finally looked into her eyes and saw a definite problem with her heart. So I had her drink some hot water with cayenne in it. I said, "If you feel better in less then 10 minutes, your problem is your heart." Five minutes later she came back in with a big smile. She was feeling great. I asked her, "Of all the doctors you went to, did anyone tell you that you had a heart problem?" She replied, "No, they always said it was normal." From then on she used cayenne pepper and she was basically normal in almost every way.

### Serious Headaches Vanish

I met Michelle after giving a lecture in Tucson. She made an appointment with me and was soon discussing her problem. She said, "I have had the most excruciating headaches, I do not know how I have survived. They never go away and though I am a strict vegetarian, I do take drugs for relief. I know that the drugs are giving me temporary relief and at the same time causing other problems, probably with a cumulative effect. Do you think that you can help me?" I looked at her eyes and could easily see that her elimination systems were far from normal and her body was accumulating more and more toxic debris. Also, her digestive system was below normal. Soon she was cleansing with two meals and after 10 days went on the full cleanse with no meals for 10 days. About every other day the headaches lessened. She began to lose some unnecessary weight and she gradually looked alive and vibrant. Before her cleanse was over she told me the headaches were, for the first time in years, completely gone. She became vibrant, outgoing, and started to enjoy life in a way that had been impossible up to that time. To give you the idea just how effective herbs can be, I'll relate this story about the same lady, just before she started the cleanse. One afternoon I went to her house to drop something off. She was lying on her bed immobilized. She called faintly to me and though barely able to talk, explained that she was in the midst of one of those bad headaches. She was in deep, deep pain. She asked me if I knew anything that could help. I brightly said, "Sure, be back in a minute." I went into her kitchen, heated some water and added some tincture of Lobelia, Gotu Kola, and Osha, brought it in to her and helped her drink it. I said, "Fifteen minutes and you should have relief." About 5 minutes later I heard her yelling. I went back into her room and she said, "I can't believe it, the famous Rich Anderson was wrong." I said, "What do you mean I was wrong?" With a great big smile she replied, "You said it would take 15 minutes and it only took 5." We laughed and talked while I rubbed some tinctures into her temples and the back of her lower skull. Soon she said, in astonishment, that her head hadn't felt so good in years.

### Sinus Problems

Robert Cronin wrote me: "Dear Rich: I am writing to encourage you to keep up the great work you are doing. I have used your products and think they are the best. I have suffered for years from **sinus problems and virtually all of my troubles were cleared up after my first cleanse**. I am more alert, alive and energetic."

### Brain Tumor in the Intestines?

I went to the health food store in Tucson and happened to run into a lady who had come to me almost two years earlier. She had terrible headaches, depression, lack of energy, and was certain that a tumor was eating away her brain. She had been on the cleanse once by the time she met with me. After careful iris analysis, I could see a toxic accumulation in her brain area; and I suggested that she start using the brain formula, take certain other products, keep on cleansing, and between cleanses eat mostly raw foods. She told me this, **"After five weeks on the brain formula, my headaches got worse; but I was completely convinced that you were sent to me by God; and that I must keep on following your suggestions**, as I might be feeling the effects of the tumor dissolving. **Several months went by and while on another cleanse, I passed something that looked like an old piece of corn on the cob**. It was about 7 or 8 inches long, looked like it was all wrapped up in white sheets and was hard. **As soon as that happened, my headaches disappeared and so did my depression**. I felt like a new person. Now I want to start cleansing again and see if I can remove all my mental blocks and move into a much higher state of living."

### 35-Year Rash Virtually Disappears

A Tucson nurse, who had suffered from a rash covering both of her legs for 35 years, purchased my cleansing products. Later she visited and reported that after using the combination herbs that I prepared for the cleanse for several weeks, all of the rash except for two small spots, had vanished. She said that she had not even gone on the cleanse, but had used only two herbal formulas that are part of the cleanse. She also told us that she had spent thousands of dollars, gone to many doctors and tried everything she could think of to no avail. Naturally, when she talked to us and showed us the two spots which were all that was left of the rash, she was ecstatic.

## An 80-Year Young Lady Regains Her Strength and Energy

This lovely lady in California had gone on many types of cleanses, as well as using a "mucusless diet" which she said had cured her arthritis in a few weeks but when she reached her 80th year, she wasn't feeling as well as she would like. Having bought all the ingredients for my cleanse program, she decided to go on the cleanse with two meals and she stayed on it religiously for nearly two months. She told her daughter that she felt good again and was doing all the things that she had done before - shopping, playing the organ, taking trips with friends, etc. She was thrilled to relate that a constipation problem, which had been plaguing her for many years, was gone. She said that she felt like a new person, is continuing to eat only an alkaline diet, while taking my two herbal formulas, and has given up all acid foods!

## Getting Pregnant

Christine shared with us: "My health has generally been good. However, 2 years ago **I was diagnosed with endometriosis and was told I would not conceive.** Doctors began with a 9-month course of birth control to be followed by Danocryn, which I refused. Symptoms worsened so I turned to holistic treatments with herbs and magnets. Shortly after that I was introduced to your cleanse program by Charles Baltzell. I completed it last March with great success. My whole life changed for the better. Since then I have continued to cleanse and eat raw foods. The great news is that yesterday I found out **I'm pregnant! I have had no morning sickness. I truly believe I got pregnant because I cleaned out a lot of old toxins that were preventing me from carrying a baby in a safe environment.** I feel so blessed to have done the cleanse. I feel it's the greatest gift I have ever given myself."

## The Average Testimonies

People report more energy (the most common), feeling better, feeling closer to God, pain gone, skin looking better, lumps disappearing, having better emotional control and feeling happier and more optimistic.

## The Happiest Testimony I've Ever Heard

From My Own Mother, Dee Anderson of Seattle: I just got off the phone with her and she has informed me that she has finished her third cleanse with 2-1/2 meals per day - a very mild phase of cleansing. Here is what she said, "I have so much more energy. Even when I first get out of bed, I feel good. For so many years I didn't feel good until I had a cup of coffee. Now I feel good without it. Last Sunday we were with... (here she listed a group of old friends about - mile long). They all started to comment how much younger I looked, and how my skin seemed so smooth, with less wrinkles." I asked about her arthritic pain. "Well, now, I haven't thought much about it, but yes, I do have less pain." Then I told her that even with my cleanse, she cannot expect to eliminate all her pain until she stops eating all the acid foods and gets onto alkaline foods, at least until she builds up her alkaline reserve. Then I asked her about her mind and memory. She replied, "It's funny you asked that, because just a few days ago Connie" (my sister) "and I were talking about an airline crash that occurred awhile back which had a flight attendant and a pilot on it that we all knew. When we got finished with the conversation, Connie said, 'My gosh, Mother, your memory is twice as good as mine. I just can't believe it.' Oh, my mind is much more clear." I then asked her what her best testimony was. She said, "I just plain feel better. Since all those operations, I had never felt good, but now I do." She was 83 years old, had had hip surgery and a triple by-pass heart surgery.

# Most Common Results of Digestive Cleansing

## 1. Absorption of Nutrients

The theory is that **the cleaner our bowels are, the more efficiently they can function and the better our bodies can absorb the nutrients from the food we eat**. Some people are surprised at how little food they need after a few good clean outs. I know a woman who ate only one small meal every other day for two years. She reported that never had she felt so mentally alert and so good, physically. Her mind was incredible. Some people, before cleansing, absorb only a tiny portion of the nutrients in their food - no matter how nutritious the food and how much they eat.

I do not believe that we can maintain an adequate supply of minerals by eating commercially grown produce. I strongly recommend that people eat only organically grown produce. In general, **organically grown fruits and vegetables have twice the minerals and other nutrients of regular commercially grown produce and they are still not what they should be**[327]. Even many organic farms are deficient and over-used. That's why people need to supplement their diets with the highest quality nutritional supplements. The only way we can be sure of getting

---

[327] Heltman, pg. 12.

the maximum nutrients from our food is to grow our own food in rich soil. If that is not possible, then let's support health food stores. They deserve it, whereas the average supermarket merely supports the disease industry.

## 2. Increased Peristaltic Action

After we have cleansed completely, effectively replanted the digestive tract with the correct bacteria, and we eat the right foods and drink enough liquids, food may have a shorter transit period when moving through the digestive tract. As long as this continues, we may never be constipated again, and we will not continue to build up mucoid plaque. Under the above conditions, food should move through more quickly, and will no longer lose its moisture, becoming sticky and hard. This means we have removed the cause of the formation of bowel pockets, bulges, diverticulitis, prolapsus, and a host of other colon problems and diseases. Not everyone who has a history of constipation will eliminate the problem on the first cleanse.

## 3. Removal of the Source of Disease

If we have thoroughly cleansed and are continuously eating fresh alkaline food, we may have eliminated the cause of putrefaction and reduced fermentation. Thus we have **eliminated the breeding environment of billions of disease bacteria, germs, and parasites**; therefore, the blood and every cell of the body is no longer being poisoned. Major organs are no longer being overloaded and working overtime. Our bodies are constantly working to correct and eliminate the problems caused by toxins; this requires a great deal of energy. Once the body is cleaned out, it **can rapidly repair the damage done in the past, and the miracle of the body is that it can repair itself when it has a chance**. All it requires is freedom from congestion and the proper nutrients.

**When our energy is no longer spent on repairs, it can flow to the mind or higher centers. Marvelous ideas, clear thinking, joy, and Love can predominate.**

## 4. Prolapsus Adjustment

Oftentimes the weight and pressure of a congested bowel, coupled with gravity and poor nutritional habits, have caused prolapsus of the transverse colon. The stomach may have dropped into what is called a "fishhook" position and cause further digestive problems. When the stomach and transverse colon drops, they exert pressure on the lower organs and are the main cause of bladder, urinary, and sometimes prostate problems, causing various imbalances of the nerve centers, prostate ailments, and most uterus and female problems. All of these conditions can repair themselves, after the removal of the mucoid plaque, and through the use of certain herbs and exercises. Here I would like to issue a warning: **While on the cleanse please do not jump on the trampoline or jog**. Jogging up and down with all the weight of psyllium shakes, could cause further prolapsus. Swim, walk, or do some stretching if you want, but be careful of jogging and bouncing.

## 5. Improvement of Nerve Flow

Following are further reasons why cleansing helps the back and other areas of the body. There are certain areas in the bowels that are directly associated with every other part of the body via the nerves and life force meridians. For an example, there are certain areas in the bowel that affect the muscles in the back. This is one reason why many people have found their back problems eliminated or significantly improved after doing my cleanse program. It is well known that millions of nerves pass through the spinal column. When a vertebrae is out of place, a pinched nerve may develop, seriously affecting the area of that nerve attachment. Similarly, but not so dramatically, there are nerve reflex points in other parts of the body, such as the hands, the feet, and the intestines. When the intestinal tract is no longer coated with fecal and mucoid impaction, the nerve supply is no longer in danger of short-circuiting. For nerves always have two ends. If either end short-circuits, nerve energy to cells, tissues and organs is reduced.

It has been my observation over many years that most subluxations of the spine and back are caused by the settling of toxic matter in the muscle that is attached to the area of subluxation. These toxic settlements form little pockets, usually along the spine, which weaken the muscles on one side or the other. This can cause pain. It can also throw the vertebrae out of alignment because the muscles along the spine are imbalanced.

After removing these pockets of toxic substance from the back by cleansing, deep tissue massage, or diet, pain decreases and the spine will stay in place after proper adjustments. Many people have toxins stored deep in the muscles and they need more help getting these out. I have found that within these toxic hard muscle pockets are also stored emotional accumulations.

# 6. Obliteration of Obesity

Obesity is usually associated with excessive acids and toxicity that are stored in the lymph. Many people have experienced the result of eating too much salt, and next morning find the bags under their eyes swollen, and sometimes their ankles, as well. This occurs because the body couldn't get rid of the salt fast enough and temporarily stored the excess salt in safe areas of the lymphatic system. Similarly, the body stores dangerous acids and toxins in the lymphatic system, surrounded by liquids, when it has lost the ability to remove them safely.

During deep cleansing, *if the body has a full supply of electrolytes,* the body will begin to eliminate those toxic elements. Many people who cleanse lose these toxins, along with the excess fluids that were required to store them, and they quickly trim down to normal.

This type of weight loss does not involve losing muscle mass. Anyone who loses muscle mass while cleansing or fasting is probably dealing with a chronic or degenerative condition, or some kind of infection such as a parasite infection. These conditions put the liver in great stress; it is forced to extract L-glutamine from the muscles for the making of glutathione. Glutathione is essential for life, and the body uses it to make enzymes that are necessary to keep the liver functioning.

## Chapter 8

# HOW TO DETERMINE IF YOU NEED A CLEANSING PROGRAM

*Indeed, most doctors fail to offer hope because they do not have confidence in their own treatments. In that lack of hope lies the seeds of death.. Perhaps it is for the patient to be his/her own doctor, and to seek for the cure until it is found. Pythagoras said, "Physician heal thyself", and I say, "Patient heal thyself, through the powers of purity, Love and intuition."*

- Dr. Richard Anderson

*"There are men so conservative they believe **nothing** should be done for the first time."*

- Alexander Smith

## Conditions Indicating You Need to Cleanse

If you've been living on raw fruits and vegetables all your life, and very seldom get upset, then, chances are you don't need to cleanse. However, if you have eaten the standard American diet (SAD) and get upset from time to time like most of us, you are most likely in serious need of intestinal cleansing. The following chart will help you identify indications that you need to cleanse. If you have *any* of the following conditions, you will want to pluck up your courage, and throw Alexander Smith's observation to the winds. The adventure of Cleansing and Purifying ourselves is one of the best features showing, and you'll never regret a minute of it, unless you fear it.

## Signs that Intestinal Digestive Cleansing is Needed

- over-acidity or over-alkalinity (see pH tests in the Appendix)
- any disease or malfunction of the body
- constipation[328]
- bad breath
- overweight or underweight
- have taken antibiotics[329]
- flatulence (gas)
- offensive body odor
- negative emotions and thoughts
- dry and hard stools (they should be soft and break up when you flush the toilet)
- foul-smelling stools (they should not have bad odor and should be light brown)[330]
- evacuations that take more than 30 seconds or require pushing or grunting (it should be quick and easy)
- dark spots inside the autonomic nerve wreath in the iris of the eye

---

[328] Constipation: a person should have a bowel movement the first thing each morning and within 30 minutes after each meal. If three meals a day are eaten, there should be four movements a day even with light meals. Anything less than that is inclining toward constipation. A tendency toward diarrhea is also a sign of constipation - because the body uses emergency procedures to overcome the problem, diarrhea is often the result.

[329] Antibiotics usually destroy all the friendly intestinal flora and most people never get it back. Once this is gone, a major defense of the immune process is wiped out. Without the friendly bacteria, we are open to all sorts of destructive bacteria, yeast, and other infections. People with AIDS, for an example, have lost their friendly bacteria before they got AIDS.

[330] Guyton, pg. 840.

# Reading the Eye:  Iridology

## Examining the Digestive System Through the Eye[331]

Looking at the iris, there is usually a thin line circling the iris about 1/5 of the way from the pupil to the outer edge of the iris.  This is the autonomic nerve wreath.  Everything within this line marks the digestive tract.  If this area is darker than the rest of  the iris, or if there are dark spots, or dark spokes or lines (radii solaris) coming from this area, then there are digestive disorders in either the stomach, small intestine, or colon.  These dark areas indicate mucoid plaque pockets and congestion.  The darker they are, the longer the congestion has been in the body and the more serious the condition.  Black indicates a degenerative state.  Any darkness in these areas also indicates the perfect environment for worms, parasites, and possibly diverticulitis.  However, it is not proof of parasites.  The iris reflects nerve responses.  When the cells are abnormal, the iris reflects that condition.  The iris can only reflect cell structure, it cannot reflect foreign objects such as parasites.  See the Chart on Iridology below, and note the area from the pupil to the autonomic nervous wreath; this is the area we are talking about.

The chart of the iris of the eyes, "Iris-1," serves as a map.  Each point of the iris reveals the condition of its corresponding part of the body.  It reflects the various stages of degeneration and conditions of cell tissue.  Before cleansing, it is fun and informative to study your iris, or better yet, have a photo of your iris taken.

It is important to note that some people with a strong constitution and blue eyes, have little or no dark crypts or radii solaris.  Yet most of these people still do remove large amounts of mucoid plaque.  My theory is that with these people, the mucoid plaque has not contaminated any cells which are attached to nerves.  Therefore, problems may be developing, as with many people, but their nerves remain unaffected and their eyes do not indicate a problem.  But for most people, iridology can be an effective means of gauging the need to cleanse.  Within three to five weeks after completing a few cleanses, your irises should reflect improvements in your body's condition.

---

[331] See Dr. Leonard Mehlmauer for Iridology information and readings. Sclerology is the ancient art of reading the whites of the eyes.  Dr. Mehlmauer has refined this into a cutting edge tool for today's health evaluation.  Dr. Mehlmauer may be contacted as follows: (805) 484-8686 OR 1000 Paseo Camarillo, Suite 140, Camarillo, CA 93010.

# IRIS-1
## (Iridology)

©June 1996 by LEONARD MEHLMAUER, HP
Cammarillo, California, USA • 805-484-8686
e-mail: grandmedicine@vcnet.com

A hybrid stylized projection map of the human body using the irises of the eye as a chart to physical conditions; developed by LEONARD MEHLMAUER, HP, after Deck, Jensen, Wolf, Kriege, et al.

- The Perineum is at 1 in the right Iris, 2 in the left
- The arm areas show frontal aspect of shoulder only

- PNP = Pulmonary Nerve Plexes
- C.A. = Coronary Arteries

- Vas/FT = Vas Deferens/Fallopian Tubes
- 1 - 7 = the chakras

**Left Eye, Cancer Patient**
(Slide from Dr. Richard Anderson)

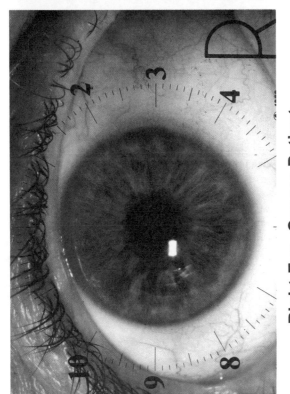

**Right Eye, Cancer Patient**
(Slide from Dr. Richard Anderson)

# Colon Reflex Points

The following diagram is a chart of the colon and its reflex points. When bowel pockets accumulate, you will generally have problems in the areas indicated at the various reflex points. Do you have any soreness in the colon area? Check the reflex points on this chart. If you have problems in the areas indicated, you now know the cause. And you can be sure that cleansing the colon (as well as the entire intestinal tract) will be one of the best ways to get rid of those problems. An example I have seen many times is with people having heart problems. Usually their iris will reveal a tiny dark spot in the left eye, at 3 o'clock, just on the outside of the autonomic nerve wreath. Whenever I would see this, I would ask the person to poke their fingers into their left side in the descending colon area, and feel for soreness. Usually it is very tender there. After the cleanse, this soreness disappears.

# Cleansing Can Be Easy — You Can Do It!

Ironically, I have found that **the people who need to cleanse the most have the most resistance to the idea.** And even when they choose to go forward with cleansing, they still often express great fear about it. But it is important to remember that the beginning phases are gentle and easy to accomplish, yet still quite effective.

Many people want to jump right into the full cleanse with fasting and forget about doing the gentler cleansing first. This is a great mistake as is discussed in Chapter 9: Facts About an Optimal Cleansing Program, under "Four Phases of Cleansing." These people tend to underestimate just how effective a gentler cleanse really can be. For example, when my mother finally did the cleanse, she did the mildest phase (with three meals each day). It was an easy cleanse, but what it did for her mind was incredible. Her testimony is in Chapter 7, but what I realize now, that I didn't realize when I related her testimony, is that not only did her memory come back to full, but she took on an entirely new concept of life. She developed a wisdom that she never had before. Her mind became aware of things that she had never been aware of before her cleanse. Now when my mother and I are conversing, I listen with both ears (before I only listened with one ear), for she now comes up with concepts that are truly astounding and accurate.

# Reflex Points of the Colon

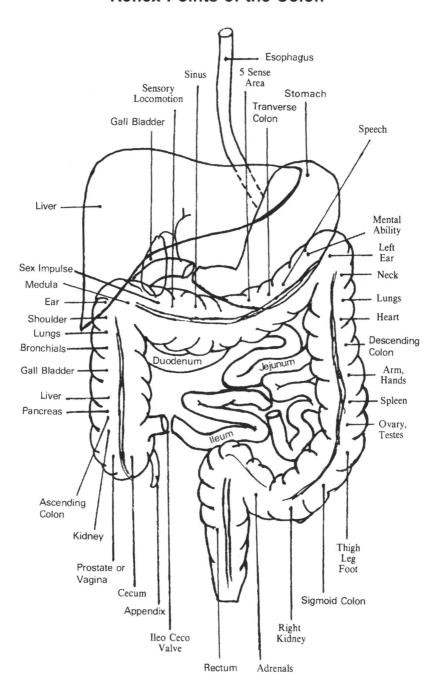

8-187

Here is a testimony from a person who had remarkable results on her third day **of gentle cleansing**. Barbara Havens from Chula Vista, California wrote:

>"About five years ago I was diagnosed with Epstein Barr, sinus and allergy problems due to large polyps in my nasal passage, I was a whopping 200 lbs. and on antibiotics every month. The last diagnosis that was suggested to me was that I see a 'shrink' and get help. The final diagnosis that the doctors gave me (to see a shrink) was the best news I could have heard because I knew that I wasn't crazy. Lo and behold, I was introduced to the book Cleanse & Purify Thyself. I read the book and in the first chapter I knew that this was my answer to my problems. So my husband and I went on the Power Phase and on the third day of the cleanse, I had a strange sensation in the back of my nose and shortly after this happened, I could smell things like I could never have smelled before. I asked myself what was going on and the only thing that I could come up with was that my polyps were shrinking. I went to my allergist, who suggested surgery for my polyps, and he examined me and said "they're gone". **To sum it up, I have lost about 70 lbs. and I do not have Epstein Barr symptoms any more. The best part about cleansing is about how much more you can Love.** You have to try this cleanse to really know what I am truly saying. Don't be discouraged by what doctors tell you. I always tell people; if it can be created, it can also be uncreated. One last comment, my husband and I do a couple cleanses a year because this shouldn't be a one time experience. Thanks Rich for sharing with us your knowledge... Love & Light, Barbara and Curt Havens"

# Chapter 9

# FACTS ABOUT AN OPTIMAL CLEANSING PROGRAM

*"The cures attributed to the influence of certain medicines, relics, and places are the effects of imagination and faith. The curative power is not in the spirit that is in them, it is in the spirit in which they are accepted."*

-E. W. Neville

*"Your faith has made you well."*

-Jesus of Nazareth

## The Cleanse is Potent

I have investigated most of the intestinal cleanses on the market, and by that I mean I have used them myself. I am convinced that the program I was subsequently inspired to develop is, without a single exception, the most effective, powerful, and complete intestinal cleansing program available. I say this not only because of my research and cleansing experience, but also because of many people who, after doing many other cleanses, finally did ours. With a united voice, they proclaim my program to be the most effective. Unlike most programs similar to it, this program cleanses the stomach and small intestine, as well as the colon. However, due to its unusual potency, it must be used wisely and with caution.

The key to this program's success is the combination of two herbal formulas which I designed for the cleanse. When combined, the herbs in these two formulas prepare the mucoid plaque in the stomach <u>and</u> intestines in such a way that it can easily be removed.

# How the Herb Formulas Were Developed

After I had spent years using other cleanses (usually just colon cleanses), I discovered (or was "given" through inspiration and unusual experiences), a select combination of herbs that had an incredibly powerful effect in loosening and dissolving that horrible mucoid plaque. This occurred during an herbal expedition, where a friend and I lived for almost 3 months off the land, eating only fresh herbs. After traveling from one state to another, we came to a certain meadow in the Sierras. This meadow contained key herbs that became the main part of our meals. After two days in that meadow, the mucoid plaque started to be released in 2-4 foot sections. This was while eating two large herb salads daily. Knowing what a valuable discovery this was, I was thrilled. I knew all too well how difficult it was to remove that slow death from the intestines. I knew how seriously the mucoid matter and a dysfunctional digestive system contributed to almost every disease known.

After this experience in the meadow, I had two remaining questions about those herbs pulling out the mucoid plaque:
1) These were herbs that every herbalist knew about, so why did they not know these herbs would pull out the mucoid plaque? And,
2) Could we get the same results using dried herbs as we did using the fresh herbs?

I often thought that it must be the fresh herbs that made the cleansing work so well. After all, how many people go up into the mountains and eat just the wild, fresh herbs? Maybe that is why the herbalists didn't know about it; they never tried them raw and fresh. But something kept telling me that these herbs would work in the dried state just as well as the raw state, that **it was the particular combination that made them so effective**. So I began to put together an herbal formula using dried herbs. That way I would know for sure, and not only that, but if my intuition was correct, it would become available to everyone. Without any doubt in my mind, I knew that I was being guided by a very high intelligence, far beyond my own. Perhaps it was meant to be, that I was to get this out to the world.

After our experience in that special meadow, I had to figure out which of the 15 different herbs we were eating were causing the mucoid plaque to come out so fast. I narrowed it down to about 6 herbs, and it was with these herbs that I first began to experiment. I quickly found that if we took too much of certain herbs, we had very undesirable reactions. In fact, all sorts of symptoms developed. I knew that I needed to be very careful and find the exact amounts of each herb to perfect the combination. I experimented over and over on myself. After making the necessary adjustments, I was ready to do a full cleanse. My friend was also willing to be a guinea pig, as he also felt that this was really something that could benefit our bodies. I felt confident that I finally had the right combinations, and that we were truly ready to do a full program.

We were not to eat anything during the full cleanse. Six days later, without even preparing on the gentler phases (which would have increased the amount eliminated), I had passed a total of 40 feet of unbelievably gnarly mucoid matter. My friend had passed 28 feet and this on his first cleanse. He had taken no enemas and on the fourth night of our cleanse, he got up and went downstairs and had a potato feast! Of course, this slowed him down. Even so, cleansing still did him a lot of good, and he went around telling everyone how much he got out and how wonderful he felt.

My former wife's first cleanse was just as successful. Having only done one other "cleanse" before and getting nothing out at all, she was only doing it to appease me. In seven days she passed 37 feet of the old, mucoid gunk and a few parasites. She was so thrilled she continued to cleanse about every seven weeks for the first year. She intends to keep cleansing until nothing more comes out!

## Only Highest Quality Herbs

The natural supplements industry has expanded radically in the past 10 years, and in many cases, the demand for herbs has exceeded the supply. As a result, herbs suppliers are rushed and scraping the bottom of the barrel in many cases, and the quality of many herbs has suffered in the process.

If you're going to spend the money for a product that you want to help your body, you will be wise to pay the extra and get the highest quality herbs. How can I guide you in this? It is very difficult to know for there are so many variables. Was the herb wild-crafted or organically grown? If so, was it picked properly, at the right time of the year, month, and day? Was it dried and handled properly? How was it stored? Was it picked in an area away from cities, airports, and freeways? Or was it grown with chemicals and picked in a commercial manner, by machines, etc., or even fumigated with toxic chemicals before it entered the United States?

When you examine as many herbs as we do, you learn about these things. You hear about what is going on behind the industry's polished public doors. You get educated, sometimes by hard knocks. With my own organization, I have set the highest standards possible. I have been involved with several different manufacturers. After they listened to my quality specifications, they usually tell us how refreshing it is that someone really cares about the quality of their products. They tell us that most people are only concerned about when they can get the product and how much it is going to cost. I tell them that not only do I use my own herbal products, but so do my mother, brother, wife, all my friends, everyone who works for us, plus all the thousands of other people who trust me to recommend only the finest. Someone has to have good quality and by gum, I'll do everything I can to make it happen.

# A Program Adaptable to Individual Needs: Four Phases of Cleansing

For a cleanse to be effective and health nurturing, it must be geared toward the level of strength and health available in the body. **A deeper, more powerful cleanse releases old toxins very quickly; only a body which has already achieved a significant level of strength and health can handle this type of cleansing.** When one is weak or fighting illness at the outset of cleansing, the process must be taken very slowly, lest the body's ability to remove toxins be overwhelmed, resulting in increased but unnecessary stress, and extreme cleansing reactions. Hence, I have developed four phases of cleansing which can be alternated, as needed, to meet individual needs.

**The most important rule in using the phases:** On all four phases, **we should always feel good, at least as good as before we started the cleanse.** Anyone who feels exceptionally weak, tired, or just plain lousy, should first take an enema. If that doesn't help, take a coffee enema.[332] If that doesn't help, the person should go back to any of the earlier phases until feeling good again, and he or she may want to take some of the foods which are indicated to slow the cleanse process, then progress again through the phases at a comfortable pace. Allowing ourselves the luxury of feeling bad, can be hard on the liver, kidneys, heart, and brain, and is simply not necessary and is not a good idea.

## Alternating Between Phases

One of the advantages of these programs is that we can alternate between the four phases, in other words, switch back and forth from one to

---

[332] Coffee enema - **See Appendix III: How to Take Enemas and Implants.**

the other, as needed. **It is in this way that we can keep cleansing reactions to a minimum, boost our energy when needed, and keep feeling good while cleansing.** It's great for those who just do not have the will power to do the full cleanse (no meals), who have to work full-time, have an exceptionally heavy work schedule, have social obligations, have to deal with a great amount of toxicity, or have energy problems. Most people who do an ideal cleansing program, work full-time while they are doing the program. **Alternating between phases makes it possible for a person to work and still be in top condition.**

Example: let's say a person begins to pre-cleanse with two meals per day for four weeks, then spends a few days on the intermediate phase (one meal per day), and then progresses on to the final phase of the cleanse. Three days into the final phase, he starts feeling weak and it affects his work. Then it is a good idea to switch back to the intermediate phase, eating a meal once a day. Perhaps that perked him up and the next day he goes back to the final phase. If not, it may be a good idea to stay on the intermediate phase for a while or go back to one of the gentler phases. **Eating meals slows down the cleansing, and the toxic flow is lessened.** By the week-end or on his days off work, he may feel OK to use the full cleanse again. Then Monday he can go back to the one of the other phases again, if needed. It is good to be flexible.

Someone who is very ill or can't pass the pH tests, can alternate between the alternate beginning phase with 2-1/2 meals and the gentle phase with two meals. The point is that a person can control how he or she feels by switching from one phase to another,[333] still obtain maximum nutrition, and keep cleansing reactions to a minimum. **Yet, those who cannot pass the pH tests should not go beyond the mildest phase, until they have sufficiently boosted their electrolyte reserves so that they can pass the pH tests. To accomplish this, they should be sure to drink plenty of fresh, raw, organic vegetable juices and take natural electrolyte supplements made with vegetable juice concentrates and goat whey.** I have designed one which is available to supplement an ideal cleansing program. I have also designed another supplement to accomplish the same purpose for those who have sugar problems, such as diabetes, hypoglycemia, Candidiasis, etc.

---

[333] It is not normally a good idea to take a day off, or even water fast in the middle of cleansing, because the herbs have momentum. It's better to continue cleansing with two and one-half meals per day.

# Four Phases of Cleansing

## The Mildest Phase (Alternate Beginning)

This phase was developed to make cleansing possible for those who are significantly weak or ill when beginning cleansing. pH tests are used to determine if a person has the necessary electrolyte reserves to safely accomplish cleansing. If one cannot pass the pH tests, only this phase should be used. While cleansing on this phase, the cleanser may continue to check pH readings to determine when to increase intake of alkalizing mineral supplements, and also to determine when it is wise to proceed on to the next phase. When using this phase, the cleanser takes two and one-half alkaline-forming meals each day, in addition to a regimen of cleansing herbs and shakes. This phase is very gentle on the body, and yet can be a very effective aid towards increased strength and health for someone who starts in a weakened condition, or for those who simply want to take their cleansing at a more gradual pace. Once cleansers have achieved a level of stability with this regimen, that is, they are able to maintain it without uncomfortable cleansing reactions, they may safely progress on to the next phase of cleansing. Whenever cleansing reactions are experienced, the cleanser should 1) increase intake of alkaline minerals (which the body needs to remove toxins), 2) do enemas *if elimination is sluggish*, 3) increase intake of the two herbal formulas to achieve 3-4 easy eliminations daily, and 4) may take more foods which are indicated to slow down the cleanse process, such as potatoes.[334] On this phase and the gentle phase, use enemas only as needed. Many persons do not need any enemas during these phases.

## The Gentle Phase (Beginning)

The phase should be used as the beginning phase by most persons. **Some people try to skip this phase, thinking they don't need it. This is a mistake.** Even when your body is relatively healthy, **this phase is needed to give the herbs time to prepare and soften up mucoid plaque for most effective removal.** Some persons will find plenty of challenge and reward in this phase alone, and choose to do only the gentle phase in their first cleanse or two. This phase involves eating two alkaline-forming meals per day, and all the fresh carrot/celery/beet[335]

---

[334] **See the chart on Alkaline Foods before the Suggested Reading List in the back of this book.**

[335] Those with significant sugar sensitivity should avoid all sweet juices, both fruit and vegetable. However, they may want to take other fresh organic vegetable juices.

juice one desires, along with a complementary regimen of herbs and shakes. **After a cleanser has reached a level of stability where he or she can maintain the gentle phase comfortably, with no cleansing reactions, then that person may safely progress on to the next deeper phase of cleansing.** If cleansing reactions should persist *during any phase of cleansing*, even after following the steps outlined for handling cleansing reactions under the mildest phase, the cleanser should return to a milder phase of cleansing to slow the cleanse down and make it easier on the body.

## The Power Phase (Intermediate)

This phase demands more commitment, strength and body vitality. As you progress in this sequence of phases of cleansing, your body should steadily gain strength and vitality. Periods of feeling weak, nauseous or tired are usually indications of toxins being released faster than your body is able to eliminate them. This indicates either electrolyte deficiency or sluggish liver and/or kidney function. To resolve cleansing reactions, you may increase your intake of alkalizing minerals, do enemas as needed, and if they still persist, you may need to revert back to a less challenging phase of cleansing until your body regains its balance, and you feel better.[336] Many people will use the power phase as a test to determine whether they are really ready to do the master phase. After being on the power phase for two or three days without cleansing reactions, then they know they are ready for the master phase. Some people may stay on the power phase longer if they choose. On the power phase, the cleanser takes one alkaline-forming meal per day, and all the fresh juices one desires, along with a complementary regimen of herbs and shakes. As the amount of solid food intake is decreased, the body is freed more and more from its usual digestive tasks, and can devote increased attention to its cleansing priorities.

Note: *While on the power and master phases, pH tests are of no use, because the body will be removing so many acids that the tests will not reflect true electrolyte reserve levels.*

---

[336] **See Chapter 9: Facts About An Ideal Cleansing Program** for more information on cleansing reactions.

## The Master Phase (Final)

During this final phase of cleansing, no meals are taken. A regular regimen of herbs and shakes are taken to help the body remove sometimes astounding amounts of mucoid plaque. Fresh, organic fruit and vegetable juices, as well as high quality green superfood drinks may be taken for additional nourishment during this phase, which typically lasts one week. This phase is obviously the most challenging, and many also testify it is the most rewarding. Stories of seemingly miraculous healing are reported by cleansers who accomplish this phase of cleansing.

# Fresh, Organic Juices and Water Essential for Health and Cleansing

Drinking fresh juices from organically grown fruits and vegetables, on a daily basis, is one of the wisest and most effective things anyone can do to achieve and maintain good health. Organically grown foods have, on the average, double the nutritional value of commercially grown foods.[337] We need nutrition to be healthy; fresh juices supply concentrated levels of that nutrition. Not only that, but they are full of life-force! I suggest reading further books on juicing and fresh, organic juices.

One of the best aids to a powerful cleanse is the generous use of fresh, organic juices. They offer a concentrated source of live enzymes, as well as easily assimilated minerals and vitamins. These further prompt and strengthen the body's cleansing activity. **I encourage everyone who cleanses to obtain a good juicer and make their own fresh, organic vegetable juices.** Fruit juices are excellent, too. The citrus juices have the strongest cleansing effect, and should only be used with moderation (if at all) by those who have a high level of toxicity, and a tendency toward low pH. The only exception to my encouragement to use juices is that those with sugar sensitivity should avoid all sweet juices. Fresh organic juices are especially important during the final phase of cleansing when no solid food is taken.

The more juices we drink, the less water we desire. However, while cleansing and drinking juices it is essential to drink water, too. If you take 3 quarts of juice, take an additional 32 ounces a day of water (if you drink less juice, take more water). This should be pure, non-chlorinated water, preferably distilled which is stored in glass or extra high-grade plastic containers; not the standard supermarket grade plastic container.

---

[337] Heltman, pg. 12.

Water used for drinking should be fresh and pure, and free from all contaminants, including chemicals such as Chlorine and Fluoride. It may be clean well or spring water, water purified with a solid carbon block or other high quality unit, or distilled water. Many advocate distilled water for its added cleansing effects; it helps extract inorganic minerals and toxic waste from the body.

Some people have expressed concern about distilled water pulling out the body's electrolytes or organic minerals. About the only time this may appear to happen is when the body is already depleted of these elements. This condition would indicate that there is a problem in digestion, assimilation, or diet. It might also indicate a malfunction of the body, or an environmental problem. Dr. Walker had been drinking distilled water since 1930, and was in good health at the ripe age of 116! An interesting fact is that the liquids in fruit are identical to distilled water. That's one of the reasons why fruits are so cleansing and can succeed in helping the body repair itself, when all else fails. Drinking lots of juices obviously provides the body with some water.

Water is critical while cleansing because without enough water, elimination is slowed and cleansing reactions worsened. On a hot summer day, the average size person should drink about a gallon of water a day while cleansing (if no juices are taken); that is, about one ounce of water for each pound of body weight. On cooler days, at least 2 quarts of water are needed, but it is important to realize that it is better to have too much water than not enough.

# Super Results of the Final Phase

People doing my gentler cleansing regimen get wonderful results. They remove a great deal of toxicity from their bodies. **But, it is on the full cleanse, with adequate preparation on the beginning phases, that people obtain the miraculous results**. There is something about going without food that has incredible transformative powers. It seems to work on all levels of our being: the mental, emotional, spiritual, and the physical.

On the physical level, **when we stop eating, our bodies begin to seek out the *excess* proteins that are stored in our livers and kidneys, and even in our cells.**[338] **These are the proteins that are killing us**. Excess proteins not only acidify our bodies, because protein foods are acid foods, but they can clog everything up, and create mucus and congestion. That is one of the reasons that our livers and kidneys malfunction. When we fast, the stored proteins are attacked by our bodies and degraded into

---

[338] The liver can store large quantities of proteins; this is also true of the kidney and the intestinal mucosa (Mucoid Plaque), Guyton, pg. 831.

amino acids, [339] then deaminated and oxidized, and used just as though we were still eating.[340] We're like camels, only instead of storing large amounts of water to save our lives, we store proteins which are killing us. Fasting is not starvation. Proper fasting never attacks the proteins we need; only the ones we don't need. Congestion is the primary cause of disease on the physical level. Fasting removes congestion. **Imagine, removing all this excess protein and everything else that is clogging up our systems!**

Talk about relief! As of the time of this writing, all persons I know of who accomplished my cleanse and had critical high blood pressure, found their blood pressure normal before they finished the intermediate phase. There was only one exception to this - a man doing the cleanse in the hospital. He had suffered a great deal because of the equipment attached within him. Even so, his blood pressure improved by 50%. People with bone cancer pain (about the worst pain of all), found 75% of their pain gone within 6 days.[341] We have many testimonies of people with severe back pain gone, or greatly reduced, before finishing the cleanse. Hundreds of people have reported their pains disappearing while cleansing. What do you suppose is happening to our bodies when we get relief so quickly like this?

Several years back I received a call from a RN. She wanted me to see a man who had liver cancer and cirrhosis of the liver. "I can't see him right now." I said. "I just returned from traveling and I am missing some parts to my microscope." She begged me to see him. "He is in a great deal of pain and the medical doctors have completely given up on him and they say there is nothing they can do." Reluctantly I let him come in. The parts missing in my microscope were for taking photographs, and oh, how I wished I had them. If you ever have seen red blood cells (RBC) from a cirrhosis patient, you would faint. They look something like stars in stark contrast to the circular shapes of normal blood cells. This man had almost no normal blood cells. I finished my analysis and offered my suggestions. Two days later she called to tell me his pain was completely gone. Two

---

[339] Parasites and bacteria are also made of mostly protein. Imagine on a long fast what might happen to these guys. Ahh, we have the picture now. So maybe this is why the greatest and most incredible individuals who ever walked the earth, fasted so many times. Fasting cleans up the body, mind, emotions, and spirit. However, in this day and age, we have exceptionally over-polluted bodies, which are saturated with large amounts of chemicals and drugs, and **we cannot fast like they used to without intelligent preparation**.

[340] Guyton, pg. 833.

[341] These persons used coffee enemas, along with the regular cleanse program.

days later he came in again. The normal RBC's were substantially increased and the star shapes reduced significantly. His edema was less. About two weeks later, his energy had significantly improved, he didn't need his cane anymore, no pain, his skin was brighter and looked more alive, his edema was much less. The nurse wept while in my office. "Why oh why are medical doctors so resistant to cleansing, diet, nutrition, and everything else you teach us?" After 30 days from our first meeting, all his edema was gone, his cane was history, he was talking about going back to work, only about 20% of his red blood cells were still star shaped, his face and skin looked entirely different, and he was feeling much more energetic.

What was this man doing that made him improve so much? He was doing a partial cleanse, using enemas, alkalizing his body through supplements, diet, and juices, taking nutritional supplements such as antioxidants, minerals, enzymes, etc., herbs, visualizing, doing breathing exercises, chiropractic, acupuncture, etc. Did he live? I had to go back to Mt. Shasta and lost touch with him. I do not know how he fared. There was still much more that needed to be done. However, naturopaths cannot be licensed in California and I will not practice here. Not only that, but the authorities do not look kindly on people using methods that deal with the cause of disease. They constantly look for ways to get rid of people like me. They even set up traps.[342] It is very risky business to practice true healing in the United States unless you use drugs, radiation, and surgery. Everything effective is seriously frowned upon. And now that I am so well known, I don't dare treat anyone, even on the phone. Now you know why so many doctors leave the country and why so many people leave the country to be treated.

I have a friend, the sweetest person you ever saw, who spent 2 years in prison because she was helping people with cancer. People would call her and ask where they could go to be treated for cancer. She told them about clinics in Mexico that she felt were effective in treating cancer. She developed a reputation and people were calling her from all over America and she helped the best she knew how. All she wanted was to help people. It cost her two years in prison.

At the time of this writing I have several lawyers working for me to make certain that I do not say anything, do anything, or write anything that can get me in trouble. When I do say things I make certain that I word everything just right. **I hope that you will begin a campaign and get people to write to their congressman, senators, governors, and president and demand medical and health freedom. Demand to allow**

---

[342] Lynes, pg. 35.

naturopaths to practice in your state. **Demand that the FDA and AMA be investigated.**[343]

# How Long Do I Stay on the Cleanse?

An ideal cleanse program for the average person is suggested to last four weeks, with two and one half weeks on the gentle phase, one half week on the power, and one week to 10 days on the master phase. This guideline should be modified and tailored to meet individual body needs, according to how each person's body responds while cleansing. That is, a person who has high levels of toxicity to deal with will take the program more slowly, spending more time on the gentler phases in preparation for accomplishing the final phase at a point where the body can handle it without serious cleansing reactions.

**There are no instructions that can give everyone the perfect suggestions for their unique conditions. You are the one responsible for your own body. ALWAYS USE YOUR OWN INTUTION AND COMMON SENSE.** When on the two most gentle phases of my cleanse program, we can continue cleansing as long as we feel good about it - exceptions are for the very weak and sick. Regardless of which phase we're on, we should always remember to take the bacteria at least one hour before bedtime (an hour or more after the last set of herbs in the evening).

## Never Feel Hungry

Many people do not believe us when we say that while on the cleanse you won't feel hungry. You will be so full of herbs and juices that you really won't. Some may still struggle with the desire to eat, nonetheless, because of old habits. This desire is not necessarily related to hunger.

People would be amazed how little food they really need. Most people eat about four times more food than they really need and this causes problems. Going without food once in awhile helps to tone up the body, and gives it a chance to eliminate a great deal of unwanted substance. When people do eat, they need to eat good quality food. They also need the ability to digest and assimilate it. I also strongly believe that people need to get in touch with their own bodies and learn to know what it needs and

---

[343] Ibid., See Chapters 2 and 3, and especially pg. 33 and 34. Also, **See Chapter 1 under "Facts of Medical History," and Chapter 5: The Intentional Development of Modern Disease.**

when. We need to be able to distinguish the difference between food desires and real bodily needs. We need to practice being still and to feel deeply what our bodies are trying to tell us. **Two common problems prompt many people to overeat**: 1) failure to eat nourishing, organically grown foods (This causes the body to be constantly hungry because it never gets the nutrients it needs, and 2) inability to digest and assimilate food properly. One of the main causes of over eating in this country occurs when parents tell their children to clean up their plates. This destroys their own innate knowingness of when to stop. **Healthy people do not need to eat very much**. As long as parents are feeding their children top quality food, organically grown foods, they seldom need to be concerned whether or not they are getting enough.

# How Often Can I Cleanse?

For the enthusiast, **every seven to ten weeks** is recommended if using the full cleansing program, and as long as you have passed the pH tests. Most people receive terrific benefits cleansing once every six months. That is my recommendation for the average person. If only using one or both of the two most gentle phases of the cleanse, you may do whatever feels right, and as long as good, nutritious eating habits are followed. In two to three years many people could achieve a state of health that would absolutely delight them. This has been found to be true of people even in their 80's, and it certainly was for me. Many people are rather amazed at me, especially when they try to keep up with me in climbing a mountain; and even more so, when they consider how sick I was when I started cleansing. I should also tell you that I haven't developed the most perfect eating habits either. I still have my periods of pig-outs and bad meals. At least I know what to do about it when I do those things. I must say, I am a researcher and I research everything that offers potential of health improvement; but I have never found anything that deserved so much attention as an ideal cleansing program, and I have never found anything that can bring a person back to health as rapidly or effectively as this can. When we combine this program with the other alternative healing methods available, I believe that we can achieve almost any degree of health imaginable. For this program will greatly enhance every other constructive healing method known and may very well make the difference between success or failure, and to some, life or death.

# How Many Cleanses are Necessary to be Completely Cleaned Out?

Every person is different. With me, it took about twelve cleanses; however, I did not have the advantages that are available now. For the first nine cleanses I used other methods, which I call "mini-cleanses" (colon cleanses). On those cleanses about 12 -14 feet was eliminated in seven days. Towards the end, after modifying them, I eventually got rid of 28 feet; and when I finally had an ideal cleansing program to use, nearly 50 feet. So people who start with an ideal cleansing program should be able to do better than I did. Dr. Jensen says that it sometimes takes several cleanses before some people can remove *any* mucoid plaque. Fortunately that is not the case with an ideal cleansing program. The vast majority of people get results right away, if the instructions are followed carefully.

If you read the Chapter (3) on Mucoid Plaque, you may have picked up my hint that many people may never get rid of their mucoid plaque because something inside the gut keeps creating more. Usually the cause of this will be undesirable microorganisms or heavy metals, or a return to too many acid-forming foods in the diet (which creates electrolyte deficiency). It is also a good idea to check the irises of your eyes both before and four weeks after cleansing to better understand the pace at which your body is able to eliminate toxic accumulations and congestion that are reflected there. If no change or only partial lightening of marks indicating distressed areas is noticeable, further cleansing and rebuilding is needed.[344]

The substance that can be removed during a seven-day period may be astounding. Most people should enjoy a noticeable improvement in their health within a few days after cleansing. I don't know a single exception to this aside from those who were either over-acid, did not follow the directions, used salt during the cleanse or had some other rare situation.[345] However, seven days of cleansing will not remove all the mucoid layers in the intestinal tract. Many, many years have been spent building layer upon layer of this substance throughout the entire alimentary canal. There is practically no limit as to how thick the layers can become. On a thin person, the layers may be one-fourth of an inch thick. A heavy person tends to accumulate more. One colon was known to be 18 inches thick in diameter and had a passageway through the center that was 1/4 of

---

[344] **See Chapter 8: How to Determine If You Need the Cleanse Thyself Program, under "Reading the Eye: Iridology."**

[345] There have been some people who complained that they didn't feel better after the Cleanse. I was shocked, and so I investigated. I found that each person with that complaint (the average was less than 1 out of 100), had modified the Cleanse in various ways which made it something other than our program, and those people did not follow instructions for replenishing their friendly bacteria. Later I found some people who did everything right but felt worse after the Cleanse. I discovered that they were very acid, but after alkalizing their bodies they felt better than they had in many years.

an inch!  Six to eight weeks after the first cleanse, another seven-day cleanse may be taken.  (**Note:** if you are following either of the two most gentle phases of an ideal cleansing program, you can cleanse much more often and for much longer periods.)  If this program is followed and nutritious eating habits are maintained, within two to three years, a state of health can be achieved that will amaze even the greatest skeptics.  Again, this depends on the following.

### Factors Affecting Long Term Cleanse Results

♦ the condition you are presently in, including your attitudes and subconscious patterns
♦ how closely you follow the cleansing instructions
♦ how well you eat between cleanses
♦ which phases of the cleanse you follow

# Motivation for Cleansing

Right now you may be thinking - I'm not even sure I want to do one cleanse, let alone one every six to eight weeks!  To you, my friend, let me simply encourage you to try it for the first time.  Even if you only did a cleanse once a year, you would be giving your body enormous relief, saving it from the tiresome task of spending all its energy digesting and protecting itself from the overload of proteins and toxic matter we thoughtlessly dump into it three times a day (this doesn't even include snacking and coffee breaks). How much is your health worth to you?  This once-a-year vacation would give the body a chance to take a breather and devote its energy to healing itself.  Besides, you may change your mind once you make it through the first time.  The most important thing is to muster your courage and venture a first step into the unknown.

It's true, not everyone can do this.  You will be distinguishing yourself from most of mankind who accept ill-health as a cruel twist of fate and unconsciously struggle blindly through life, or who have neither the wisdom nor the courage to remove causes of potential suffering and disease.  These kinds of people will not take responsibility for their lives, have victimized themselves and have become totally dependent upon others for their security.  Not only will you be saved from their fate, but after you have completed your first cleanse, you won't be made of the same old stuff anymore and not only will you know this from experience, but you will be mighty pleased.  You will be proud of yourself, and realize that **the stuff of which you are now really made** *is* **better than what you were made of before you took the cleanse!**

# Iris Reflects Health Improvement after Cleansing, Eye Color May Even Change

Some cleansers have reported significant changes in their iridology, which reflect improvements in their physical condition, after cleansing. Markings indicating congested or stressed areas will lighten and sometimes disappear. As noted in Chapter 8, it is wise to have a reading of one's iridology before cleansing, and again 3-5 weeks after completion of your cleanse.[346]

My friend Jonni Sue Perlman's eyes changed dramatically after cleansing. They went from brown like her mother's, to greenish hazel. We both expect her eyes will soon be a beautiful blue. When she started cleansing, she was already in excellent health. She is always exercising and has been a vegetarian for more than 20 years. So the strength of her body is capable of making rapid changes.

# How Long Will It Take to Really Get Well?

This depends on the constitutional strength of the individual, the length of any disease or affliction, what the problems were, the mental and emotional attitudes, the dietary habits, how closely the person follows the cleanse instructions, etc. Dr. Jensen says that it generally takes about ten years to bring a sick person back to truly good health. I think he was very realistic, based upon his techniques. However, I believe that with an ideal cleansing program, the use of certain herbal formulas, an exceptional diet of energizing raw foods and juices, and the use of other new, advanced products that are available which he didn't have back when he had his sanitarium, we can cut it down from ten to about three years.

However, most people cannot switch to a completely raw food diet immediately and maintain it without difficulty. They must alter their diet more gradually. The problem is that the standard American diet, which most of us were raised on, weakened our digestive strength. It takes time to develop the ability to digest and assimilate raw foods efficiently. Many people lack the hydrochloric acid, enzymes, minerals, and necessary

---

[346] **See Chapter 8: How to Determine if You Need the Cleanse Thyself Program, under "Reading the Eye: Iridology,"** for a chart of the irises of the eye, and some basic guidelines to help you understand markings you may find in your irises.

bacteria. Our bodies are so used to doing things a certain way that it takes time and specific stimuli to gradually rebuild our enzyme production and switch our bacteria into the healthy balance required to thrive on raw foods. Not only that, but if the mucoid plaque has been altered to a certain degree or we have too much mucoid plaque, we may not be able to assimilate raw food efficiently.

**Of course the length of time the entire cleansing process takes depends mainly on how quickly the cleanser can change his or her belief system, for that is the primary factor.** It also depends upon the self-control, will, and determination of a person. Most people who just take the cleanse once have incredible results. For others they usually know that wonderful progress was made, and more needs to be done. One of the keys is what we do between cleanses. But most important of all is the past programming of our subconscious mind and how quickly that can be changed. Many people are programmed to sabotage their health. This must be changed.

# Cleansing Reactions

**A cleansing reaction or cleansing response IS NOT the same as either a disease crisis or a healing crisis.** A cleansing reaction is merely a noticeable reaction from too many toxins getting into the bloodstream. It could cause a temporary headache, dizziness, nausea, brain fog, weakness, lack of energy, discharges, sneezing, skin eruption, ringing in the ears, coughing or pain, or a reappearance of other old symptoms. Depending on the toxicity of the body, there may be various cleansing reactions. These cleansing reactions differ from person to person. If people do an ideal cleanse properly, they never need to feel badly. Some, however, don't follow the directions; they go right into the final phases without adequate preparation. They may have failed to use the pH tests and build their electrolyte reserves. These people may have serious challenges. **The weaker or more toxic a person is, or the more foul the intestinal tract, the greater the likelihood there will be cleansing reactions; and the more these reactions are experienced, the more the body is crying out to be cleansed.**[347]

---

[347] Ironically, the worse off a person is, the less likely they are to cleanse, fast or even change their diet. Not only does this type of person have less energy available for making *any* changes in his/her life, but he/she also demonstrates a weak will and lower intelligence; these characteristics may likely also contribute to the physical troubles. Most of the people who cleanse are highly intelligent and express a significant degree of spiritual awareness.

For most people, the most serious cleansing reactions may occur when they stand up after lying or sitting down. When toxins are coming out of our bodies, some of them enter the bloodstream in the form of excess mucus and proteins. This can cause a temporary thickening of the blood. This is normal and is necessary for the toxins to work their way out. However, this condition can slow the circulation to the point that standing up too fast can cause a pause in the oxygen getting to the brain. Some people may find that when they stand up, they get dizzy. I know two cases where people even passed out. Though this does not occur too often, people should be aware that this could happen. If you find this is beginning to happen, then **make yourself stand up slowly. Keep your head down and be careful.** This used to happen to me. When I would go to stand up, I moved slowly. When I was in a hurry, I walked bent over for a few seconds, until I felt normal. After several cleanses, this symptom stopped.

People with Candidiasis are more prone to feel weak or tired while cleansing. When people fall into this category, I sincerely hope they will not let that stop them. I had Candida, and on my first ten cleanses, I didn't feel too well - not all that bad, but weak. In those early days I did not have the good sense to do bacterial implants, nor to avoid fruit, fruit juices and even carrot and beet juice. That was a serious mistake and at times the Candida became worse after the Cleanse. In most cases, this problem can be easily avoided if one takes large amounts of bacteria during the cleanse.[348] After my second time on my cleanse program, I knew what to avoid and experienced almost no cleansing reactions; I even felt better on the Cleanse than while eating. Not only that, but the Candida symptoms gradually disappeared until they were all gone. Now I recommend that people with Candidiasis take bacteria three or four times a day during the cleanse and after cleansing take it three times daily with double dosages. They must avoid all sweet fruit and vegetable juices, and should consult with a practitioner familiar with their condition, and with digestive cleansing.

Most reactions to cleansing fall into three general categories. **Meat-eaters** have more reactions than vegetarians, only because as a rule, they have much more filth to eliminate due to devouring already-used, toxic dead animal proteins; plus the steroids, antibiotics, and other drugs they ingest from eating the poor animals. For cattle and other domesticated farm animals are given unbelievable amounts of drugs during their short

---

[348] Bacteria in the gut help keep Candida and other yeast in check. This is why antibiotics cause so much Candidiasis. Any effective cleanse will remove bacteria and yeast. However, it will remove bacteria first, and yeast symptoms could accelerate. Therefore, it is important that anyone who has any kind of yeast infection should take extra bacteria while cleansing.

lives. Another group of people who can have some powerful cleansing reactions are those who have used a great deal of drugs. **Drugs** are not always eliminated from the body. Often they are stored somewhere and with intense cleansing, they can be reactivated. However, when used according to the cleansing directions, the action of bentonite in the psyllium shake tends to immediately absorb any drug that was stored in the intestinal tract, and most people have almost no noticeable effects. Some people do claim to taste the old drug when it surfaces during cleansing, but it does not cause any further difficulty than that. Another group of people who should be alerted to any severe or unusual cleansing reactions are those who may have been exposed to **heavy metal toxicity**. To my knowledge, no one using my cleanse program has ever experienced this type of toxicity being released in a way that caused any problem. And I have been in touch with thousands of people using my cleanse. However, anyone attempting water fasting (a more advanced cleansing method, as **discussed in Chapter 14: Secrets of Super Health**) should be alerted to this issue. Lead and mercury seem to be the worst. Lead especially can accumulate in the body for years. If lead deposits are released by the body during water fasting, the results can be dangerous. This happened to me during some intense water fasting and I was very ill for quite some time. I finally went on my cleanse again and used nutritional products and homeopathics to clear it all out. It worked very well.[349]

There are many who have "**leaky bowel syndrome**". This means that the bowel wall has stretched and become more porous, so larger materials can pass through the wall. Occasionally, a very toxic mucoid layer may loosen from the intestinal wall and its toxic debris will flood the system with toxic waste. If this occurs, one may have allergy-like reactions, feel nauseous or simply weak. That's the time for an extra enema or colonic, as these help to get rid of the toxins quickly. As soon as the toxic substance is eliminated, we'll feel better immediately. If after an enema a person does not feel better, it may indicate that the liver is unable to deal with the toxic elimination fast enough. A coffee enema may offer impressive relief. See the tonsils - no, I mean the Appendix, in the back of the book.[350]

During the first few cleanses, it is somewhat common to **feel stuffed or bloated** - something a little beyond full. As the herbs soften the mucoid plaque, it swells slightly and we feel bloated. We can also feel stuffed because we have so much psyllium in us. The bloating diminishes more and more as the mucoid plaque is eliminated. I never feel bloated anymore, no matter how much psyllium I take, but I can feel stuffed.

---

[349] **See the section on "Heavy Metals" at the end of this Chapter.**

[350] **See Appendix III: How to Take Enemas and Implants.**

With the very **sick, elderly, weak, or those who are extremely over-acid**, caution is very much advised. Almost everyone needs to eliminate more, but some are too weak to eliminate rapidly. When we begin to use cleansing herbs, the body may click into high gear and start eliminating from anywhere and everywhere. This causes what some would consider alarming symptoms. These individuals should ease into herbal programs more cautiously (following one of the beginning phases with two and one half or two meals per day, for several months), possibly with the supervision of a health professional who has had a lot of experience in herbal cleansing, as well as the equipment to test the body's conditions. If you can find such a rare health professional, you will be fortunate indeed. Their successes being so high, they are often under constant suspicion and the watchful eye of the AMA and FDA. In fact, the moment they have even a tiny slip-up, they are jailed immediately. Many of the great healers or promoters of alternative approaches to health have been illegally imprisoned; Dr. Christopher, V.E. Irons, Dr. Reams, Stanley Burroughs, and even Dr. Jensen,[351] to name a few of some of the most caring, beautiful people that have blessed our country. The truth is they got off easy. Many other doctors fared far worse.

# Healing Crisis

The healing crisis can be a scary experience for uninformed individuals. When we finally do things right, like cleanse, fast, and eat right, we will draw back out of us the toxins, poisons, and emotions that we have put in and which have made us sick. When these things surface we sometimes think that we are getting worse instead of better. In that process we can easily lose our common sense and stop doing the things that are making us well. This often occurs when friends or relatives are not informed about the benefits and actions of cleansing. Well-intentioned relatives have persuaded many people to stop cleansing or fasting, even though it was the best thing for their health. Therefore, it is important to understand the healing crisis.

**The healing crisis is a great blessing. It is something we enthusiastically work toward.** When it happens we should rejoice, knowing that we have eliminated some more causes of disease. It means that we have cleansed and purified our bodies from unwanted toxic waste which was poisoning the body, mind, and feelings, causing weakness and

---

[351] According to Dr. Jensen, every time they put him in jail, they did it on a Friday evening so he could not contact the bank for bail money. It was always harassment; he never did anything wrong, and was always released.

potential disease. **After the healing crisis we are always stronger than before, for the darkness is replaced with the light**.

This process is the exact opposite of what allopathic medicine does with its drugs. Drugs suppress and block, driving disease into deeper levels or into other areas of the body. This temporarily changes the focus of symptoms and gives the false appearance of getting well. The truth is, the cause is still there and will erupt at a later time, possibly at a more critical time when we are less capable of coping with it. Cleansing, fasting, herbs, and changing consciousness **can bring the disease causing agents to the surface, and eliminate the cause of disease and symptoms permanently**. The right diet and a positive attitude rebuilds.

**The experience of going through a healing crisis will seem very much like having a disease crisis. It is important to know the difference**. If we are going through a healing crisis we need to know that **it will soon pass** and that we are just getting rid of the cause of disease.

Joe Schecter of Tucson had accomplished about 9 Cleanses and started working on his gallbladder. One day he called. "Rich, how could it be that with all the cleansing I have done, that I could get asthma?"

"What do you mean?" I asked.
"I have all the symptoms - wheezing, coughing, and breathing is shallow."
"Well", I said, "when did you have asthma before?"
"When I was in grade school."
"Expect it to last for about 3 days. If it lasts longer than that, call me."
I didn't hear from him for a couple of weeks and when he came in I said, "How long did your asthma last?"
"My what? Oh, I forgot about that. Yeah, it went away in 3 days just like you said."

My former wife had gone on the cleanse three times in a seven-month period. On her third cleanse (having never had any cleansing reactions before), she finished the seven days as usual and then, for the first time, began to eat only raw fruits and vegetables. (She would usually just go back to her regular diet, which included some cooked foods.) Then the cleansing reactions set in. She had every symptom of the walking pneumonia and bronchitis she had suffered in her childhood and early 20's. However, this time she rejoiced, for she knew that she was ridding herself of those symptoms forever. After ten days of telling herself and certain well-meaning individuals (who kept insisting that she had abused her body with "that fast") that she was just experiencing a valuable "healing crisis," her health returned bringing a beautiful gift. Before the cleanse, every time she exercised or even climbed stairs, she would wheeze and feel a heavy congestion being stirred up in her chest. After that ten-day period, those symptoms disappeared and now they do not recur even when she's back-packing or playing tennis.

# What is a Disease Crisis?

**A disease crisis is the opposite of a healing crisis**. Instead of getting better, one gets worse. A disease crisis is a condition in which the disease has developed to the point in which it has become noticeable and uncomfortable. It has the potential of causing damage to metabolic function.

**Note**: The common cold is not a disease crisis. It is a cleansing response. The good old American cold occurs after we have abused the body and the body dumps the overload of toxins. The cold is a good thing. No one should ever attempt to stop it with drugs, but instead, assist the body in eliminating its congestion through enemas, baths, herbal teas, and eating pure foods, such as vegetable juices and broths. Allowing a cold to finish its cycle ALWAYS results in people feeling better and stronger. Stopping a cold with drugs ALWAYS results in future health problems.

# How To Know If It is a Healing Crisis or a Disease Crisis

**The healing crisis is the opposite of the disease crisis**. The healing crisis is gaining health - eliminating disease. The disease crisis is losing health.

**Disease Crisis - The Curse of Bad Habits**

* Comes with the warning of not feeling right
* Caused by not taking care of our bodies, bad diet, stress, poor living habits
* **Body has become consistently weaker and weaker - body vitality lowered**
* Eliminative process is usually sluggish and incomplete
* The iris of the eye will usually show white areas **rising above** the iris
* These acute lines are usually **straight or parallel** to the trabeculae
* Acute lines are usually raised above the trabeculae and as they go down they become darker
* Usually lasts 3 or 7 days, but can be much longer

* **Usually comes with the warning of feeling terrific the day before the crisis!**
* Caused by taking good care of body, good diet, rest, good living habits
* **Body vitality has become consistently stronger**
* Elimination is usually improved
* Healing is usually rapid
* The iris may show **white criss-crossed** "healing lines" (calcium luteum lines) **below the normal iris level**
* These criss-crossing healing lines are **not parallel** to the trabeculae [352]
* Usually lasts 3 days, but can be longer or shorter
* Often during the crisis people remember having had the same problem at some time in the past.

# Summary of Healing Crisis

**No one has ever died from a healing crisis**. The body never makes a mistake and will not develop a healing crisis until the body is strong enough to handle it. **The day prior to a healing crisis we usually will feel terrific**. Lots of energy. Apparently, the body uses that energy to release something out of itself, for it usually occurs after we hit the peak of energy; the next day is usually the day it starts. A healing crisis **usually** lasts only three days. However, it can last much longer, depending upon what is being released and how long it has been there, vitality, strength of the elimination organs, etc. **A person may need to go through many small healing crises before going through the final one.** As the cleansing or healing crises occur, they usually follow a certain order. This order is called Hering's Law Of Cure.

# Hering's Law of Cure

1. Cure from within out.
2. From head down.
3. And in reverse order as disease has developed.

I have given several examples of the healing crisis, but Dr. Jensen tops all of mine. Here is a good example of a healing crisis from his book *Doctor-Patient Handbook.*[353] "Years ago I put a man, **almost blind and**

---

[352] For illustrations on many conditions see Iridology: The Science and Practice of the Healing Arts, Vol. II, Ed. 1, pg. 122.

**with heart trouble**, on a regular health routine of diet, exercise, and rest. About three months after starting treatment, I was called to his home. This man was having a heart crisis. His heart was beating so forcibly that his bed was moving on its casters. I knew this was a crisis and that he would come through all right. His crisis lasted twelve hours. **Almost immediately afterward he was able to read the newspaper for the first time in years. Later he was able to read fine print, and in about two months he attended a motion picture show.**"

**Usually people forget what pain, injuries, or disease they had in the past, until they're having a healing crisis.** Then as they are experiencing the trouble, they remember that "this has happened before."

Another good example comes from the *Doctor-Patient Handbook:* "... had an extreme curvature of the spine. As her healing progressed, she developed a severe 'cold' which lasted 15 or 20 days. It was necessary to assist her eliminative process with frequent eliminative treatments. During one of these treatments, she underwent the retracing of an experience she had gone through in an accident 15 years previously. For a few moments, she seemed to go all to pieces. **Her tongue swelled and she could hardly talk. For 15 minutes or so her body shook all over. She seemed to be in a critical condition,** but after this experience was over, the spinal tension disappeared, the curvature was decreased, and there was constant improvement in the spine throughout the following year. She felt better than she had in many years."[354]

# The Tongue

Many people notice that as they cleanse, their tongues turn whitish gray and filmy and the breath is foul. This somewhat reflects what is happening inside the digestive canal. As they use the herbs and drink fresh juice, mucoid layers will soften some, and they may notice that the abdomen swells. As more and more mucoid layers are removed, the swelling will go down, and the tongue becomes more and more clear. This is a good gauge as to how clean a person is becoming, **for when you are totally clean, the tongue will be shiny red (just like a newborn baby's). It will be free of all whiteness or film and the breath will be**

---

[353] Jensen, D.C., N.D., Ph.D., *Doctor-Patient Handbook*, (Escondido, CA: Bernard Jensen Publishing, 1976), pg. 54. For greater inspiration and more information, I suggest that everyone read Dr. Bernard Jensen's books. They are all good, but the *Doctor-Patient Handbook* explains the healing crisis very well.

[354] Jensen, D.C., N.D., Ph.D., ibid., pg. 54.

**permanently sweet** (unless we eat onions, garlic or dairy products). Even the bowel movements can become sweet-smelling, though poor eating will cause odors to return. Let this be a goal: to have a pleasant fragrance throughout.

# Identifying the Origin of Mucoid Plaque[355]

The cleanse I have developed is more than a colon cleanse. It can cleanse the entire gastrointestinal tract or alimentary canal - all the way from the tip of the tongue to the anus. This facilitates the lymph system to drain its toxic back-up, which allows all our elimination systems to function better. *It is critical to remember that proper diet and electrolyte levels must be maintained before, during and after removing mucoid plaque.* Although the colon tends to accumulate thicker layers than the other areas, the majority of what people will see coming out of them will be from the small intestine. Due to the way the intestinal wall is formed and because the mucoid layers have been adhering to the walls of the intestines for so many years, the mucoid layers naturally take on the same shapes and creases as the area where they were formed.

Those who have cleansed have seen these striations in their mucoid plaque, plus you can also see them in the pictures. Studying the photos in Chapter 3: Mucoid Plaque, and reading the following descriptions may help you to identify the locality, or source, of your evacuations. This could be of interest if there were certain problems that you wanted to correct. When we can identify where the plaque is from, we may be able to determine if some of our problems are about to be flushed down the toilet. In that case, hurrah!

## Descriptions of Plaque from
## Different Portions of the Digestive Tract

When the plaque comes from **the stomach**, it has no striations, generally looking like amorphous globs of rubbery mucus. When plaque comes from the upper small intestines, it normally has definite striations. Generally these striations are easily seen. **The duodenum is the first portion**, located just below the stomach. About 10 inches in length, here important digestive juices from the gall bladder and pancreas enter the intestines. It is also in the duodenum where important digestive enzymatic activities should occur to prepare food for proper digestion. The striations or folds of the duodenum are marked and multi-directional, flowing out

---

[355] **See photos of mucoid plaque in Chapter 3: Mucoid Plaque, following the section, "What is Mucoid Plaque?"**

from and around small circles which reveal the locations of pancreatic and bile ducts. The **jejunum is located just below the duodenum**. About eight and 1/2 feet long, here the special cells of the intestinal wall secrete various chemicals to be combined with gall bladder and pancreatic juices. In this manner, the small intestine controls the digestive process. The majority of nutrients are assimilated here, and in the ileum. The folds in the jejunum are large, closely packed and run in one direction. **The upper ileum is found just below the jejunum**. About 12 feet in length with the lower ileum, assimilation is its major function. The folds are shallower and fade away as it approaches the colon. The striations disappear in the plaque from the **lower ileum**; this plaque is smooth in texture and usually shiny with no bumps, striations, or curvy shapes. **The colon** has no striations, but does have definite bumpy shapes and overlaps caused by its accordion-like haustrations.

## Results of Mucoid Plaque in Specific Locations

The following is hypothetical and I would like to be able to put in more study to discover the realities of this theory, but, let's say someone had thyroid trouble. While on the cleanse, she was able to identify the source of the plaque as coming from the jejunum area of the small intestine. This is where the Peyer's patches are located. The Peyer's patches may have a direct effect upon the thyroid. If mucoid plaque were in the Peyer's patches area, then by nerve reflex, the thyroid could be affected. Elimination of plaque from that area is a good clue that her thyroid may improve.

Another example: If a person has pancreatic trouble or digestive problems due to lick of bile salts or lack of digestive enzymes, and we identified a segment of mucoid plaque as having come from the duodenum area, chances are that his/her problem will improve. In this case, any plaque buildup in the duodenum area could have an effect upon the function of the pancreatic and bile ducts. Interference with these ducts could affect digestion. It's fun to try and identify these pieces. If we are fortunate, and we use an ideal cleansing program, our first cleanse will eliminate obstructions in this area. If not on the first cleanse, it is important to persevere with repeated cleanses (allowing a minimum of 4-6 weeks between each cleanse), until the duodenum area is freed up; for if this area is covered with layers of mucoid plaque, the secretions from the digestive glands would just flow under the mucoid matter, never even reaching our food! If the mucoid layers exerted sufficient pressure, a back-up could occur in these glands, causing sluggish activity or even a possible shut-down of them.

In summary, it may be enlightening to identify the physical origins of mucoid plaque; it can help us know which organs may need special attention with post-cleanse rebuilding, and confirm the cause of physical improvements we notice while cleansing. But it is even more enlightening to identify the emotional origin! Sometimes there are problems that hang on, no matter how much cleansing and fasting we do, and usually there will be some old sections of mucoid plaque that do not get released. Why? I believe it is due to certain deep-seated emotions that seem to hold related mucoid plaque in place. Many times I have seen the mucoid plaque suddenly release while on the mildest phase, within 12 hours after a core emotion and its cause was transformed. Not long ago I worked hard on the cause of an old emotional pattern. It was finally transformed and I told my wife that mucoid plaque would probably come out in the morning. It did.

# Psyllium or Mucoid Plaque?

Many have questioned whether they were indeed eliminating the mucoid plaque or just the psyllium. Here is how to tell: The psyllium, after passing through the body, is *never* evenly formed, never smooth, and never consistent in size or shape. It never has even lumps, creases, overlaps, smoothness, or striations, and it is never shiny like plaque usually is.

If you look carefully at the psyllium with a magnifying glass, it looks like miniature pollywog eggs. It has very tiny, egg-like centers with a jelly-like substance surrounding it (about 1/64 of an inch). You have to really scrutinize it to see that, but it's there. If you don't see it, then you are looking at mucoid plaque. However, the mucoid plaque may not always have (though it usually has some) striations, smoothness, overlaps, and creases. But it never looks like psyllium. The plaque is usually somewhat shiny and often looks like thin or thick pieces of leather or rubber.

Another way to identify plaque is to cut the eliminated material apart. It can usually be broken and examined. If you see a definite mass inside that is different from the outside, either in color or texture, then you know for sure that you have removed a mucoid layer.[356] The larger pieces usually look like hunks of leather or rubber rope. The psyllium is always on the inside and looks different from the plaque. Sometimes mucoid plaque comes out without the psyllium medium. Identifying these pieces is easy.

## No Mucoid Plaque!

Several years ago, I met the first person who claimed that no mucoid plaque came out of him during the cleanse. I asked him one

---

[356] The only exception is when we're on the intermediate or one of the beginning phases and still eliminating food, the inner part may be regular feces.

question after another to find out if he, like many other people, just didn't know how to identify mucoid plaque. Yes, he had followed the instructions perfectly. Indeed, his description of what was coming out of him did sound like psyllium. It turns out this man had been raised as a vegetarian from birth, on a farm in Germany, miles from the nearest city. They eat almost entirely from their own farm and most of it was raw. **He had never been sick in a day in this life**. He actually was brought up under what I would call, ideal conditions. I have never seen anyone else like him. His skin looked as though he were from another planet. It was 100% blemish and wrinkle free, smooth, soft, and radiant. His skin and hair glowed to such a degree that he looked a little unusual. He was extremely harmonious, confident, and happy, which was revealed in his mannerisms. I couldn't help but envy him a bit. I asked him if he had any benefits from the cleanse. He said that during the cleanse he felt spiritually elevated, but he had no physical benefits that he could tell. He felt perfect before the cleanse and felt perfect after the cleanse. When you're perfect, you can't get better.

## If Only Liquids or Small Pieces are Removed

Some people just get the small pieces out, maybe from microscopic to four or five inches, that look like little pieces of leather. Some of these people have complained that they are getting nothing out at all. One lady called from Phoenix. She said that she had been pre-cleansing for ten days and nothing had been eliminated. That was 30 psyllium shakes with nothing coming out! I knew that something was wrong, because if nothing was being removed, then she was the size of a rhinoceros and just as mean. Finally, she admitted that black liquids were coming out. So the next question was, how many herbs was she taking? She was taking tablets, 50 of each herbal formula a day, and the liquids were black. I explained to her that the herbs were pulverizing and liquefying the mucoid plaque. She kept waiting to see big chunks being removed and they were, but in liquid form. Unfortunately, we can't measure how much comes out that way, but I think it's considerable.

One doctor gave me a full day-by-day report of his cleanse. He took 40 tablets of one herbal formula a day, which caused him to eliminate the plaque in liquid form, but he felt he was getting rid of more that way and was not concerned about cutting back on the herbs and watching for the big pieces. One advantage to this method is that you don't need to take enemas, as there will likely be several eliminations a day. However, it is important to remember that each person is unique and responses to the same amounts of herbs may vary widely. Not only that, but our bodies change as we cleanse, and our needs change. In addition, the herbs themselves vary sometimes because of differences in where and how they were grown.

# Cleansing and Candida

Those who have Candidiasis and are planning to do my cleanse program should have very good results if they follow the guidelines below and use the friendly bacteria (probiotic) supplements correctly. However, those with advanced cases of Candida are strongly advised to secure the help of a qualified health practitioner who is familiar with digestive cleansing and with treating Candida. This practitioner should monitor their progress while cleansing, and adapt the program to meet their individual needs. **This is particularly important with Candida because it has so many complicating factors**.

Following are five important guidelines for cleansers who have Candida. 1. Do not have fruit juice on the cleanse. Use only water with the psyllium/bentonite shakes. 2. Take a high quality general use probiotic formula (with bacteria which are more alkaline-forming, including B. Infantis) at least 1 hour before bedtime throughout all phases of cleansing, one-half hour after each set of herbs and one-half hour after each meal. 3. Take ample amounts of a general use probiotic supplement orally, as well as doing rectal implants with it, as described in Appendix III: How to Take Enemas and Implants. 4. Begin using a second probiotic formula I designed specifically to help end yeast problems during the last week of the cleanse, and continue using the main probiotic formula. 5. Begin use of the formula for renewing or rebuilding the bowel wall approximately 3 hours after the last psyllium shake.[357]

In addition, since there is a strong emotional component with Candida overgrowth, it is critical to do some honest self-evaluation while cleansing, and make a strong effort to apply the mental and emotional cleansing principles discussed in Chapter 10: Optimize Your Cleanse. You may also want to secure the assistance of a trained professional who can guide you through an emotionally focused body cleansing practice such as breathwork. Unresolved emotions alone may precipitate a Candida outbreak, even if all other cleanse instructions are followed to the letter.

# Friendly Bacteria Essential

Failure to replace bacteria *after cleansing, fasting, or after using strong laxatives or antibiotics* can cause an overgrowth of pathogenic microorganisms that may already be present in the bowel. **This is so**

---

[357] Note: Because I continue to do research, formulas and suggestions change. Therefore contact my office for updates.

critical that I developed a general use probiotic formula especially for cleansers to use during and after cleansing. It may also be used any time you sense that your friendly bacteria may have been weakened due to improper diet, stress or even when you have been exposed to a "bug" you don't want to catch! Even when persons have started to 'come down' with something, using this formula has been reported to speed recovery time. With today's diet and lifestyles, using the correct bacterial formula is essential for good health. What is the correct friendly bacteria?[358]

Some persons have taken large amounts of *acidophilus*, thinking they were helping their bodies. Yet even doctors disagree about the uses of *Lactobacillus acidophilus*. In my opinion, *acidophilus* should be used as an agent to remove pathogenic bacteria, or sparingly, in combination with other bacteria that produce a higher pH. Everyone agrees that *lactobacillus*, such as *acidophilus*, has an important role in the treatment of pathogenic bacteria such as *E. coli*, *Salmonella*, etc.[359] However, it also produces an acid by-product with a pH between 4.5 and 3.9. Because of this extreme acidity, bowel problems are likely to occur if a more alkaline formula such as one containing bifidobacterium is not used after *acidophilus*.

**My experience indicates that the best *general probiotic formula* consists of *Bifidobacterium infantis*, along with a variety of other bifidobacteria, as well as a <u>small</u> percentage of *acidophilus*.** Bifidobacterium infantis is found in healthy, breast-fed infants, and is possibly the basic foundational bacteria for the human species. Since I began using this new bacteria, my health has moved up another notch. It is designed to replenish the normal, healthy bacteria and should be used any time your system has been weakened due to stress, poor diet, use of antibiotics, birth control pills, or other medical treatments.

I have also created a ***second probiotic formula*** to be used when we have symptoms indicating the presence of pathogenic microorganisms. Symptoms indicating a need for the second formula may include excessive gas, food poisoning, nutritional deficiencies, candida albicans, bacterial

---

[358] **See Chapter 14: Secrets to Super Health, under "Friendly Bacteria," and "The Perfect Bacteria" for more in depth information.**

[359] *Lactobacillus acidophilus* strain DDS-1, which is the preferred *acidophilus*, has proven to be the most effective natural intestinal antibiotic of which I am aware. Khem Shahani, Ph.D., "Antibiotic Acidophilin and Process of Preparing the Same," U.S. Patent 3,689,640, (Lincoln, NE: University of Nebraska, 1972).

infections, systemic toxicity, and a weakened immune system. The bacteria I include in the second formula are known to stimulate the production of immunologic factors.[360] This includes interlukin-1a, and tumor necrosis factor-1 by microphages.[361] They are also known to help eliminate various species of pathogenic bacteria, including: *Staphylococcus, Salmonella, Pseudomonas, Shigelfla, Klebsiella pneumoniae,* and *Sarcina lutea, Vibrio comma (Asiatic cholera),* and *Escherichia coli.*[362, 363] The second formula is specifically for yeast problems, as well as for addressing specific pathogenic bacteria such as those listed above.[364]

# Avoid Salt When Cleansing - If You Want It All Removed

I received a phone call once from one of our distributors. She told me that one of her customers had just taken the cleanse and nothing was eliminated. I knew who the person was. I knew that he had plenty of it in there, and that he must have been doing something very unusual to stop the cleansing process, and I wanted to know what it was, so I asked the distributor to get the facts. Later, during another phone call, she told me that he had followed the instructions in the book exactly. I again told her to dig deeper, find out everything, since he must have done something to keep the herbs from working. Soon I received another call. She said that the only thing that might be unusual is that he used salt water when taking the enemas.

---

[360] *Facts & Fallacies About Probiotics*, Dr. Khem M. Shahani, Professor, Food Science & Technology, University of Nebraska, Lincoln, NE 68583-0919.

[361] N. Rangavajhyala, K.M. Shahani, G. Sridevi, and S. Srikumaran. *Nonlipopolysaccharide Components(s) of Lactobacillus acidophilus Stimulate(s) the Production of Interleukin-a and Tumor Necrosis Factor-q by Murine Macrophages.* Nutrition and Cancer, Vol. 27 or 28 (2). 130-134.

[362] Khem M. Shahani, Jayantkumar R. Vakil, Rarnesh Chandra Chandan, United States Patent # 3,689,640, Sept. 5, 1972.

[363] K.M. Shahani, J.R. Vakil, and A. Kilara, *Natural Antibotic Activity of Lactobacillus acidophilus and Bulgaricus,* Department of Food Sciences and Technology, University of Nebraska, Lincoln, Nebraska 68583.

[364] **See Chapter 12: Rebuilding Vital Organs, under "Fight Candida and Pathogenic Bacteria."**

I was raised in Western Washington. In the summer evenings our yard always had slippery, slimy, slithering slugs, seriously searching for a succulent supper. Anyway, they look like dark, slimy rotten bananas. Their skin looks and feels like a mucous membrane, and they respond similarly. When we were kids, we were not taught to respect other life forms, nor to consider that other life forms had feelings. These slugs did terrible damage to my mother's garden and flowers, and our job was to eliminate these critters any way that we could. We used salt. Cruelly, we thought it was fun to pour salt on those guys and watch them dry up, crinkle, contract, crystallize, and die right in front of our eyes. Within seconds after pouring salt on them, they shriveled, calcified, and they never moved again.

This is exactly what happens when we put too much salt into our bodies. Salt shrivels, hardens, and crystallizes the healthy mucous membranes in our alimentary canal. Is this only my idea? No.

One day I was in the University of Arizona Medical Library gathering medical facts about AIDS. I was looking for a certain book, walked down an aisle containing thousands of medical books and just happened to go by the gastrointestinal section. I thought, "Just can't get away from the guts." I intended to walk right on by, when suddenly my hand reached out and grabbed a book. It was called *Mechanisms of Mucosal Protection of the Upper Gastrointestinal Tract.*[365] It had an article about clinical studies of the effect salt had on the intestinal wall. It supplied the scientific proof that table salt was extremely harmful to the digestive tract.

What we did with slugs is a good example of what sodium chloride (inorganic salt) does to our mucosa membranes. Using salt orally or rectally is one of the worst things people can do to themselves. It is a shock to the alimentary canal. Less mucoid plaque is eliminated by those who eat salt. The more salt they eat, the more calcified their mucoid plaque is, and the more difficult it is the remove it. Salt has been used to embalm cadavers and cure hams. It sucks moisture and dries everything out including the healthy intestinal mucosa. Salt is good for a few things - killing slugs and curing hams. It's also good for making mummies and tanning hides.

Organic sodium, on the other hand, actually softens. It helps keep calcium soft and usable. Many people have stiff and sore joints. This is caused by two conditions: acids and organic sodium deficiency. The body cannot use sodium chloride. It can only use organic sodium.

---

[365] Allen, et al., "Mechanisms of Mucosal Protection of the Upper Gastrointestinal Tract," pg. 317.

## "Cell Talk"

# Salt and the Athlete - The Illusion Is Shattered

As much as 5 to 10 pounds of weight loss has been recorded in athletes in a period of 1 hour during athletic events under hot and humid conditions. We all know that sweat contains large amounts of salt, but what kind of salt? Many athletes and even soldiers in the military have been known to indulge in large amounts of sodium chloride and/or tablets of salt to make up for the amount of salt lost in sweat. Many athletes are afraid that if they do not get enough salt when they exercise, they may cause serious harm to themselves. This is absolutely true if they run low on organic sodium, but not true if they run out of inorganic sodium. Heavy sodium chloride intake has caused far more harm than not getting enough.[366]

Why does the body sweat with exercise? We have all been trained to think that it keeps us cool. I'm not going to argue with that, but why does all that salt come out when exercising? No one seems to know the answer to that. But did you know that very little salt is excreted by healthy vegetarians who stay away from sodium chloride? So what is the story? Possible explanation: The average person who eats so much salt usually sweats enormous amounts of sodium chloride, and that is fortunate for them, because it is a good way to get rid of it quickly before it does any more harm. Yes, the body wants to be rid of it, but the truth is that organic sodium is retained even during heavy exercise. Sweat glands have the ability to reabsorb organic sodium from the sweat before it issues forth onto the surface of the skin. Medical science has recognized that the greatest danger with exercise is the loss of organic potassium, which is never a problem for vegetarians unless they fail to eat or their digestive systems were destroyed - which is very unlikely for vegetarians.[367] In addition, as was stated earlier, it is almost impossible to become potassium deficient unless you are deficient in organic sodium. And, sodium chloride can actually contribute to a deficiency of organic sodium.

---

[366] Guyton, pg. 1017.

[367] Guyton, pg. 1018.

# Shrinking the Abdomen

Mucoid plaque may eventually stretch the intestinal wall, especially the colon. Those people boasting the famous "beer belly" (and others whose stomachs fold over the belt), or those who cannot see their feet when they stand up straight, can be sure that they have a thick and dangerous mucoid buildup in the intestinal tract.[368]

Once the mucoid layers are removed, the seriously-stretched intestines are still soft and flabby. But there is hope for a normal and healthy look - blessed are herbs! After cleansing, the herbs white oak bark and ginger root, when used together, can help to draw the flesh back to its original position. Using these and other herbs, I developed a very effective formula to help rebuild the bowel wall.[369]

# Heavy Metals

Many people have heavy metals stored in their cells. If anyone suspects they are experiencing symptoms due to heavy metals toxicity, they should immediately stop whatever they have been doing and contact my office for information on detoxing from heavy metals. I have been in contact with thousands of persons using an ideal cleansing program, and have never heard a report of an adverse heavy metals reaction while cleansing. However, I have seen heavy metals toxicity surface with water fasting in combination with enzyme therapy, as discussed in Chapter 14.[370] I have developed a program that works very well to cleanse the body of heavy metals toxicity. Heavy metals are dangerous. They can do a great deal of damage, and detoxing should be handled with great care, and immediacy, whenever the need arises.

---

[368] This stretching may cause a **"Leaky Bowel Syndrome," which is discussed in Chapter 6: Impaired Digestion and It's Outcomes.**

[369] **See Appendix II: Essential Elements for Effective Cleansing and Rebuilding.**

[370] Further information on heavy metals is covered in **Chapter 14: Secrets of Super Health, under "Water Fasting, Enzyme Therapy and Heavy Metals."**

# Chapter 10

# OPTIMIZE YOUR CLEANSE

*The environment you fashion out of your thoughts, your beliefs, your ideals, your philosophy, is the only one you will ever live in.*

## - O.S. Marden

*The real voyage of discovery consists not in seeking new landscapes, but in having new eyes.*

## - Marcel Proust

*If we are not laughing or at least chuckling to ourselves every few minutes, then we can be certain that we are suffering from illusion.*

*The fulfillment of all hopes is love.*

*Joy is Love in action.*

*The most important effort anyone can ever make to obtain success, happiness, and health, is to establish the habit of unconditional love for everyone and everything. No greater aspirations exist.*

## - Dr. Richard Anderson

# An Optimal Time

**While the body is cleansing, it is an optimal time to also start changing negative thoughts, feelings, and habits, which have caused us poor health, unhappiness, and failure in our lives.** Often they spontaneously transform while cleansing, and all that is needed is to reinforce the new habits we wish to cultivate. Any time we cleanse, **it is essential to keep our attention upon the things we want rather than the things we do not want.** We must focus on the thoughts, feelings and habits that move us toward perfect health, vitality, success and love. This process provides an incredible practice which can help us create increasing health, joy, unconditional Love, and success in our everyday lives.

To some, cleansing is seen simply as a means to remove toxicity from their bodies in hopes of achieving more energy and better health. Though an ideal cleansing program does help many accomplish this, it can become even more powerful and effective when it is also used as a catalyst for the release of negative emotions, memories and habits that are stored in the plaque and other areas of the body, which caused toxicity. I cannot emphasize this enough. By using the cleanse in this way, we are able to address the energetic cause behind the physical cause, further erasing any underlying tendencies for problems to recur.

After more than 30 years of study in the field of etiology,[371] there is not the slightest doubt in my mind that negative emotions are **the base cause of disease in the mind and body,** as well as the cause **of failures in achieving goals.** Just about every doctor and person with whom I am associated agrees. **Every feeling or emotion has a profound and direct effect upon our glands and nerves, which trigger hormones. The hormones then control every physiological process in our bodies.**

The great key to transforming our emotions is found in the practice of unconditional Love which many cleansers report is strengthened while cleansing. **It significantly helps to consciously establish the intent to choose the practice of unconditional love as a focus while cleansing.** Many have also found cleansing breath practice[372] particularly helpful in shifting emotion, especially when used in conjunction with an ideal cleansing program. These procedures significantly help to increase our ability to focus more positively and visualize more effectively, as inner conflicts are resolved and energy draining emotions are released. Many have then experienced a growing ability to direct their lives and bodies

---

[371] The science and study of the causes of disease.

[372] Breathwork is a well-known cleansing process which involves breathing practice with the assistance of a trained guide.

towards any experience they choose, and that includes being in perfect health.

As the emotional body cleanses, uncovering its own innate wisdom, the tongue naturally becomes quieter, a more steady reflection of an ever purer heart. We may also exercise the will to refuse to speak or think in negative ways. However, this discipline must be exercised carefully and thoroughly, with full honesty and awareness of possible denials. We must not allow suppression of symptoms of deeper hurt that may still be festering, and still require deeper cleansing and healing to be fully released.

**The truth is** many of us **have become victims of our own mental and emotional processes to the point that we have lost control of them and they now control us.** The unconscious mind (that part of our thought process not currently controlled by conscious awareness) stores these automatic thought patterns. These patterns direct our health and many other parts of our lives without any conscious choices on our part. But our conscious mind has the ability to change these automatic thought patterns. Unfortunately, most people have failed to realize this and have allowed their unconscious minds to run wild and rampant, secretly sabotaging their health and affairs. In this wild state, the unconscious acts as an indiscriminate sponge, absorbing whatever mental/emotional patterns surround it, whether they are helpful or not. In this way, the unconscious copies from others at random and may create undesirable conditions in our lives.

**With proper intent, discipline, training and cleansing, we can recreate our lives to become the way we want them to be.** Many people are so totally out of control that all the suggestions that could make their dreams come true go unheeded, because they are so blocked by emotional habits which are anchored in physical garbage. To change our lives, we must become free of those old habits of mental and emotional illusions. Here is a story I like to use in some of my lectures, which illustrates how emotional thought forms affect us.

# Mop-hildegarde

Mop-hildegarde, a welfare worker, pulls her car up to the curb. She pauses for a moment before getting out of the car. She ponders about the last time she was here - about the child who is so beautiful, so sweet, so touching. Sweet little Polly Anna is barely 3 years old and is the most lovely child Mop-hildegarde has ever seen. As she thinks of her, little Polly Anna walks out the front door and is carrying something. Mop-hildegarde gets out of the car and walks through the gate and up to the porch. Little Polly Anna is still on the porch, holding her cat - a black cat. Mop-hildegarde, all 240 pounds of her, gently as she can, walks up the steps to the little Polly Anna, who is still holding the black cat. Mop-hildegarde is touched with the purity and sweetness of little Polly Anna, who is so sweet and innocent, with her beautiful golden curls. Sweet little Polly Anna has just enough shyness to bring out Mop-hildegarde's gentle spirit. And as like attracts like, all the sweetness and goodness of Mop-hildegarde floods forth, and she bends down to kiss little Polly Anna on the forehead. As she does, the black cat responds quickly; claws lash out and scratch big Mop-hildegarde on the face, drawing hot blood. Big Mop-hildegarde recoils and in the process, automatically strikes at the cat, knocking both the cat and little Polly Anna down the steps. Little Polly Anna goes flying all the way down. The cat jumps off and lands safely, but poor Polly Anna smashes into rocks below. Big Mop-hildegarde seeing what she has done, stands there in shock. But, it is too late. The damage is done.

## Interpretation

The question is: Who is at fault? Is it the fault of Big Mop-hildegarde who was only trying to be kind and loving? Was it Little Polly Anna, who was always sweet, innocent, and never did anything wrong? Or was it the black cat, who seemed to be minding his own business and merely lashed out in self-defense?

The analogical symbolisms may be understood as follows: through our thoughts and feelings we create many conditions which have various forms. These forms, though invisible to most people's limited sight, nevertheless are real and solid in the realm of thought and feeling. These forms become our habits and patterns in life. As they accumulate, they exert greater and greater force and influence in our lives. They become so automatic that they cause us to react almost instinctively, repeating patterns that are not always helpful - in the same way that the black cat reacted when lashing out at Mop-hildegarde.

Our personalities, for example, are an accumulation of the created forms of our thoughts and feelings. We are totally influenced by them. In fact, they are so powerful that they tend to turn on us and control us - they influence every thought, act, and the way we respond to every person. In a sense, we have become our thoughts and feelings. These thought forms seep into our bodies and even influence our cell structure, our glands, hormones, and nerves. The black cat represents these thought forms, which become our belief systems and automatic thought and emotional patterns. Indeed, our personalities are nothing more than the sum of our thoughts and feelings of the past. We have all created undesirable forms by consistently dwelling upon negative thoughts and feelings.

Have you ever met someone who said: "This is just the way I am. Don't expect me to change." What they are really saying is: "I've created myself to be this way, but don't realize it and I don't want to change." The truth is however, we all are changing constantly with every single thought we think. **But, there are two kinds of people: those who have no control over the way they change and those who consciously choose the ways they change.**

Sweet little Polly Anna represents the spiritual beings we truly are: immortal, incapable of permanent injury, and a pure focal point of life, yet very capable of thinking and feeling, and of becoming a victim of self-created thought processes. Many people tend to think that we *are* the things we have created. We've forgotten who and what we are, and the power we really have to change.

**As we cleanse out the physical accumulation (toxins and mucoid plaque) from our bodies, and the associated emotions arise and symptoms are released, it is possible to rediscover the mental/emotional process which initiated the physical problems.** This benefits us in three major ways: 1) we learn how we create our experiences and this lesson helps us gain greater control, 2) the cleansing itself helps to uncreate the patterns and momentum we had developed which caused us difficulty, and 3) we gain greater confidence to exercise our creative power, affecting our own destinies in a helpful way. Even though we originally, in most cases, were unaware of what we were doing to cause our problems, once we become aware, we can choose to change those things which we previously felt victimized us.

In the effort to accurately discern the truth of how our problems were created, and own up to our past mistakes and their physical results, **it is critical to regard ourselves with unconditional love rather than harsh judgment and guilt.** Such judgment only increases a sense of mental separation from the Oneness of all life, prolongs any suffering, delays necessary releases, and adds darkness to ourselves and the world. And further, dwelling upon harsh judgment leads to another debilitating state of mind — guilt.

It is important to notice that the mental/emotional process which initially created the suffering also involved a sense of separation, in some form, from the Oneness of all life. This illusion of separation then led to insensitivity or lack of awareness about truth or information critical to our own well-being - also known as '**ignore-ance.**' Ignorance is an automatic result of '**deni-all.**' In reality, **all suffering is an automatic result of denying the Oneness of all life.** The killing of any life form, in other words, eating meat, is another dynamic act of forgetfulness of the Oneness.

**People who eat meat perpetuate suffering, not only for themselves, but for other innocent life forms**.

It is the unwise use of our own mental powers which creates the illusion of separation and thereby the experience of 'ignore-ance.' A person caught in this trap might say in all innocence, 'I didn't know if I threw garbage over there that it would affect the whole system and come back to me over here - I didn't know it was all one!' Such a person is ignoring their intuitive awareness of the inherent connectedness of all things. It is wise to remember a simple saying that holds profound truth: **"Everything affects everything!"**

It is through mental separation from the oneness of all life that we are capable of creating suffering. **And that suffering is never caused by anything but ourselves, through the unwise use of our mental powers**. So, although the process of cleansing mentally, emotionally and physically may involve some temporary discomfort, particularly if we take the process too quickly, the ultimate result of this cleansing is to free us from creating ongoing pain and suffering.

Big Mop-hildegarde represents the law of cause and effect responding to our self-created, automatic as well as consciously-chosen thought patterns. How does this law work in this context? Thought is the seed. Emotion follows, nourishing and magnifying the seed; and in time, the physical results take root and flourish accordingly.

So, the answer to the question: who is at fault? Is it the black cat? Or the sweet, innocent Polly Anna, who represents the beautiful innocent child within us? No matter what, she always remains pure and good, but she has the ability to create things that are not good. The black cat represents one of her creations. Sweet little Polly Anna did not really mean to create the defensive black cat which was responsible for the terrible hurt, but because little Polly Anna didn't know what she was doing, she went right ahead and created it, **like we all do. It was her creation that caused the hurt; her misuse of her own mental faculties**. Should we blame and judge her for making this error? As Jesus of Nazareth counseled, "Let he who is without error cast the first stone." **Don't we learn from our mistakes? Then at some level it was good and worth the mistakes, for if we made no mistakes we would never grow.**

Her body is lying smashed upon the rocks, but the truth is that little Polly Anna, her real self (the soul), can never really be hurt. She may think that she can, and create/attract that physical reality. Yet that physical reality (and all physical reality) is but a passing illusion from the eternal point of view of Spirit. But in this physical world, we experience ourselves as the products of our own emotions, thoughts, and illusions. And when we create them, they take on a form that can be seen by those who have the sight to see. Yes, thoughts and feelings are real causes in the physical world and have a profound effect upon our bodies and affairs. The good news is that we can direct them to our advantage and use them in perfect harmony with the laws of the Universe. How do we know that we are doing this? What can we use as a measurement to gauge if we are on the right track? Love! **For the degree that we love is the degree to which we are on the right track.** As long as we are loving without judgment.

# Thought is Creative

*There is an old story that has been told in several ways. It basically goes like this: A merchant set out from a city to make a trip to a nearby village. He got up early in the morning and set out about his business. On his way out of the city, he met 'The Plague.' He asked 'The Plague' what it was doing, and 'The Plague' replied, "I have come to take 10,000 people from the city." The merchant was horrified, but continued on his way. Later that day, as he was returning to the city, he met people leaving who told him that more than 30,000 people had died that day in the city. As he journeyed on, he met 'The Plague' itself, as it was leaving the city. He said to 'The Plague,' "I thought you told me you were only going to take 10,000 people?" 'The Plague' replied, "I did. Fear took the rest."*

Our lives are a by-product of our habitual and conscious thought processes; it is through our thoughts and feelings that we have created all sorts of experiences in our lives. Many are good, and many are not, but all are a result of our mental and emotional processes. The more we place our attention upon these thought forms, the more they gain greater and greater power to affect us and others; they act like invisible magnets, attracting the experiences which fit our inner pictures. It is these thought patterns that form our personalities. I am convinced that negative feelings are the number one cause of disease, old age and death. **Our attitudes reflect our thought forms and this is what either brings us to greater freedom or greater bondage; to either health or disease**, success or failure. Once we establish them as unconscious habit patterns, **they control us.** Until now, we may not have realized that **when we created resentment, jealousy, self-pity, guilt, anger, and hate, that these were creative energy forms that would stick around and haunt us - making our lives miserable.** Until now, we may not have realized that our black cats would some day seep into our bodies and cause disease, or seep into our emotions and victimize us by altering our personalities to the point that they would rearrange our lives, mentally, physically, socially, financially and spiritually.

How do we know if we are really suffering from these things? If we are not, then we would be blazing bright with unconditional love, joy, health, and success, 100% of the time. There would be no disease, no failures, no disappointments, and no attachments. The awareness of who we are and what we are would dominate our consciousness, for we would constantly be in the presence of our own true being which is radiantly loving.

Sometimes we wonder why we get so angry over such little things or so hurt from unimportant comments. We wonder why someone else had all the opportunities and we hardly had a chance. We wonder why people think about us the way they do, and we should consider why we think about others the way we do. We wonder why we are so hung-up on sex, lovers, certain foods, drinks, money, power, or beliefs.

All these attitudes are nothing more than an accumulation of mental/emotional energy that we have been storing up since the beginning of our existence: the emotional counterpart of mucoid plaque. Too bad that we usually don't remember what we did to cause them; but we did cause them. Yes, we are responsible for everything that has ever happened to us. It's not our parents, husband or wife, school teachers, brothers or sisters - not even our government. **We are the ones** who **made the choices about how we were going to feel and act**. This is the key, and it is a creative use of our capacity to judge or discern the truth in situations. **Yet, many of our choices may have been based on mis-perception initially or later were largely made without *any* thought, for we had already become victims of our unconscious mental/emotional habit patterns a long time ago. And once these patterns were established, they significantly impaired our ability to accurately perceive the truth in any situation.**

# Reclaim Creative Power

**Those who blame others or other things for their conditions are never in charge of their lives, and never will be until they face up to the fact, that we are all responsible for everything that has ever happened, or ever will happen, in our lives.** Only then can we reclaim our creative power.

Too bad we were never taught that our outer lives are nothing but a reflection of our inner selves. Too bad we were not taught how to think and feel in ways that would bring us joy, success, and love. Oh yes, we were told to love God, but we didn't realize that God was everywhere, even in our friends and enemies.[373] Yes, we were told to love our enemies, but we didn't realize that we were our own worst enemy. Yes, we were even told to love ourselves, but we didn't spend the time to discover who or what we were. Now some of us even think that we *are* the black cats that we created. Some even think that we *are* our bodies or minds. Imagine not even knowing what we are! We even fail to see that we truly are the sweet, innocent, beautiful child. We are children of the Universe, who are forever and ever, who never die, but only change forms, and have the power to be like Angels in Heaven.[374] Yet because of the way we direct our attention, we create undesirable emotions. This forces us to become caught into our own personal selves, and that means forget who and what we are.[375] Therefore we live as miserable worms, our bodies destined to rot and decay as food for humble bacteria. In a sense, we have become that which we are not. As the leaves of the trees change with the season, we change with our emotional seasons.

So now this leads us to explaining one of the most important things I have ever found to be true. **Though we have all made many mistakes, we are not those mistakes.** Though we have all created quite a mess for ourselves, we are not those things we created and that includes our bodies. We simply didn't know any better. We don't even need to feel guilty about it all, **for in the process of creating, we were also learning, and that is what it is all about.** However, we are responsible for all that we have created. **The trick now is to stop worrying about it all, give up our guilt and anger, and undo the mess.** How do we do that? **WE MUST PLUCK OUT OF OUR CONSCIOUSNESS (THOUGHTS**

---

[373] " 'Master, which is the greatest commandment in the law?' Jesus said unto him, 'Thou shalt love thy lord thy God with all thy heart, and with all thy soul, and with all thy mind. This is the first and greatest commandment. And the second is like unto it, Thou shalt love thy neighbor as thyself.' " *The Holy Bible*, Matthew 22:36.

[374] "For in the resurrection they neither marry, nor are given in marriage, but are as the angels of God in heaven." Ibid., Matthew 22:30.

[375] This is something to think about. For are we not all the sons of God? "I have said, Ye are gods; and all of you are children of the most High." Ibid., Psalm 82:6 "Behold, what manner of love the Father hath bestowed upon us, that we should be called the sons of God." Ibid., 1 John 3:1. "For as many as are led by the spirit of God, they are the sons of God." Ibid., Romans 8:14. Jesus answered them, "Is it not written in your law, I said, YE ARE GODS?" Ibid., John 10:34. Wouldn't it be a good question to ask: "What is a son of God?" What are we?

**AND EMOTIONS) EVERYTHING THAT HAS ANY POTENTIAL OF CAUSING HARM TO ANYONE.**

So it is a two-fold procedure. One, we remove the old thoughts and feelings that have held us captive, and two, set the new patterns or images that create our new self — the self we want to be — that which will bring love and joy. For those feelings bring us the happiness we all desire. So how do we begin?

First, we must decide upon what it is that we really want. We should assume that we can become anything we want and have anything we want, **for the universe contains everything we could ever need or desire, and we never have to take it from another to have it.** But that is another story. We need to realize that **however we see ourselves or others, we are both reinforcing and becoming. Whatever anyone feels from us, they tend to become; we share in that creation, and it reflects back into us, as well.** So we create something in them and we create the same thing in ourselves. Indeed, the accuser becomes the accused; a simple mathematical consequence of cosmic law. **Whether feeling or visualizing, we are telling our subconscious mind that this is what we want, and the subconscious mind will activate the Universe and bring it into our lives.** And that is exactly what we have been doing all along. It is that easy. But to make things happen by our own design is difficult, because of all the emotional stuff we have created which may create blockages to moving forward. Yes, it is a mess inside, don't you think? There will be some who don't think so, but either they are perfect, or in denial. We need to clean it up. It is mostly the emotions and the worst kind are the unconscious ones. **But once we start the process of cleaning up the mess by seeing ourselves in a new way, the conscious and unconscious emotions will surface, as they must if they are to come out.**

# Cleanse and Purify

When we do an ideal cleansing program, we open up the lid to the box of stored emotions and we begin to let them out. In other words, emotions actually get stuck in our cell tissues and nothing short of Divine Lightning bolts can remove them except cleansing and fasting, or the fire of suffering. More needs to be said about the many ways to transform those undesirable emotions. But right now, please be satisfied with what will be given in the following pages; it will be highly effective in getting started with cleaning up the undesirable emotions and releasing the causes of disease via this cleansing program.

To acquire the full benefits of an ideal cleansing program, **we need to know how (while we cleanse) to extract and replace the mental** and emotional substance that has interfered with our goals in life. I am talking about ways other than just cleansing and fasting. I have referred to this previously. Now I will address it in more detail.

The mental and feeling techniques which are about to be described, I feel are exceedingly important in achieving the greatest possible success of what this program has to offer. **If we do not use them properly, we can just as easily recreate the very things that we are trying to get rid of or transform.** Doing it right, can easily make the difference between outstanding achievement or mediocre success or failure. These mental and feeling exercises have *work*ed incredible miracles for many thousands of people. Many books have been written about them. However, they have not worked so well for the majority of people who have tried them. Why?

**Those who <u>were</u> successful using only the following techniques had less confusion, less clutter, less mental and emotional fears, worries, hate, etc. than most people.** They simply had less interference to begin with, so the momentum of their energy was more easily shifted. As I have said before, I have seen few excellent results with the majority of people using only various *mental* methods or techniques to eliminate their negative emotions. **It is through cleansing and later fasting, that we can quickly remove the physical accumulation which has anchored various mental and emotional patterns.** Yes, the following techniques become infinitely more powerful when we combine them with the intestinal cleansing program offered in these pages.

I must admit that this deep inner cleansing is not really for everyone. It is not for those who look for easy hand-outs, and are willing to harm or take from another to get it. It is only for the strong, the fearless, the more aware individuals, the ones who are willing to do more than their share, the ones who have the wisdom and strength and desire to go to the trouble to eliminate their self-created blockages. It is for those who have the courage to face their creations and stop denying them. It is for those who are willing to take responsibility for their lives and not look for someone else to do for them what they can do for themselves. And most of all, it is only for those who are unselfish enough to want to help their brothers and sisters out there, and that includes our animals, birds, and plant friends, and the earth as well.

# Setting Goals

Assuming that one of our goals is to obtain better health and vitality, we should ask ourselves: Do we really want to be strong and healthy? Are we willing to do what is necessary to get that way? Some people may need to be sick for awhile longer. Some people even have a secret death wish. Many people love to talk about their ills; it is a major part of their fun in life, and they don't really want to get well, even though they say they do. Being aware of where we really stand helps us to gain control over our lives and achieve our goals. We never get far while living in denial, nor do we get far when we are unwilling to face our fears.[376]

To achieve any goal it is important to see the goal clearly. The practice of seeing our goal fulfilled is called visualization. **It is important to be consistent in what we visualize.** To write down our goals on paper is one of the most effective methods of being consistent. **The process of consistent visualization is a method which allows us to transmit our desires to the unconscious mind. Once the unconscious mind picks it up and believes it, then we will have it.** This is the method that creates "faith". "According to your faith, it is done unto you."[377] Our unconscious mind is the direct link to Universal or Innate Intelligence. **When we link the two together through purification, visualization, love,** and by agreeing that it has come to pass (believing), we can have anything we choose. This is very powerful. **We must be careful not to write down what we don't want, but only what we do want, and most important of all, we must be certain that whatever we visualize will not take from or harm another part of life.**

# Instructions

Step 1. Get some paper and a pen and write down your goals. Then pick out that goal you think is the one you want to obtain right away. Condense this goal into one sentence, which will embody your total concept of achieving your goal.

Step 2. Every night just before bed and every morning before you get dressed, read this goal to yourself. When you have memorized the words, destroy the paper.

Step 3. Now begin to act or pretend that your request has been answered. Do little things that verify that you have already achieved the answer to your desire. **We must arrive at a point where we fully accept its**

---

[376] Fear defeats more people than any other thing, and it is the fear, not the thing we fear, that causes failure. "Face the thing you fear and death of fear is certain." - Ralph W. Emerson.

[377] "Be not deceived; God is not mocked: for whatsoever a man soweth, that shall he also reap." *The Holy Bible*, Galatians 6:7. In other words, for every action there is a reaction, and it applies to thoughts and feelings as much as anything else.

**fulfillment as already manifested. Until we do, we short-circuit or interfere with its manifestation.**

If you practice prayer and meditation, you can greatly enhance the above procedures. Prayer, visualization, meditation, and consciously directed feeling are powerful acts that can manifest a miracle. These are skills that require clarity and self-control. The main requirement is to make the request clear. Then, after writing it down, we can assist this process by reading it several times a day, and holding in our minds how we would act if we had fulfilled our goal. Then, to the best of your ability, **act as though it were fulfilled**. If you cannot do this, then your goal is too high. Choose a lesser goal. **Never choose a goal that is beyond your ability to believe. Your goal must be in agreement with your belief system.** Set easy goals at first. After a series of successes, you can reach higher.

Through prayer, making affirmations, visualizing our goals as already fulfilled, and acting as though they have manifested in our lives **now, not in the future**, we plant the creative seeds into the unlimited supply and power of our friend, the Universe. It is best to incorporate all of these techniques, but **the most vital, most important part of all is to see, feel, and act as though our goals are complete — now!** That is trusting in God. Many people pray to God for this and that, but few believe that their prayer will be fulfilled. The Great Master Jesus said: "Therefore I say unto you, What things so ever ye desire, when ye pray, believe that ye receive them, and ye shall have them.[378]

# Making Ourselves Believe

The process of acting as though we are, even right now, the fulfillment of our desire, becomes even more powerful when we realize that **this pretending process is an extremely effective transmission which allows the unconscious mind to believe it.** Some may feel that this

---

[378] "For verily I say unto you, That whosoever shall say unto this mountain, Be thou removed and be thou cast into the sea; and shall not doubt in his heart, but shall believe that those things which he saith shall come to pass; he shall have whatsoever he saith. Therefore I say unto you, What things soever ye desire, when ye pray, believe that ye receive them, and ye shall have them." Ibid., Mark 11:23. Jesus said unto him, 'If thou canst believe, all things are possible to him that believeth." Ibid., Mark 9:22. Also check out Matt 21:22.

How does anyone believe that we have the power within to do these incredible things, when we have never seen any evidence that it can be done? In the Christian world, unbelief is the common denominator, but in the East, in the world of the Yogis, there is ample evidence. The point is, examples do exist.

pretending is a lie and it may go against their nature, and they simply do not want to do it. **We need to understand that this process is a way of communicating with our subconscious mind and the universe.** It is in this way that we are putting in our request for a change. The unconscious mind doesn't know the difference between what we think is real and what we imagine as real. **Our unconscious mind doesn't function in limitation, only our conscious mind does that.**

Visualizing the way we want things to be, even though they do not appear that way on the outside, is telling the unconscious mind that "this is the way it's going to be, so get to work and get it done". **You see the unconscious mind has already created our life to be the way it is now, because we programmed it to be that way.** We have become a by-product of our past thinking and feeling. And if you dig deep enough, you will realize that the thoughts and feelings which created your present reality were also created by illusionary thoughts and feelings! So let us make visualization an art. **The process of visualization stimulates our glandular system in a very positive way. We can even change our DNA structure and greatly enhance our immune system.**[379]

The unconscious mind cannot tell the difference between an imagined experience and a real experience. In truth, when we visualize ourselves in ways that appear to us as not yet being real, we are not lying. We are only feeding the unconscious mind the seeds that will cause it to be reprogrammed according to our will. **The unconscious mind doesn't care what seeds we give it, nor what it will manifest for us. Its fruits will always be from the seeds we planted within it.** It reacts appropriately to what we think, feel, or imagine to be true *every single time - it cannot do otherwise.*

What I have just said is important, for it reveals one of the secrets of how we got into our situations in the first place, and how we can get back into a more favorable life. It also reveals the need to Cleanse & Purify. It tells us to get rid of all that is within us which is interfering with our joy in life and to start programming ourselves to be what we want to be. It affirms the great Master Jesus' request, "Sin no more." Let us train ourselves to accept only thoughts and feelings that bring the fulfillment of our desires. Why not give it a try? **To see ourselves at a better level,**

---

[379] Medical science has proven that using visualization techniques can substantially improve the immune system. Visualization can totally alter the glandular system and affect the DNA. Read: *Getting Well Again*, by O. Carl Simonton, M.D., Stephanie Matthews-Simonton, and James L. Creighton (New York, NY: Bantam Books, 1978); See also: *Love, Medicine and Miracles*, by Bernie Siegel, M.D., and all of Deepak Chopra's books.

certainly will not hurt anybody, and it won't interfere with anyone's choices or freedom.

So let us start now, during this cleansing activity, by writing down our goals, by praying, visualizing, seeing, and affirming that which we want, as our reality. **Let us see ourselves the way we want to be. Let us, to the very best of our ability, act as though we are now that which we want to be.** Start writing down your goals right now and absolutely do not let anyone see them.[380] And never question whether or not it will work. Refuse to submit to negatives or failure. Reject all thoughts of failure. Our lives are the result of what we have done in the past, our lives in the future are formed by what we think, feel and do now. Continued effort after what may appear to be failure produces the greatest growth. "The season of failure is the best time for sowing the seeds of success!!" - Yogananda.

# Mental and Emotional Cleansing Reactions

The following is an extremely important concept in achieving health and success. Please think carefully about what I am about to say. **When we begin to practice these exercises, all the negative thoughts and feelings that interfere with our desired goals will begin to rise to the surface.** And if we allow it, the negativity will stop our new creation. This negativity or karma, may be reflected in our bodies, our social life, finances, or our environment, but mostly it will be obvious in our attitudes. **It is important to know that this will happen,** for it surely will. When we know that it must happen, then when it does, we will be in much better control of ourselves. **It is far easier on us to have these old undesirable substances surface during a cleanse, and be eliminated from our beings quickly, than to allow them to slowly manifest themselves through our daily lives, interfering with our happiness, our goals, and our health, for a period of years or lifetimes.** No matter what is said by others, no matter what we see in the mirror or feel as pain, weakness, or any outer condition or inner experience, we should attempt to remain unaffected, except to know that the old is now gone, or at least is moving out, and the new has arrived, even though the seeming reality is that the old is sticking up its ugly head to be released once and for all. This is the critical time to reaffirm our new reality.

It is similar to when the toxins are surfacing during cleansing or fasting. We can do the cleansing now and get it over with quickly, or we

---

[380] "All that we are is the result of what we have thought." - Buddha

can let those old toxins stay there and destroy our bodies. To me it is best to get it out now while we still have the strength and ability to do it. Similarly, **when we visualize ourselves the way we want to be, the interfering mental and emotional toxins seep up to the surface of our consciousness, almost like a challenge**. Then we re-experience them again. It is important to keep in mind that this is going to happen; that it *has* to happen for them to come out forever; **that it will soon pass**, and; that if we keep holding our goal in mind and heart to the best of our ability, then we will be successful. We cannot fail unless we give up. It is in this way that we release out of us the substance, be it physical, mental, or emotional, that prevents the health, success, happiness, and love from manifesting through us.

These mental exercises plus cleansing, speed up our success a hundred-fold. So let's write down our goals now! (See I knew you didn't do it the first time I asked.) **Let's put notes on our mirror, bed stand, in the kitchen, in the car, and anywhere else to remind us to keep seeing ourselves as the fulfillment of those goals**. But the main goals must be kept silent. Tell no one. Use your notes as a reminder to yourself. If anyone asks you what all those notes are, just say that you are trying to be more positive. Absolutely do not discuss your main goal, for that may nullify it. For if anyone doubts your ability, that will create more resistance you will have to push through.

One of the most important considerations in achieving any goal is to **watch that our attention does not become fixed on the things we do not want**. To do this is to nullify or short-circuit our creation, not to mention creating an undesired result!

As long as negative conditions are still inside, improvement may be slow, but not impossible. **Our greatest victory is when we can rise above the situation while still in the midst of it.**[381] Then we make the greatest progress and we gain the greatest strength. There will be times that being positive will be difficult. That is expected. Sometimes, when these troublesome thoughts/feelings surface, that is all we can think about for awhile; we must remember that they are only surfacing so they can be gone forever. Don't let it scare you. There are times that we must allow them to be released, and sometimes expressed, dynamically! Never deny or suppress your feelings as they surface. However, the second the negative thoughts let up, go immediately back to thinking and feeling that which we want, knowing that we just erased forever those old, undesirable creations. Yes, we can "Arise & Shine."

---

[381] "The season of failure is the best time for sowing the seeds of success." - Paramahansa Yogananda.

Let us always remember that these creative processes have always been at work through us. We have unconsciously been using these creative processes since the beginning of our existence. Behold, our lives - the struggle, the pain - a result of our wrong thinking and emotions.

The only thing that will ever bring us permanent health, success, joy and love, is the habit of giving love. **For what we give or do to other parts of life we force into ourselves.** As the Great Master said, "Whatsoever ye do unto the least of my brethren you do unto me." We can also say it this way: "Whatsoever we do to the least of our brethren, we also do to ourselves." That is the Law of Life - the Law of Success and Health- the Law of Oneness. This is why killing and supporting meat eating has a very negative effect on our inner consciousness. This is why the dark forces have always promoted flesh eating. This is why Jesus and all the great teachers of mankind were vegetarians.[382]

# Helpful Guidelines

**Health, success, and joy in life on a consistent basis, is very much dependent:**

1. upon the willingness to take full responsibility for our lives;
2. upon the willingness to face all our fear, anger, guilt, pain and denial;
3. upon the willingness to completely forgive everyone and everything, including ourselves, no matter what; and
4. upon the desire to **love everyone and everything unconditionally.**

Notice the word willingness. It doesn't mean that we have to be there now, but we must be willing to get there. I believe that the number one reason patients fail to conquer cancer or any other serious disease, is because they were unwilling to forgive and forget. They held onto resentment, anger, guilt, and doubt, and that is what killed them. Chemotherapy and radiation only helped them die faster and with greater pain. Maybe that was but the fulfillment of the law of cause and effect.

We must give up our guilt. That is a big one for many people. We all have things to feel guilty about. Admitting that we were wrong is a noble thing! Once we get out of denial it becomes easier and we can set out correcting the cause. Sometimes, the damage done is unable to be repaired,

---

[382] Was Jesus Christ a vegetarian? Did he really teach this? Read the *Gospel of the Holy Twelve,* which is an Essene book giving one account of New Testament events as it was before it was modified to suit those who sought control over the Christians.

but even then we must let it go. If you can change something, there is no need to worry. If you can't change something, there is still no benefit in worry! However, we can change the motive or mental condition that caused the problem in the first place. Then we can attempt to improve the outer conditions the best we can. That's all we need to do. After that, there is no more need for guilt. Guilt was designed to correct internal attitudes. Once we have accomplished that, we can but trust in our friend the Universe (God) to balance the scales, and that we can always count on. But why contaminate the world with any more feelings of guilt, self-pity, or any other negative feelings? How we see others or ourselves is a creative blueprint containing powerful self-programming forces. **If we want perfection, we absolutely must see perfection in others as well as ourselves.**

As one of my teachers once told me: **"If you do not see perfection, if you see other than God's perfection, then you contribute to the darkness of the world;**[383] therefore, you are as guilty as any other. And should we judge and condemn others for being a little more wrong than we? Indeed, some crimes are worse than others, and with each crime against life, there comes an automatic reaction, a penalty, so to speak, a synchronization process to bring the creator back into balance. This process usually is identified with as pain, but let God be the judge. Why condemn yourself because another has make a mistake? Who hasn't made mistakes?" **Judging the mistakes of others binds us to them.**

My teacher continued, "If you desire freedom, if you wish for the manifestation of God in your life, then see everyone as God, for every other conscious or subconscious act is incorrect judgment." Earlier this teacher said: "When people are confused and they wonder what they should do, then see light, visualize light, and feel love. If you have trouble doing this, then 'Cleanse & Purify', for **it is the darkness in your own consciousness that deflects God's light, God's perfect plan.**"[384]

---

[383] Thoughts and feelings accumulate into the atmosphere. The accumulated consciousness in certain areas is quite different from one area to another. When we travel, we can feel the difference. This is one reason why people find it so difficult to get out of their ruts. They are affected by the consciousness around them. I remember when as a young man I first came back to my parents house after being gone for two years. I had changed a great deal during that time, but the moment I walked into my parents' house, I became the same person I had been two years before. It was challenging.

[384] "Jesus saith unto her, 'Said I not unto thee, that, if thou wouldest believe, thou shouldest see the glory of God?'" *The Holy Bible*, John 11:40.
Sometimes we must force ourselves to see, to believe.

My teacher further explained to me that when we see ourselves and others as perfect, that whatever inhibits or has blocked the perfection from manifesting will surface. Then we must continue to visualize or see the perfection we desire. At the same time, we work on dissolving the old substance through cleansing, fasting, visualization, and other techniques. It is in this way that we can completely purify ourselves.[385] I believe his wisdom, for truly, he has accomplished these things himself. He's quite a fella!

I think it was in Richard Bach's book, *Illusions*, where it was said: "The original sin was limiting the Is". I think that a greater understanding is: **The original sin is egotism.** Egotism, be it inflated or deflated, is seeing ourselves separate from God or the oneness of all life everywhere. That is an illusion. "I and my father are one", said the Great Master, and the same holds true with us, for God is love and God is everywhere (omnipresent).

All the negative feelings are in reality, based upon fear. Think about it. Anger, hate, resentment, etc. are emotions resulting from the fear of not having things the way we wanted or expected. Guilt is fear that we did something wrong. Lack of forgiveness is a feeling based upon selfishness and judgment, with a touch of fear and distrust in the Infinite. The antidote for such fear is to focus attention upon being safe and protected by divine love and intelligence. **To learn to completely trust in Divine Intelligence is sheer power.** This is the state of consciousness that every great Master and Saint lived in. **Any other response contributes to greater darkness in the world and especially to our own internal darkness.**

Who are we to know why things happen the way they do? We do not know the forces behind people's acts. We do not know the "inner" reason for things. **To be upset about things is a deliberate choice to bring more negativity into the world and is also distrust in the divine intelligence which governs all things.**

People say they trust and believe in God. The test is complete forgiveness, unending joy, and love for everyone and everything. **To be**

---

Jesus answered them, "Is it not written in your law, I said, YE ARE GODS?" *Ibid.,* John 10:34.

[385] "Blessed are the pure in heart: For they shall see God." *The Holy Bible,* Matthew. 5:8. Ahh, now we know why so few people have seen God! And some are so impure that they do not think such a thing is even possible. But, those who have attained, know. And those who have not attained, think they might know, but do not.

**upset about a single thing is proof that our trust in God is lacking**. We should always have faith that the Infinite is in control of every situation on the planet regardless of appearances. When we activate that kind of trust, incredible things happen.

We're all in the same boat. We really need to forgive everyone and also ourselves. Why shouldn't we forgive others? After all, how many mistakes have we made? How many mistakes has everyone else made? Let's clear the slate; let's forgive everyone. We have to, if we want to get well and fulfill our highest potential.

Therefore, let us practice the attitudes that bring forth love. **I challenge everyone reading these words to practice gratitude, appreciation, and non-judgment, for these bring forth love like nothing else does.** They strengthen our immune systems, glandular systems, and even our muscles and endurance. Try finding the good about everything we see and appreciate it. With everyone we talk to, we should think of that person as a lesson in life, a gift from our friend the Universe, someone who is Divinely teaching us exactly what we need to experience or hear.

Author E. W. Neville said, **"Every dream could be realized by those self-disciplined enough to believe it. ... The world, and all within it, is man's conditioned consciousness objectified."**[386]

Remember that our bodies are an extension of our own consciousness, and so is every other aspect of our lives.

"Disregard appearances and subjectively affirm as true that which you wish to be true. **Assume the feeling of your wish fulfilled and continue feeling that it is fulfilled, until that which you feel objectifies itself."**[387] - E. W. Neville

"Men are disturbed, not by the things that happen, but by their opinion of the things that happen." - Maxwell Maltz, M.D.

---

[386] E. W. Neville, *The Resurrection*, (Marina del Ray, CA: DeVorss & Co., 1966), pg. 71.

[387] Ibid.

# How to Increase Your Success

Several years ago, my friend Dr. Bernard Jensen came to visit me while I was in Tucson. We spent four hours talking about health and the mind. He told me the following story that I think the world should hear about. "Many years ago, when I was still a young man, there were rumors that the Virgin Mary had been appearing at Fatima and that many people were being healed. I wanted to see if this were true, so I went there. While I was there, there was also another doctor visiting, a very famous doctor, one who had won a Nobel prize. **Dr. Alexis Carrel had received the Nobel prize for proving that the cell, when properly nourished and cleansed, was essentially immortal.** He was conducting a study to try and determine why some people were being healed and others were not. For there had been thousands of people who traveled there for healings. Some people couldn't walk, some were blind, others had incurable diseases. Only a small percentage received healings and those healings were considerable, far beyond anything that science could explain.

Dr. Carrel had designed a questionnaire that had more than a hundred questions. He gave this questionnaire to everyone who received a healing; and apparently there were hundreds. **There was one question that everyone answered with the same response.** That question was: What were you thinking when you received the healing? Now get this, for this is important. Thousands of people asked for a healing; only a small percentage got a healing. Everyone who got a healing answered this one question with the exact same answer. **'What were you thinking when you received the healing?' The answer was: 'I was praying for someone else to be healed.'**

There is something that happens within ourselves when we are unselfish. **When we are willing to sacrifice our self for another, we initiate awesome power.** In fact, this is one of the things that all the great Masters have in common: they are completely unselfish. **When we are willing to pluck out all our selfishness, we take on a new energy, a new attitude. Let us become unselfish and not only to humans, but to all life as well.**

# Chapter 11

# WHEN THE UNEXPECTED HAPPENS

*Success always comes to those who persevere, but let us do it wisely.*

- Dr. Richard Anderson

## Questions and Answers

Q - I was on my second day of the beginning phase of cleansing and followed the directions to the letter. I felt pain in my lower stomach. It continued to get worse and by the third day I had to stop cleansing, for the nausea and pain had become unbearable. I had passed a lot of the mucoid fecal matter, so I know that it is in there. I want to keep cleansing. What should I do?

A - You did the right thing by stopping cleansing. Having seen the iris of your eyes and knowing what you just went through, it is likely that you have some serious parasite activity. You're fortunate to have discovered it at such a young age. If I were you, I would postpone doing an ideal cleansing program and follow the anti-parasite program I have developed.

**Note**: That is exactly what this person did. After the parasites program, she went back on an ideal cleansing program, and she never had another problem.

---

Q - I take that "psyllium shake" and my stomach hurts!

A - Usually this problem is caused by taking too much psyllium. Are you using teaspoons or tablespoons when following the directions? Even if you followed the directions, then I suggest taking less. Try half the amount or even less, and then gradually build back up to the proper amounts. This has worked well for those who had this problem.

Q - I am so skinny, I'm afraid to cleanse because I might lose even more weight. Will I?

A - Obese people often lose quite a load while on the program and usually most of it remains off, unless they go back to the eating habits that caused the obesity in the first place. Thin people usually gain whatever they lose within three or four days after finishing an ideal cleansing program (minus whatever mucoid layers they passed). Sometimes thin people will continue to put on weight after cleansing, because their digestion and assimilation works better. They may even put on weight during the mild phases of cleansing. However, many thin people have many other problems that they may need to deal with, such as liver, thyroid, kidneys, heart, mucoid plaque, over-acidity, attitudes, protein digestion, enzyme deficiency, and bacteria imbalance. Cleansing, in my opinion, is the first step in improving all the other problems. Some people are too thin because they are over-acid, and digestion is impaired; check your pH. If your muscles are soft and flabby, an L-Glutamine deficiency may be the problem.

---

Q - I am only 5 feet 5 and weigh 227 pounds. I lost almost 20 pounds while on an ideal cleansing program, but now I am gaining weight again. What is wrong?

A - I have found that most obese people eat far too much acid food. As I mentioned earlier, we cannot continue eating acid foods and expect to be healthy. So far, in my experience, all obese people who have come to me and gone on an alkaline diet, have lost weight without starving themselves (one exception). In fact, they can eat all they want and still have success, but they must eat the right foods. But there can be other factors such as the glands. When people have tried everything and nothing works for long, they need to look deep within themselves, root out the old consciousness, and replace it with the new image. Especially look for resentments, unforgiveness, and fear, especially fear of what others will think of you. If an obese person has fear of being obese, (conscious or unconscious) because they are afraid of what people will think of them, the subconscious will activate their glands to make it happen. Look within.

Q - Is it okay to take a colema or colonic?

A - Absolutely. Both are good methods for those who are able to get the liquid to flow all the way to the ileocecal and back out while resting on the back. But for some people, it doesn't work very well. I am one of them, and therefore must stick to using the enema, but I would prefer the other methods and would recommend either over the enema. Colonics are rather expensive, but are well worth it because they can remove an incredible amount of loosened waste material. The main difference between the colema or colonic and the enema is that the colema and colonic allow the use of much more water, plus it's easier to massage the abdomen while on the back. There are many thousands of people who can testify to the incredible benefits of colonics.

For those who have a prolapsus of the transverse colon, a board can be a great advantage.[388] After we have flushed out the colon and we are lying on our backs, we are in a great position to pull the fallen colon back up. Imagine just lying there with white oak bark tea swishing in your colon. Gently pull up that hunk of gut back up into position. Just dig in the lower abdomen with the fingers and gently nudge the guts upwards, over and over. This will help. Lying on a slant board will help even more. The white oak bark will assist the tissues in shrinking back to normal and staying that way. Doing this exercise several times a week can really help.

---

Q - Can the enema water flow into the small intestine?

A - If your ileocecal valve was somehow stuck open, it could, but that is a rare malfunction of the body which is most likely caused by too much mucoid plaque. I can't think of anything better to help a condition like that than an ideal cleansing program. Can you?

---

Q - Will the bowel cleansing remove diverticuli?

A - I believe it is possible, and is probably the only thing that could, but it would take the use of several cleanses, proper eating habits, exercise, enemas, and herbs on a consistent basis.

---

[388] One of the best colema boards available may be obtained from Ultimate Trends, Inc. 7835 S. 1300 East, Sandy, Utah 84093, 801-638-2554, 800-745-3191.

Q - I get sick to my stomach when on an ideal cleansing program. Is this because of worms?

A - There are only three reasons you have nausea while on an ideal cleansing program:
1. Toxins
2. Old drugs being released
3. Parasites

If it's because of toxins, you may want to go back to one of the gentler phases, until you're more cleaned out. But, I suggest switching back and forth through the various phases. This should help you. Another thing that can help, is take a heaping teaspoon of slippery elm in a small glass of water. Drinking peppermint tea or ginger/fennel tea, will also help eliminate nausea. Taking an enema may help more than anything. As you may have discovered, purification is not for the average individual. If it's due to parasites, use the anti-parasite program I have developed.

---

Q - I don't want to take enemas anymore. They make me feel weak.

A - That happened to me a couple of times. Again, it's usually because of the toxins. Leaky bowel syndrome could cause this condition. Remember, sometimes things must get stirred up before they can be removed. I stuck through it and never regretted it. Remove the toxins quickly with an enema, and you'll perk up for sure.[389] One man I know was very, very ill. He also became extremely weak from taking enemas. He was certain that he was losing electrolytes by using the enemas. I kept assuring him that was not his problem, that it was toxins causing his weakness. He didn't believe me. Several months went by and in his desperation, he decided that if I were right, then taking more enemas instead of less would help. He started using as much as 3 to 5 gallons during his enema sessions. It worked! His energy got better each time. The only regret he had was not doing this sooner. A colonic therapist would probably have solved this problem the first time. Read the appendix on coffee enemas. Weakness after an enema indicates a sluggish, toxic liver. A coffee enema may work magic by eliminating large amounts of toxins and freeing up the liver. Leaky bowel syndrome could also cause this condition.[390]

---

[389] For weakness after enemas: Jonni Sue suggests lying down for at least several minutes after each enema. Schedule time for a short nap after enemas. Also, a glass of fruit juice may help.

[390] **See Chapter 8: How to Determine if You Need a Cleansing Program, under "Cleansing Reactions."**

Q - Boy, do I have a lot of gas!  What can I do?

A - When you have too much gas, or a headache, or any other pains, take an enema.  Taking more enemas is really the best thing you can do.  Ginger/fennel tea is very effective in reducing gas.  Also, take the pro-biotic formula as indicated above.  If you are still eating, take enzymes.  After deep enough cleansing, you should not experience any gas while cleansing.

---

Q - Rich, I think I've just lost part of my intestines.  Maybe I'd better go to a doctor.  You should see what just came out of me!

A - CONGRATULATIONS!  You just passed a layer of mucoid plaque.  When it first happened to me, I thought the very same thing.  Remember, according to Dr. Robert S. Mendelsohn, M.D.,[391] going to the doctor may be hazardous to your health.  He explains that once the doctor

---

[391] Dr. Robert Mendelsohn, M.D. authored: *Confessions of a Medical Heretic, Mal e Practice, How Doctors Manipulate Women*, and *How to Raise a Healthy Child...in Spite of Your Doctor*.  He was the national medical director of Project Head Start and chairman of the Medical Licensure Committee for the state of Illinois.  He was also associate professor at the University of Illinois Medical School and a director of Chicago's Michael Reese Hospital. Dr. Mendelsohn viciously, but accurately, attacked the medical religion.  (Now you know where I got the idea to use "medical religion".)  He referred to doctors as medical priests.  His books are full of truth, as well as humor.  He makes incredible statements and backs them all up.  For an example, he points out that "Doctor-prescribed sacramental drugs of Modern Medicine kill more people than illegal street drugs." (about 25,000 a year)  ..."The risk of being killed by drug therapy was better than one in 1,000 in American hospitals".  It is four in 1,000 for those who have serious chronic diseases, such as cancer, heart disease, and alcoholic cirrhosis.  He points out that five percent of the people in American and British hospitals are there because of adverse reactions to drugs, and that the income of just this one situation is over $3 billion.  Another example is a doctor's records that he knows about, which show 300 cases of vaginal or cervical cancer in babies whose mothers were treated with DES.  He points out that even though they know that DES definitely causes cancer, the FDA still allows the use of DES in contraceptive pills.  A few more: "Historically, when doctors have gone on strike, the mortality rate has dropped."  "Approximately 2.4 million operations performed every year are unnecessary and cost about 12,000 lives."  His books should be mandatory reading in high schools and colleges.

has you in his office, your life is in danger. You are likely to unnecessarily lose some of your body parts; and the least, of what might happen, is you may be poisoned by drugs.

---

Q - What's the big deal about what water I use in the enema? After all, it's just going in and coming right back out with all that garbage!

A - During your enema you will always absorb some of the liquid. Unless you live in an area that has very pure water, beware of chlorine and sodium fluoride in water. Sodium fluoride is a waste product from aluminum milling companies. By selling it for 1.5 cents a pound, they made a $15,000,000-a-year profit. That was many years ago. The reason they ever managed to sell it in the first place is that in certain areas of the country where calcium fluoride was abundant in water, there was little tooth decay. Unfortunately, and evidently without complete investigation, the FDA approved its use and **sodium (not calcium) fluoride went into the water systems of major American cities**. Eventually the truth came out: the use of sodium fluoride in tap water led to an increase of tooth decay, a 12% increase of Mongoloid children, and a massive increase of Alzheimer's disease. Isn't the FDA something? **Sodium fluoride is a deadly poison that is used to kill rats by destroying the digestive system**. Keep in mind that sodium fluoride and calcium fluoride are not at all the same thing. Using R.O. (reverse osmosis) water will not remove fluoride; only distilling water can do that.

---

Q - Should I continue to take my medication while on an ideal cleansing program?

A - I really cannot advise you on that one. Use your own discretion or talk to an experienced doctor about it. Read *World Without Cancer*. Get the facts, but, this I should say: **the cleaner you get, the more impact the drugs have**. So it may be wise to watch carefully for any signs that you are getting too much of a drug during an ideal cleansing program. Many diabetics have dropped their insulin intake by half, during and after an ideal cleansing program, because they find they do not need it.

---

Q - While on an ideal cleansing program, I notice that I sometimes feel dizzy when I stand up. What is happening?

A - This is a common occurrence. The stirred-up toxins are the cause. The circulation gets gummed up and it takes longer for oxygen to get to the brain. After cleansing the body of the toxins, the dizziness will go away and even if you should fast in the future, this condition will become less and less. If you are prone to this condition, always stand up slowly and keep the head down until you are sure you won't faint.

---

Q - I'm pregnant and would like to start cleansing. Is it okay?

A - No. Ask for our tape on infants. You may also want to read about Red Raspberry tea in some herb books; it will make your delivery much, much easier. Also, avoid impure water, especially water containing chlorine and sodium fluoride. I also suggest you drink carrot/celery juice every day.

---

Q - I've been told by my doctor that I have a spastic colon and that I'd better be careful with colon cleansing. What do you think?

A - I agree. Be careful. If I had your condition (which could cause pain), I would cut down on the recommended dosages of psyllium. I would use catnip tea enemas, made with distilled water, to relax the colon. I would be very generous with the catnip. Believe me, though, if I had a spastic colon I sure wouldn't hesitate to cleanse. I would do anything and everything I could to repair that area now and not wait until it got worse. You may find it better to stay on the beginning phase for a longer period of time. But realize this, if you can eat food, you can cleanse. I would also suggest working on renewing your bowel wall. I have designed a supplement specifically for that purpose.

---

Q - What about using bentonite in my enemas?

A - I do not recommend it. You must be careful with bentonite enemas. Clay, especially bentonite, is an excellent healer for the outside of the body. It can be used for all sorts of things - sores, wounds, rashes, cysts, and anything that has toxins which need to be drained. It may be effective as an enema against protozoan and bacterial infections. I have experimented by adding about 2 to 4 ounces of extra thick hydrated bentonite per gallon. Mix well and inject. Keep the solution in for about fifteen minutes. If you use too much bentonite, it could affect the mucosa lining of the colon and it may even pull out too many electrolytes and damage the mucosa. If this occurred, you would find yourself becoming very weak for several hours. So, don't do it, unless your intuition is strong in favor of doing it. If you do it, use small amounts at first. Gradually increase. You will know if you used too much. Again, I would only do this if I had a serious protozoan infection, and nothing else worked.

---

Q - Is it true that friendly bacteria can be destroyed when you take a colonic?

A - Yes and no. If there is chlorine in the water, yes. But chances are, if you need a colonic, the friendly bacteria in your colon has already been overrun by the harmful bacteria. **I would always recommend taking a general use pro-biotic formula as part of an ideal cleansing program whenever you take enemas or colonics.**

---

Q - My menstrual periods have changed since I've been cleansing. Is that normal?

A - It is normal for those who have had a problem with their menstruation. After cleansing, the body is more able to adjust itself to a better pattern. The cleaner you get, the more apt you will be to find changes. Rarely, someone may find that their menstrual cycle changes for the worse. This is a sign that the person stopped cleansing too soon. She should return to cleansing. Contrary to popular belief, I am convinced that menstrual discharges are normal only for those who do not eat the natural diet intended for the human species. Fruitarian women who have cleansed themselves through fasting and a fruitarian diet usually do not have the discharge. The more pure a woman's body becomes, the less there will be, until eventually there will be none at all. I have a friend who had been on a raw food diet for three-and-a-half years, then she was on only fruit for another one-and-a-half years, and at last found she no longer had any menstrual periods. People used to guess her age to be 23 to 29 years young when she was 44!

---

Q - If I eat yogurt, do I need the pro-biotic formula you recommend for the program?

A - Yes, you do. Yogurt will not be able to replenish the intestines with the correct type of flora or the correct amounts of flora. If the yogurt were made from fresh, raw goat's milk, it might be good for you, providing you had the necessary enzymes to digest it. Even then I would add a general use pro-biotic formula to any yogurt.

Q - Someone told me to drink carrot juice while on an ideal cleansing program because it would help with the feeding and strengthening of the constructive mucous lining of the intestines.

A - It probably will. Carrot juice is one of the best food substances there is. It is very high in nutrients, especially calcium and other electrolytes. It is also high in life-force. Make certain that the carrots you juice are organically grown. Add some celery, beet and ginger root for even more benefit. Do not add fruit.

---

Q - Do you recommend an ideal cleansing program for all diseases?

A - WARNING: Those with tuberculosis, cancer, emphysema, diabetes, and other serious, life-threatening degenerative diseases should be assisted by expert health professionals who have a high success rate in those areas. But, to answer your question, if I were suffering from one of those diseases, I would most certainly cleanse. How do you think people get those diseases in the first place? Those are filth related diseases. These people are congested - gummed up, clogged up and jam packed full of mucus, toxins and all the microorganisms that feed on all their filth. What do you think we should do with mucoid plaque in the body? Get rid of it! Once we get rid of the mucoid plaque in our bodies, we can start getting out the rest of the garbage - cleansing all the organs on a cellular level. The diet, thinking and emotions must be addressed as well.

---

Q - I've heard skin brushing is a good way to cleanse. Do you agree?

A - Absolutely! Skin brushing is actually better than using soap. Soap will not clean your skin as well as skin brushing with a natural bristle brush. (Avoid nylon brushes.) Soap removes only a small portion of the dead skin, while skin brushing removes far more of the dead skin and dirt with it. Soap often clogs the skin's pores and inhibits its ability to eliminate; it dries your skin. Skin brushing removes acids from the body and stimulates the skin by causing new blood to flow and circulate through this major elimination organ. Skin brushing helps the lymphatic system, and brushing just two minutes a day before you shower will stimulate and strengthen it.

Q - Do you recommend using digestive aids when I'm not on an ideal cleansing program?

A - Yes, if you feel that you need it. When you eat, proteins require special digestive enzymes, designed to digest amino acids. When you eat carbohydrates, you should take enzymes designed for their digestion. The fruit of the mature green papaya is the best natural source of enzymes.

---

Q - Does it cause any problems to have liquid minerals and bentonite in plastic containers?

A - The plastic used should be a food-grade plastic. Liquid minerals in this plastic may coat the plastic with minerals, but the minerals will not leach the plastic. However, it is possible that bentonite could leach toxic substance from the plastic bottles, although food-grade plastic bottles are not supposed to allow that. I recommend that when keeping bentonite for a long period of time, to either keep it refrigerated or store it in a glass container. Throw away any bentonite stored in a plastic bottle at room temperature for more than 6 months.

---

Q - I have Candida. Is there anything I should know about before Cleansing?

A - Do not use any fruit juices. Take psyllium shakes with pure water. Be sure to re-read this book, especially the sections on Candida, bacteria, and plucking out all negative emotions.

---

Q - What do you recommend for PMS?

A - Cleanse, eat pure foods, and use good herbs to help the situation. Make sure you have adequate electrolytes. Take mineral supplements, a full spectrum of antioxidants and other nutritional supplements. Be sure to avoid being constipated, especially the few days before and during menstruation. Stay away from salt, meat, dairy, sugar and wheat products. We may research this subject in the future. Stay in touch.

Q - I have a weak heart. I notice that while cleansing it pounds a lot.

A - I used to have a weak heart too. Because of rheumatic fever I had bad valves and an enlarged heart. It used to pound occasionally, while I was cleansing. If the body is releasing drugs and other toxins, they can cause anyone's heart to do that; however, it doesn't happen to me anymore. If you are really concerned, take cayenne pepper in capsules and hawthorn berries in tincture form.

---

Q - I heard that cayenne is good for the heart. What's the story?

A - Let me tell you about my mother and cayenne. She is one of the neatest people you could ever meet - she gets straight A's in personality. She has always marveled at the wonders of science - particularly medical science - and has always trusted the AMA's treat-the-symptom syndrome. Her faith in that area has dwindled to a low ebb, but only after watching her mother die a horrible, unnecessary, slow, painful death after following medical advice, and having seen so many of her friends and relatives suffer needlessly. However, when her hip started giving her trouble she began to hope for a bionic hip. I did my best to try to convince her to first try healing herself Nature's way - with herbs and diet. My efforts were in vain. It was like talking to a brick wall. She eventually got her wish and had a metal hip put in. She loved it! But after her operation she never could seem to enjoy her original active condition. Her heart was always bothering her. She kept taking all of the concoctions her doctor gave her, to no avail. Finally, one day I left her just a few cayenne capsules saying, "Mother, it can't hurt you! It's just food. There's nothing better for your heart! Just take two and see what happens." She said, "Well, maybe," as I left.

A few weeks later she was again very tired. She was just going to take a mid-morning nap on the couch. She went into the kitchen for some more coffee, saw those cayenne capsules on the counter, and decided to try just one (even though I had told her to try two). She swallowed it down and went to get a book to read, went upstairs to the bathroom, and headed for the couch. She started to lie down, suddenly stopped, and said to herself, "Wait a minute! I'm feeling pretty good!" Not only did she dispense with the nap, she ended up spending the whole day working in the yard and called to tell me to order her a large bottle of cayenne. She was so impressed that she was willing to take my advice one more time. I suggested that she take hawthorn along with the cayenne. She has been taking them ever since.

Even though, at that time, I had not been able to get her to change her acid diet to an alkaline diet, she continued to feel pretty good. A few years later, a family problem caused her a great deal of stress and she had a heart attack. The doctors ran some tests and found that three of the arteries leading to her heart were completely blocked and one more artery was almost blocked. They felt that her life depended upon a triple by-pass surgery and right away. But due to her age, the nicotine in her body, and the large amounts of aspirin in her blood (she was taking for her arthritis), they were not certain she would survive; so they did further tests and to their absolute surprise, they found out that my mother had an incredibly strong heart, so they performed the operation. A week later I arrived and she wasn't feeling good at all. I looked at the drugs they were giving her and said that her problems were related to one particular drug and recommended that she not take it; it was what was making her feel badly. She wouldn't listen. About a week later, she went in for a check-up and the doctor told her to double her intake of that drug. Three days later she was back in the emergency room. This time some other doctors advised that she quit taking that drug. A week later she felt renewed. A year later she started cleansing, which helped her so much that she can hardly believe it.

She did the mildest phase (with 2-1/2 meals per day). And the results were fantastic. Not only did she greatly increase her energy, but her memory came back to full. Her skin looked so much better that all her friends asked her what kind of cream she was using on her skin. Not bad for someone who ate mostly acid foods, smoked like the reincarnation of a forest fire, drank beer everyday, and took heavy amounts of aspirin daily for 60 years. She was more than 80 years old.

## Chapter 12

# REBUILDING VITAL ORGANS: ESSENTIAL CLEANSE FOLLOW-UP

*He who says it cannot be done, get out of the way of he
who is doing it.
According to your faith it is done unto you.*

-Anonymous

## Remove It!??

Several years ago a lady approached me and asked me to try and talk her sister out of having an operation she was planning to have. The doctors told this lady that if they did not remove her decaying adrenal gland that she would probably die. We have to have at least one adrenal to survive and apparently one of them was so bad that it if it didn't come out, it would rot and cause a life-threatening situation. Have you ever wondered why medical doctors are such awesome salesmen? They simply scare people so much that they are afraid of doing anything else. Car salesmen can't do this, but doctors do it everyday. Anyway, I told her that if her sister asked my opinion, I would give it, but I wouldn't volunteer to try and convince her to listen to me if she didn't want to. So she ended up having the operation. Oops, they cut out the wrong one! Oh well, we all make mistakes now and then, right?

I cannot tell you how many times I have heard stories like this. Not long ago we read in the paper that doctors had cut the wrong leg off a patient. The point that I want to make is that there are alternatives. Dr. Jensen wrote me a message one time. "Wisdom is the ability to discover an alternative." **Wisdom is not something we find very much of in this world, because most people are always looking outside of themselves for the answers that can only be found within**. People are so used to having someone else think for them that they seldom seek alternatives. Millions of people die every year because they cannot discover an alternative. In this chapter, I will present some alternatives. Although I believe that cleansing the alimentary canal is one of the most important places to start, it is only the beginning. This chapter brings you to the next step.[392]

# Address the Cause Behind the Cause: Renew Digestive Capacity with Proper Diet

I am convinced that our bodies were originally designed to partake of raw foods only.[393] However, as much as I believe in eating only raw foods, I am also very aware that most people have weakened their digestive tracts to the point where they cannot efficiently eat a raw-food diet for long periods of time.

There are several reasons for this: 1. Most people's digestive systems are so weak that they cannot produce or maintain the elements for adequate digestive chemistry: hydrochloric acid, enzymes, electrolytes, bicarbonate, bacteria, alkaline bile, etc. 2. Raw foods are pure clean foods with abundant life force. This means that they help cleanse the body. **Eating raw foods** can cause people to eliminate large amounts of toxic debris and this **can cause stress on any organ that is weak**; the liver, kidneys, etc. **In other words, it is common for people to experience cleansing reactions, until those organs have become strengthened.** How long will that take? It depends on how long it takes to clear out the toxic thought forms that are affecting those organs. 3. Attitudes: a sour attitude will cause sour digestion; thus people who have chronic habits of negative thinking are not likely to do well on raw foods. 4. Though people receive much more life force from raw foods, it also takes more life force to digest them. Many people lack the necessary life force to digest raw foods. 5. In addition, **the extra life force entering the system from raw foods will bring up emotional issues much more quickly.** Very few people are prepared for this. Further, our society and medical system basically deny such things, and totally fail to offer support for people dealing with these situations.

**We must cleanse and rebuild our digestive systems before we can consistently eat raw foods.** This includes restoring the liver, kidneys, and bowel, as well as the glands, including: thyroid, adrenal, pituitary, and pancreatic functions. And most important of all, we must

---

[392] While reading this chapter you may also want to **consult the Appendix titled: "Essential Elements for Effective Cleansing and Rebuilding."**

[393] **See Chapter 14: Secrets of Super Health, under "Why Raw Foods are the Perfect Foods."**

continue to apply the principles discussed in Chapter 10: Optimize Your Cleanse, to remove the suppressed negative emotions that cause those defects. This chapter addresses rebuilding the organs. The glands are best re-vitalized and healed by embracing creative and healing emotions, beliefs and points of view, as their functions are directly controlled by thought and feeling.

# Liver and the Gall Bladder

The health and vitality of all organs, glands, and cells, are dependent upon the liver. **Even our intelligence, attitudes, emotions and vitality are largely related to the liver**. This is why cleansing the liver can be a very emotional as well as a physical process. Our ability to repel disease or recover from disease is also very much associated with this incredible organ. **There are more than five hundred known functions that the liver performs, most of which are essential for life**. Along with the heart and brain, the liver is among the most important organs in the body. **No one can be healthy without a strong, clean liver**. The liver is so important that if you cut off a chunk of it, it will grow back every time.

Notice: Live-er. The name itself gives us an idea of how important this organ really is. It is the largest gland in the body, weighing about 4 pounds. Some people believe that at least 90% of the Western World's population have sluggish livers. 100% of people with cancer, AIDS, diabetes, heart problems, yeast infections, digestive problems, parasites, immune problems, etc. have liver problems. Yet how many doctors help their patients cleanse and strengthen the liver?

There are more than 500 different known functions of the liver. Following are just a few of them. Note the ones you think are essential for life.

### *JUST A FEW* KNOWN FUNCTIONS OF THE LIVER

Stores protein.
Stores glycogen.
Degrades proteins into energy or into fats.
Converts ammonia into urea.
Forms one half of all the lymph.
Formulates lipoproteins.
Synthesizes cholesterol and phospholipids.
Converts carbohydrates and proteins to fat.
Metabolizes protein, carbohydrates, fats.
Stores vitamins A, B-12, and D.
Stores copper and iron.

Detoxifies body from drugs.
Neutralizes certain poisons.
Metabolizes vitamins and minerals.
Converts galactose and fructose to glucose.
Helps to maintain alkaline pH of bowel.
Excretes excess calcium from blood into bile.
Removes dying red blood cells from blood.
Produces bile for digestion and assimilation of fats.
Converts L-Cysteine into Glutathione.
Maintains normal blood glucose levels between meals.
Converts the B vitamins into usable forms.
Makes Glucose Tolerance Factor (GTF).
Controls endocrine hormones.
Regulates blood clotting.
Converts vitamin D into usable form.
Formulates globulins, a necessity for immune system.
Essential for red blood cell production.
Essential for iron utilization.
Manufactures Vitamin A.
Stores sugar for future energy.
Produces important enzymes.
Supplies glucose to muscles.
Maintains equilibrium.
Formulates antibodies.
Helps to maintain alkaline pH of bowel.
Produces critical life-saving enzymes.
Controls saliva pH.

# How Liver Problems Originate

Physiologically, we develop liver weakness after we have abused our bodies by long-term eating of acid-forming foods, processed foods and other unhealthy foods. These include foods that are unnatural to the human body, like meat, sugar, white flour, white rice, foods cooked in oil, etc. Bad diet gradually weakens the digestive system, and do you know what organ takes the brunt of a bad diet? Yes, the liver. All the food that is absorbed from the small intestine, goes directly to the liver, by way of the portal vein. The liver and bowel then must deal with all the harmful chemicals from the bad food. Food colorings, preservatives, heavy metals, fried oils, partially digested proteins, etc., all take their toll upon our precious liver and digestive system. **It is for these reasons, that cleansing the bowels is absolutely the most important treatment in helping to rejuvenate the liver.**

# What Harms the Liver

Chemotherapy
Vaccines
Alcohol
Tobacco
Constipation alternating with
diarrhea
Medications and food chemicals
Cooked animal fats
Foods cooked in oil
Other drugs
Cod-liver oil
Margarine
Large amounts of meat in diet

Oils not cold pressed
Pasteurized milk
White sugar
Over eating
Coffee
Excessive fatigue
Over cooking
Fluoride from water
Chlorine from water
Salt-Sodium Chloride
Cooked wheat - especially
white bread
Lack of exercise

# Emotions Affect the Liver, Too

*More than any other organ, the liver is affected by negative thoughts and feelings.* Anger and fear, and all their emotional tributaries harm the liver more than anything else. With the exception of injury, 99% of all disease has an association with toxic waste settlement in conjunction with unconscious negative thoughts and feelings. This is why when people cleanse or take herbs to cleanse and strengthen the liver, strong emotions surface. This emotional cleansing is a key part of the process.

# A Toxic Liver Results from a Toxic Bowel, and Leads to Disease

When the bowel is overburdened with the wrong foods, and/or negative emotions cause physical stress and toxicity, the liver must work overtime to save the life of the body. Every vein from the digestive tract empties into the liver, which filters out toxins and waste. The skin and lungs are the body's first line of defense against toxins, the bowel is next, then the liver.

If the liver is unable to perform its full function, it will not only become even more toxic, but all the other organs become challenged. Prior to the first sign of disease, the effectiveness of the liver has been reduced. First come negative thoughts and feelings, then toxins from poor diet, which cause congestion and contamination, then the liver becomes overburdened until it becomes weak. This results in a lack of oxygen and nutrients to cells, and the inability of the cells to rid themselves of their waste.

## Problems Related to Liver Weakness

| | | |
|---|---|---|
| Abscesses | Anal itching | Adenoid and tonsil problems |
| Anemia | Appendicitis | Poor assimilation |
| Bad breath | Bronchitis | Cancer |
| Chills | Diabetes | Poor digestion |
| Enlarged spleen | Gas | Mental fatigue |
| Flat feet | Hemorrhoids | Dizziness and blind spells |
| Hemorrhages | Proneness to insect bites | Inability to tolerate heat or cold |
| Spasms in intestines | Migraine headaches | Problems with intestinal flora |
| Nervousness, anxiety | Obese and skinny people | Vision trouble and ear trouble |
| Red nose | Difficult sleeping | Sticky mouth when waking up |
| Sleepiness after meals | Strange yellow stool color | Sinus trouble and head colds |

Nervous depression

Jaundice-yellow coloration of the skin

Brown or dark spots on face and on back of hands

Nausea, especially if no appetite and feeling of heart trouble

Feeling of pain around the right shoulder blade and shoulder

Tongue coated with whitish, yellowish or greenish coating

Frequent urination at night (example of how a weak liver can weaken the kidneys and bladder)

Appearance of small bright red specks on various places of the body

Glandular imbalance, discomfort during menstrual period

Headaches-especially when a feeling of heaviness in the whole head, especially if pain forms a circle around upper part of head and temples

Intestinal inflammation, infections and fermentation

## The Noble Liver Deserves Cooperation

The liver keeps us alive and buffers all our lousy food decisions; it deserves the best. The secret of a strong liver is purification. Cleansing the alimentary canal is the first and most important activity to help the liver. Herbs, specific nutritional supplements such as antioxidants, diet, and visualization are very effective in helping to cleanse and rebuild the liver function. For those who have indulged in fatty foods, specific nutrients are necessary to cleanse out the congestion of fats. Same thing with various chemicals and heavy metals; specific nutrients are essential. I have been studying this subject for a long time and continue to keep up to date on the latest clinical studies. I also experiment on myself. In short, I never stop looking for better ways to improve liver function. **If you are interested in my latest formulas, you can contact the source listed at the back of the book.**

# Liver Cleansing and Rebuilding Program

An effective liver cleansing and rebuilding program needs to include all of the following:

> Specific herbs to cleanse and help rebuild the liver
> Specific nutrients to remove fats
> Specific nutrients to strengthen and protect the liver
> Proper diet.

# Liver/GallBladder Cleanse

### Do You Have Gallstones?

Medical textbooks indicate that only 20% of Americans over 65 have gallstones. However, I have found that about 80% of those who has taken the gallbladder flush find gallstones. Perhaps, the 20% they refer to have chronic biliary calculi. This means the condition has become so severe that medical doctors feel that they must remove the gallbladder. Just as medical science will not use inexpensive, but highly effective cayenne pepper to prevent and stop heart attacks, so they also will not use the inexpensive, but highly effective gallbladder flush to successfully remove gallstones.

### Compare the costs

Medical treatment for heart problems, may cost from a few thousand dollars, to a potential of twenty thousand or more, as compared to fifteen dollars or less of cayenne pepper and hawthorn berry herbs. Similarly, it may cost you about five dollars for a gallbladder flush now and then, compared to several thousand dollars for operations, not to mention the severe trauma and side effects of the drugs they will use. Perhaps we should also mention that patients who have had their gallbladders removed usually have consistent and severe health problems for the rest of the lives. Obesity, constipation, gastrointestinal problems, and diabetes to mention a few. What a racket - and they have the nerve to call doctors who do not use the conventional drug and surgery methods, quacks.

## Symptoms

Prevention of disease is a very wise process to follow. Most people who use a gallbladder flush do so to prevent future trouble. Those who wait until gallstones become a chronic condition may suffer from the following symptoms:

### Problems Related to Gallstones

| | |
|---|---|
| dyspepsia (heartburn) | ulcers |
| colic (severe pain) | fatty food intolerance |
| belching | bloating |
| fullness | nausea |
| jaundice | pancreatitis |
| infections | backaches |
| dark complexion | high blood pressure |
| slow pulse | strong appetites |
| a quick, irritable temper | coated tongue |
| constipation | headache |
| dizziness | pasty complexion |

and you can be sure, the dreaded mucoid plaque.

## The Cause of Gallstones

Although medical science has failed to recognize the cause of gallstones, it is no mystery to those who have studied physiology with the sincere desire of helping people to inexpensively solve their health problems. Gallstones are usually formed in conjunction with a deficiency of organic sodium.

When the body becomes deficient in organic sodium, it will go to another part of the body and leach out sodium to be used in blood homeostasis. The easiest place the body can extract sodium without causing serious problems is from the bile. This extracting occurs at the gallbladder. When the sodium has been removed from the gall juice, the pH of the gall juice drops. If enough sodium is withdrawn, the pH can drop to a point where the bile, which should be alkaline, becomes extremely acid, and then calcium and cholesterol hardens. As it hardens, it forms gallstones. From this understanding, it is easy to see that to correct this condition it is imperative to replenish the sodium reserves. A nearly 100% alkaline diet is absolutely essential until one can pass the pH tests. Once we can pass the pH tests, chances are the bile will also return to its natural pH levels. Using natural alkaline electrolyte supplements will assist the body in correcting the problem sooner. It is important to use the correct supplement, because when the body has been leached of its sodium, it will use up other minerals faster. Therefore, the alkaline supplement must have high levels of organic sodium. The highest source is from goat milk whey. Do not use whey from cows; yes, it is cheaper, but extremely mucus forming.

My studies indicate that due to the high protein consumption in America, it is likely that most Americans have gallstones. After flushing the gallbladder, people will find out if they have been eating too much protein — too much acid-forming food. Seeing gallstones after the treatment is a sure sign that they have been eating too much acid food.

### Instructions

For current instructions on how to accomplish a very effective gallbladder/liver flush, contact my office. These are periodically updated as new information becomes available; this allows for ongoing refinement of the process.

# The Kidneys and the Urinary Tract

The primary function of the urinary system is to help maintain homeostasis[394] by controlling the composition, volume, and pressure of blood. It does so by removing and restoring selected amounts of water and dissolved substance. There are two kidneys, two ureters, one urinary bladder, and a single urethra that comprise this necessary system.

The kidneys are about 4 to 5 inches long and weigh about 6 ounces. The body must have at least one kidney to maintain life. See the following list to understand more about what the kidneys do.

## Kidney Functions

Regulate the composition and volume of the blood.
Filter wastes products from the blood in the form of urine. The most important waste products are those generated by the breakdown of proteins.

---

[394] Homeostasis: The state of equilibrium in the body with respect to various functions and to the chemical compositions of the fluids and tissues. *Stedman's Medical Dictionary*.

Regulate electrolytes and help control proper pH levels.

Regulate liquids. If we drink too much water, the kidneys get rid of it. When we become dehydrated, the kidneys conserve water.

Help regulate blood pressure by secreting the enzyme renin.

Contribute towards the releasing of aldosterone, an adrenal hormone that helps to regulate the sodium/potassium ratio - an essential metabolic activity.

Play an essential role in metabolism by: 1) Secreting the hormone erythropoietin, which stimulates production and release of red blood cells from bone marrow. 2) Converting vitamin D into a usable hormone. 3) Performing gluconeogenesis[395] during periods of fasting or starvation.

I believe that the urinary tract plays other important roles in regulating brain and gland function. This has not been affirmed by medical science as yet. But, it is based on my observation of people who have kidney weakness. An example: I have seen people's eyesight, brain function, and attitude improve in just a few minutes using herbs for the kidneys. My intuition tells me that kidneys are more important than medical science realizes.

Along with the liver and bowel, no other organ suffers more from the consequences of the American diet. White sugar, sodium chloride (table salt), too much protein, and processed foods are very harmful to the kidneys. Heavy metals, however, affect the kidneys more than anything else, especially lead and mercury. Heavy metals seem to be attracted more to the kidneys than any other organ. Consistent intake of toxins can gradually settle in the kidneys, causing weakness, sluggishness, and poor performance.

## Signs of Possible Kidney and/or Urinary Problems

| | | |
|---|---|---|
| Bloody urine | Cloudy urine | Mucus in urine |
| Tired all the time | Weak eyesight | Pain in eyes |
| Copious urination | Incontinence | Swelling - edema or dropsy |
| Kidney stones | Hypertension | Diabetes mellitus |

Color of urine other than clear yellow
Foul-smelling or dark urine
Pain in back near lower part of rib cage
Weakness of the lower extremities
A cold sensation in the lower half of the body

---

[395] Gluconeogenesis: The formation of glucose from noncarbohydrates, such as protein or fat. *Stedman's Medical Dictionary.*

Tenseness in the lower abdomen
Burning pain on urination - usually bladder infection
Lower abdominal pain
A pale swollen tongue with a thin, white and moist coating
Pain in joints
Frequent need to urinate; excessive urge to urinate at night
Brain fog

There are herbal formulas designed to help remove mucus, toxins, and other forms of congestion from the liver and urinary system. Traditionally, the herbs for the kidneys are known to be highly effective in strengthening and tonifying the entire urinary pathway. They help to increase the flow of urine and may reduce inflammation. They may also be effective in removing uric acid and other crystal formations in the urinary system. Many times I have seen these herbs remove pain in eyes within one day and clear a foggy head. I have also known them to increase the flow of urine with those who had difficulty urinating.

# The Bowel

## Mucous Membrane and the Bowel Wall

The lining of the intestine is the most consistently damaged area in the body. The constant presence of food, fiber, bacteria, toxins, acids, and the normal activity of digestion causes large amounts of cells to "slough off". This is normal and ordinarily the body is capable of dealing with this activity. Due to the excessive indulgence of acid-forming foods such as meat, dairy, processed foods, wheat, cereals, nutrient deficient commercially grown produce etc., plus negative emotions, drugs, and alcohol, the standard American bowel has become deficient in nutrients. Without adequate nutrients, the bowel loses its ability to defend itself from acids, toxicants,[396] microorganisms, and other chemicals that damage the bowel wall. As the bowel loses its strength, poor digestion develops, which compounds the already mounting problems. Continued abuse finally forces the gut to become less and less able to defend and repair itself. Indigestion, diarrhea, constipation, and mucoid plaque are the natural result of this long term defilement. These conditions are the first signals that disease of the bowel has developed. It indicates that the bowel, as well as the rest of the body, has become vulnerable to even worse conditions.

---

[396] Herbicides, pesticides, preservatives, and other unnatural chemicals found in our food.

Unnatural bowel environment, no matter whether luminal or internal, diminishes the ability of the bowel's immune system to function. When the bowel is healthy, IgA's[397] are capable of destroying virtually every known pathogenic microorganism (including bacteria, yeast, fungus, parasites, etc.). When we lose the necessary nutrients or acquire an over-acid bowel, the IgA activity can no longer function effectively and the bowel, as well as the entire physical body becomes vulnerable to attack. Consistent attack from pathogenic microorganisms, unnatural chemicals, and acids eventually weaken the structure of the bowel and we become even more vulnerable to diseased states.

The presence of intestinal irritations such as Candida, heavy metals, colitis, ulcers, parasites, and other bowel diseases, are more signals that the breakdown of bowel tissue is occurring at a faster rate than the repair. All of the above can weaken the integrity of the bowel structure to such a degree that the bowel wall pathways (normal nutrient pathways into bloodstream) stretch beyond their normal diameters. However, any inflammation of the bowel is also likely to cause this condition. This spreading of the tissues is called "Leaky Bowel Syndrome". It is a condition which allows undesirable and often, pathogenic substance to penetrate through the bowel barrier and enter into the bloodstream. This undesirable scenario allows toxic material, such as bacterial fragments, yeast, undigested protein, fats, fecal matter, and other bowel toxins to enter the bloodstream.

When a leaky bowel develops,[398] the liver must deal with the toxic overload. The relentless flow of toxins from the bowel eventually weakens the liver. At first the liver is usually able to cope with these unhealthy conditions. However, after the unrelenting inflow of toxic matter, the liver gradually becomes more sluggish and weak. The liver then can no longer process the toxic debris, and various symptoms gradually develop as other organs, glands, and tissues become vulnerable to mucus, congestion, and unmerciful attacks from microorganisms. This is why insufficient bowel function results in variety of chronic and degenerative diseases. **Cleansing and rebuilding the bowel should be one of the most important goals of everyone who has become health conscious, for when the bowel functions optimally, then, and only then, can the liver and every**

---

[397] Ig means "immunoglobulin" which are antibodies produced by B-lymphocytes (white blood cells). IgA is a specific type which is found in the healthy and normal mucus of the gut. Tortora and Grabowski, pg. 702.

[398] **For common conditions or diseases related to leaky gut syndrome, see Chapter 6: Impaired Digestion and It's Outcomes, under "Leaky Bowel Syndrome."**

other organ have the ability to also function optimally. *It should be noted, that a perfectly functioning body is virtually invulnerable to any microorganism.*

# Repairing a Damaged Bowel Wall

A damaged bowel wall requires specific nutrients for rapid repair. There are important nutritional supplements capable of feeding the lining of the intestinal tract as it regenerates, reducing inflammation, and allowing the production of new cell tissues. These nutrients will also help to detoxify the bowel from rancid oils, free radicals and assists in reducing intestinal toxemia. Some supplements may help to neutralize chemicals, alcohol and heavy metals and may increase the effectiveness of white and red blood cell production and help to strengthen the capillary walls, cell membranes and reduce inflammation. The kinds of supplements that I recommend are designed to heal and soothe the serosa, muscularis, submucosa, and mucosa (the four anatomical sections of the bowel). Without the perfect functioning of all layers of the gut, it is impossible to achieve our fullest potential in health, mind, and spirit.

### Steps to Take to Remedy a Damaged Bowel Wall

1. Alkalize - Take pH tests and bring your electrolyte reserves up to full.
2. Cleanse the bowel - Cleanse the entire alimentary canal prior to using supplements.
3. Remove parasites and pathogenic bacteria
4. Take a diet of 80% alkaline-forming foods - Mostly fruits and vegetables. No citrus, distilled vinegar, alcohol, table salt, fried foods, processed foods such as white flour, sugar, pop, soy products, wheat products (bread, cookies, cakes, cereals etc.).
5. Use a general use probiotic formula which is more alkaline-forming and has colostrum. I believe that *Lactobacillus*, particularly *Lactobacillus acidophilus*, should not used for treating Leaky Bowel. *Lactobacillus* secretions have a pH of **approximately 4.5** and sometimes even less. Our bowel needs to have a pH of at least 6.5 and preferably between 7 to 7.5. We do not need more acid when healing the bowel wall. On the contrary, most bowel diseases are associated with acids and a lack of alkaline electrolytes.
6. Use supplements specific for bowel repair and rebuilding. Contact me for an update of the latest and most effective supplements available. **See Appendix II: Essential Elements for Effective Cleansing and Rebuilding.**
7. Detoxify the liver.

As the bowel receives needed nutrients and becomes stronger, it may "throw off" harmful particles and it is not uncommon to experience gas, unusual odors and discharges. Within 2 weeks, improved bowel performance is likely to be noticed. It is recommended that supplements be used for 3 to 6 months to assure maximum results.

# Fight Candida and Pathogenic Bacteria

An ideal probiotic formula for general use should provide a strong supplement of the friendly bacteria your bowel and other vital organs need to *stay* healthy. Any time you suspect your friendly bacteria may be weakened or challenged, you should use such a formula.[399] *A second probiotic formula (with acid bacteria) should be used **with** a general use formula (a more alkaline formula), specifically to fight infections of Candida and pathogenic bacteria which may occur following prolonged stress, poor diet, food poisoning, use of antibiotics, birth control pills, or any medical treatment which could reduce the friendly flora.*[400]

## When a Second Probiotic Formula
## May Be Helpful

The following are the most common conditions indicating the need to use an acid bacteria probiotic formula, along with a general use formula.

- Candida albicans
- Intestinal infections of *Staphylococcus*, Shigella, Kiebsiella pneumoniae, Sarcina luta, Vibrio comma, (Asiatic cholera), *Salmonella*, *Pseudomonas*, enterobacterium (consists of various bacteria including E. coli (Escherichia), and some parasites).
- Constipation, diarrhea or loose stools
- Chronic colds and frequent illnesses
- Skin disorders such as pimples, acne, or persistent blemishes
- Food poisoning
- Allergic reactions within 30 minutes of eating, such as fatigue, sneezing, or intestinal gas and bloating
- Food cravings and an abnormally excessive appetite
- Any chronic disease, especially immune deficiencies

---

[399] **See Chapter 9: Facts about Dr. Anderson's Cleansing Program, under "Friendly Bacteria."**

[400] **See Chapter 9: Facts About Dr. Anderson's Cleansing Program, under "Cleansing and Candida."**

- Post-antibiotic therapy or history of antibiotic use
- Excessive flatulence
- Cravings for sweets due to yeast
- Bowel diseases such as colitis, Crohn's disease, IBS, Candida Albicans, Leaky Bowel Syndrome
- Chronic fatigue
- Food intolerances and allergies
- High serum cholesterol levels
- Weakened immune system
- Poor digestion
- Cancer[401]

> **Note:** It is always essential to take the more alkaline, general use formula either with or following any use of the acid bacteria formula. It may be necessary for 30 days or even longer.

When we take both formulas together we may first notice rumblings in the abdomen, and some people may get gas. In about one to two weeks we may have loose stools, sometimes mild cases of diarrhea. This is not serious. It is caused because the bacteria is reducing the unfriendly bacteria (*E. coli* etc.) and Candida, etc. In a week or two this should stop. Then for a few days to two weeks we may have constipation. This is because the bad bacteria was greatly reduced and bacteria makes up about 30% or so of the stools. The new bacteria is now growing, but it's microscopic and it takes awhile before it grows enough to produce the amount needed for good bowel movements. Next we may feel bloated for a few days, and right after that, our bowels kick into gear. The bloating disappears and from then on, we should have good healthy bowel movements. This will not occur exactly in this way with everyone. Those who do not have a bacteria problem will probably not notice anything at all.[402]

**Note**: In one of my experiments, I ended up taking too much of an acid bacteria formula and it caused diarrhea. I had to stop taking it for a few days. Taking excessive amounts is not recommended.

---

[401] Dr. Khem M. Shahani, Professor, Food Science & Technology, *Facts & Fallacies About Probiotics,* University of NE, Lincoln NE 68583-0919

[402] It is possible that some people may not be entirely successful in reducing the pathogenic bacteria from their bowels on the first cleanse. Some pathogenic bacteria may continue to maintain a strong foothold even after using the main probiotic formula. Under these conditions people may continue having constipation. The second pro-biotic formula may be the answer, or maybe another cleanse will be necessary.

# Eliminate Parasites

## Medical Treatments for Parasites

Medical treatments against parasites can be dangerous. Many times they use chemotherapy drugs. Side effects from parasitic drugs may include the following items:[403]

| | | |
|---|---|---|
| abdominal pain | anorexia | arrhythmia |
| ataxia | blindness | blood |
| dyscrasiabradycardial colic | chills | cinchonism |
| colic | color vision disturbance | confusion |
| convulsions | cramps | diarrhea |
| dizziness | dyscrasia | eosinophilia |
| epigastric burning | fever | folic acid deficiency |
| headache | hemolytic anemia | hepatic/renal toxins |
| hepatic necrosis | hypotension-hypoglycemia | insomnia |
| itching | kidney impairment | leukopenia |
| liver impairment | muscle pain, joint stiffness | myocardia |
| nausea and vomiting | neutropenia | ocular damage |
| paresthesias | peripheral neuropathy | photosensitivity |
| pruritus | psychosis | rash |
| retinal injury | sedation | GI disturbance |
| shock | sweating | tachycardia |
| thyroid enlargement | tinnitus | urticaria |
| vasculitis | vertigo. | |

That is about it. They didn't list death, which was a surprise. **Modern medical science is the only organization that suggests using treatments worse than the disease.** But that is where the money is and fortunately for them, the people go along with it. People foolishly think that the disease made them victims and medical science will free them from their victimization. It is really the other way around. Would I recommend using drugs to treat parasites? I can't imagine that I would. There are certainly better methods. Would cleansing, rebuilding, strengthening all aspects of the body, including the immune system, and the use of herbs and other natural treatments work? In most cases it would.

---

[403] Ruth Leventhal, Russel Cheadle, *Medical Parasitology, A Self-Instructional Text*, 4th Edition, (Philadelphia, PA: F. A. Davis Co., 1996), pg. 152-156.

## Natural Treatments for Parasites

Generally, herbal remedies work very well in removing most varieties of parasites, as many thousands of people can testify. For protozoa, concentrated citrus seed extract has proven to be one of the most effective treatments yet devised. I recommend three additional herbal parasite-specific products to aid cleansers using an ideal cleansing program: herbal capsules,[404] concentrated green black walnut hulls extract, and concentrated citrus seed extract. Health food stores generally do not carry the concentrated citrus seed extract, but a watered down version of it.

As with any disease, it is essential to cleanse the bowels, liver, immune system and remove the negative attitudes that made the body susceptible to parasite infestation in the first place.

# Antioxidants

There has been a great deal of discussion in the last couple of years about "free radicals", their effects on health and well being, and the role that antioxidants play in ridding our bodies of free radicals and restoring health. Most people read about how good antioxidants are for us without really understanding what free radicals are, how they are formed and how antioxidants prevent their formation and repair the damage they have done. The wise use of antioxidants can help in rebuilding vital organs, preventing disease and slowing the aging process.[405]

---

[404] See Appendix II: Essential Elements for Effective Cleansing and Rebuilding.

[405] See Chapter 14: Secrets of Super Health, under "Reversing the Aging Process," "Free Radicals," and "Uses of Specific Antioxidants," for more information.

# Chapter 13

# EATING FOR GOOD HEALTH

*The end of science is not to prove a theory, but to improve mankind.*

- Manly P. Hall

*"Human improvement is from within outward."*

- Froude

*"Life in all its fullness is Mother Nature obeyed."*

- Weston Price

*It is not death that a man should fear, but he should fear never beginning to live.*

- Marcus Aurelius

**Is there any animal, bird, or fish that cooks its food? Were we issued stoves upon birth?** *Cooking food certainly was not designed by the creator. It is an art created by the dark side;* **"And he entices every one by that to which their heart is most inclined."** [406] *It is so easy for the "dark side" to manipulate people in regards to food, for almost everyone willingly gives*

---

[406] Essene Gospel of Peace, Chapter 1.

*into their lusts, appetites, and desires, and the world*
*supports them in this. Yummy, delicious, gooey*
*cooked food - we pay for it with our lives.*

- Dr. Richard Anderson, N.D., N.M.D.

# Poisons to Avoid

The true definition of a food is: a substance that nourishes or fuels the body with life-giving force and substance, thereby strengthening, energizing, and maintaining it. Food is not simply something one puts in the mouth, chews and swallows. Sawdust and rubber could be used for that. Food should not deplete or rob the body of its life essence or harm it in any way. Dead foods take an enormous toll on the body. Not only do they deplete us of valuable enzymes, but they drain life force from our bodies, and contribute towards toxicity, mucus, and that inner environment in which pathogenic bacteria, parasites, and yeasts thrive.

## The Very Worst Physiological Things We Can Do to Our Bodies are to Consume the Following Poisons

- **Drugs**: Especially antibiotics which destroy the natural, alkalizing, friendly bacteria; and aspirin which destroys the natural mucous lining and depletes electrolytes.

- **Alcohol**: Destroys the healthy mucous lining and the villi in the small intestines, as well as damaging the liver and the brain.

- **Spoiled and rancid foods:** Cause an emergency situation for the body. They create tremendous acids, extreme toxins, and an army of free radicals which cause great strain on the liver, enzyme systems, immune system and other organs, plus draining the alkaline minerals.

- **Inorganic Salt - Sodium Chloride (table salt)**: When salt contacts mucous membranes it either destroys the membrane or causes an emergency bicarbonate condition which further depletes organic sodium and other minerals.

- **Distilled Vinegar**:  Creates an extreme acid condition which causes the body great difficulty.  It forces the body to use strong buffering minerals.  It is a common ingredient in commercial salad dressings, mustard and hot sauces, read the labels and avoid those products.  If the label does not say raw cider vinegar, you can be 99% sure the vinegar is distilled vinegar.

- **Fried foods**:  The oils turn into inorganic acids, causing extreme acidity to the body.  Even vegetables fried in oils are extremely hard to digest and are extremely hard on the liver and other organs.  Nothing except drugs does more damage to the liver.  The effects of fried foods are similar to rancid foods.

- **Meat, fish, and birds**:  These are not so acid when the whole body is consumed uncooked, that is, raw!  The cooked muscles of animals are extremely acid and their constant consumption is the number-one dietary reason for poor health in the Western World today.  Eating these innocent creatures drains the alkaline minerals from our bodies faster than any other habit.[407]

- **Pasteurized Dairy products:**  Coat the gastrointestinal tract with mucus and contribute to more acids in the body.  Pasteurized cow milk depletes calcium from our bodies.[408]  Guess what they make "Elmer's Glue-all" with?  Pasteurized cow's milk even kills *calves* between 3 and 6 months of age.[409]  If we would use *raw* milk, from goats instead of cows, then it would be much better for us, but we should still be weaned as soon as we grow teeth.

- **White Sugar**:  Though the pH of sugar is neutral, it causes extreme stimulation of the metabolic processes, which does create acids.  Sugar can

---

[407]  If you want to eat animals, you should do it like any other decent meat-eating animal.  First, you should kill the animal yourself.  Second, you should never even think about cooking it.  Third, you should eat the guts first - raw.  Fourth, eat the muscles along with the skin.  Fifth, chew the bones.  If you follow the above five steps, then you can consider yourself a true meat-eater!  However, physiologically, you are still not qualified.  Sorry, your digestive system is not designed the same way that those of carnivorous animals are.

[408] Allen, et. al., "Protein-Induced Hypercalciuria: A Longer Term Study," pg. 741-749. H. M. Linkswiler, M. B. Zemel, M. Hegsted, S. Schuette, "Protein-Induced Hypercalcuria," *Federal Proceedings,* 1981; 40, pg. 2429. Cow's milk is not only a negative source of calcium, but contributes towards inhibiting calcium from being absorbed and utilized from other food sources.  No wonder vitamin D is added to cow's milk; they hope that it will help increase calcium absorption.  Maybe it helps, but it is not enough.

[409] Dr. Ted Morter, *Your Health Choice,* (Hollywood, FL: Fell Publishers and Company, Inc., 1990), pg. 167.

cause many pathogenic problems, especially involving the thyroid, adrenal glands, liver, and pancreas. No one should drink soft drinks made with white sugar or artificial sweeteners.

- **Flour products**: Wheat burns the tips of the villi, causing them to shrink. White flour not only burns the tips of the villi; it also coats the intestines with an unnatural mucous paste, which adds to the mucoid plaque. When the condition becomes serious, it is then given a name. It is called "celiac disease". It is the gluten in the wheat flour which does the damage. Wheat is by far the worst, but rye, barley, and oats can also cause problems.[410] Gluten burns tissue and then mucus flows into that area to prevent further damage. Now get this! Medical science strongly suggests that celiac disease results from a primary defect in the intestinal mucosa caused by the gluten in the wheat.[411] I suspect that white flour may be one of the factors that trigger excess mucin secretion which adds to the mucoid plaque thickness. It also may be one of the transforming factors that leads to bowel disease. The main reason I think this is that I have noticed over the years that the most sickly people eat more white flour products than the average person.

Notice that the above foods, which we consider toxic to our bodies, are all highly acid-forming foods. The ingestion of these poisons, or the creation of over-acidity in the body, drains the alkaline minerals which inhibits the intestinal fluids ability to compensate for the excessive acidic bile. It is possible however, that the body can become so drained of vital nutrients, especially electrolytes, that even the healthy protective mucoid layer cannot be formed. Crone's disease, colitis, bowel cancer and other bowel inflammations may be the result.

### What Cooked, Frozen, Canned, and Processed Foods Do

- create toxins
- cause stress, congestion, and mucus
- overwork the digestive system
- produce the ideal environment for parasites
- drain the life force from the body
- strain the glandular system
- alter the constructive bacteria in the intestines
- poison the bloodstream, thereby feeding disease
- clog the lymph system

---

410  Yamada, ed., pg. 1503.

411  Yamada, ed., pg. 1504.

- drain the enzyme reserve
- overwork and clog the elimination systems

I imagine that if all Americans stopped indulging in the detrimental foods described above, we would become one of the healthiest nations in the world within 10 years. Beyond avoiding the poisons, we can strengthen our bodies even further by gradually moving towards a diet of raw foods.

# Avoid Dairy Products

Pasteurized cow's milk in any form is the most mucus-forming of all foods. Cow's milk is **NOT** the same as human milk. Here is something that some people have not realized. **Cow's milk was designed and made for calves. Human milk was designed and made for human babies**. There is a vast difference in the chemical composition as well as the energetic character; **when cow's milk is pasteurized, it becomes a poison to our bodies and to the bodies of calves**. My definition of a poison: Something that causes harm or depletion to our bodies. **Calves fed on pasteurized cow's milk will die in three to six months**[412]. Doesn't it make sense to think that if pasteurized cow's milk is a poison to a calf for whom cow's milk was designed, then pasteurized cow's milk is also a poison to humans, for whom it was not designed? Rather amazing that people don't seem to get it!

Raw cow milk from healthy cows will also cause mucus and congestion in humans, but it does not contain the poisons and nutritional deficits that are typical of pasteurized cow milk. I believe that **pasteurized cow's milk is the number one cause of poor health and disease in children. It is the leading cause of allergies**[413] **and it sets the stage for many future diseases.** Most children who drink pasteurized cow's milk will end up on antibiotics and it is downhill from then on. The decision to force all cow milk to be pasteurized was not based upon intelligent scientific facts available at the time. I am convinced it was not initiated for the purpose of helping anyone! My reasons for saying this are as follows:

◆ Pasteurizing cow milk was never done in all the world's history, until modern times. For thousands of years people survived very well drinking milk that was not pasteurized.

---

[412] Morter, pg. 167.

[413] John A. McDougall, M.D, and Mary A. McDougal, *The McDougall Plan*, (Clinton, NJ: New Win Publishing, Inc. 1983), pg.49.

♦ Pasteurizing milk is completely unnatural and mutates its health-giving properties.

We hear propaganda that milk is good for you and that it is high in calcium. The truth is: pasteurized cow's milk is not good for anything that lives, not even for calves.[414] Yes, cow milk is high in calcium but humans will actually lose more calcium by drinking it than if they don't drink any milk at all. Indeed pasteurized cow milk is bad for all life forms that consume it. A few facts:

♦ The phosphorous in cow's milk inhibits calcium from being absorbed and utilized.[415]
♦ Cow's milk contains much more phosphorous than calcium.[416] Therefore, the body is forced to take calcium from our bones in order to achieve the proper calcium/phosphorous ratio.
♦ Pasteurization alters the bonds that hold the minerals together and may prevent the calcium from being usable by the body.[417]
♦ Because of the abundance of phosphorous, protein, and chlorides, pasteurized cow's milk is acid-forming and the body must use its own reserve of sodium, potassium, and calcium, from an already depleted supply in order to handle the excess acids.[418]
♦ Pasteurization depletes enzymes, vitamins, and life force. Not only is this milk not giving us those vital ingredients, but it has to take some from our bodies in the attempt to digest it.
♦ At least 50% of the American people tested for allergies reacted to dairy products, mainly because they lacked the lactase enzyme.[419]
♦ Eating dairy products helps to perpetuate the cruelty of the dairy industry.[420]

---

[414] Morter, pg. 167.

[415] Linkswiler, Zemel, Hegsted, Schuette, pg. 2429.

[416] Allen, et.al., "Protien-Induced Hypercalciuria: A Long Term Study," pg. 741-749.

[417] Dr. M. Ted Morter, pg. 166.

[418] Ibid., pg. 167-168

[419] Lactose intolerance is found in more than 70% of black Americans, Orientals, Arabs, Greeks, Eskimos, Indians, Africans, and in more than 50% of white Americans. Yamada, pg. 1521.

[420] This is only one example of many that I would like to share with you as to what is done to baby calves in order to make veal. This is a quote from John Robbin's book which I wish everyone would read, *Diet For A New America*, pg. 187-188. "First of all, the calf is taken away from his

mother immediately after birth. Veal producers are aware this deprives the infant calf of the colostrum in its mother's milk, and so renders the little ones very susceptible to disease. But they separate mother and child at birth anyway, because the large udder of today's dairy cow can be damaged by suckling, and the cow will produce more milk if attached to a machine. Additionally, according to Dr. Jack Albright, Professor of Animal Science at Purdue University, and consultant to the veal industry, it is important the calves do not bond with their mother, as they would if she nursed them. If the calves are taken away from their mothers after this bond develops, the cow will cause a great deal of trouble and even try to break down fences to be with her calves.

The newborn calves are taken to veal sheds, and placed in what are euphemistically called 'stalls'. These stalls will be their homes until they are slaughtered at the age of four months, unless, of course, they die first. A high percentage are not able to survive even four months, so horrid are the conditions.

The stalls have been designed to keep the calves' flesh 'tender enough to be used for baby food.' If the calves were let outside, or even kept in a pen, their frisky nature would lead them to romp around and they would soon develop muscles. This, of course, must not happen. So the infant calves are shut tightly in their stalls, and allowed no exercise whatsoever, right from the start.

Every year, one million newborn calves are shut up in such stalls in the United States to be raised for veal. These youngsters not only never have a chance to romp or play; they never even walk! Remember these are babies, only a day or so old, cut off from their mothers and imprisoned in this way.

The stalls are so tiny the animals can hardly move. They are so narrow that in order to lie down the calves must hunch into a position no cow ever normally assumes. They cannot stretch out into their natural sleeping posture. They cannot turn around. Chained around the neck, the baby calves cannot even twist their heads to lick and groom themselves with their tongues, though this is one of their most basic and innate desires. They can move only a few inches back and forth, and side to side. Their stall is as cramped as a shipping crate. As the days pass, and the calves grow, they become even more cramped, so that any movement at all becomes nearly impossible.

Calves are born with stores of iron in their bodies, primarily in the form of extra hemoglobin in the blood, with lesser amounts stored in the liver, spleen, and bone marrow. During the four months the veal calf is confined and 'special fed,' these reserves decline steadily. The veal producers are pleased to have achieved their objective: the calves' flesh remains white while they put on weight.

Producers would like to take the calves to even heavier weights, but by the time four months have passed and they have reached about 350 pounds, the calves have become so seriously anemic that those still alive would soon die in their stalls.

That's enough; you've got the picture. This insane cruelty will indeed exact a retribution, according to the Laws of Life. However, let us not forget, that it is the consumer that perpetrates this unnecessary and pitiless brutality."

Henry G. Bieler, M.D., pointed out that enlightened pediatricians know that pasteurization of cow's milk is definitely harmful for infants.[421]

Summary: There is something terribly wrong about pasteurized milk. It appears poisonous and disease-producing. If you care about your children and your own health, avoid pasteurized cow's milk - your health and lives may depend upon it.

Eskimos eat more protein than any other group. They probably also eat more calcium because they eat the fish bones. It has been estimated that Eskimos eat 250 to 400 grams of protein daily and more than 2,000 mg. of calcium. They also have one of the highest rates of osteoporosis in the world. I have heard that they also have the shortest life span.[422]

In contrast to this, a study in Africa with the Bantu natives, revealed interesting facts about people living on a low-protein vegetable diet. These people consumed 47 grams of protein and 400 mg. of calcium and they have no osteoporosis. Studies were made with their genetic relatives, a population of blacks in the United States, who consume something close to the Standard American Diet. Osteoporosis with these people is as nearly as high as it is with the average American.[423]

Clinical studies have shown the effects of calcium loss due to diet. One study summarized that high protein diets cause a negative calcium balance even in the presence of more than adequate dietary calcium. It was estimated that if the patients on this high protein diet continue to consume that same amount of protein, which, by the way, was less than the American average, they would lose approximately 4% of total skeletal calcium per year.[424]

Dr. Bernard Jensen explains: "Significant losses of vitamin B-6 occur during the processing of milk. During pasteurization, enzymes are killed and much of the vitamin B-12 is lost. With the enzymes and vitamin losses, the protein, fats and minerals are less well digested and assimilated. Boiled milk is almost nutritionally worthless. Sixty-five percent of the milk used in the world is from goats. **Goat milk is comparable to cow milk in flavor (when both are fresh) and in**

---

[421] Henry G. Bieler, M.D., Food is Your Best Medicine, (New York, NY: Ballantine Books, 1965), pg. 198.

[422] McDougall, pg. 102.

[423] Ibid.

[424] Allen, et. al., "Protein-Induced Hypercalciuria: A Long Term Study," pg. 741-749.

**nutrients, but is much more digestible, possibly because the fat particles are much smaller**. ...I have seen fresh, foaming, warm goat milk practically bring people back from the dead. (the vital force in the milk diminishes rapidly from the time the animal is milked and is gone in four hours).... Most children and adults who have trouble with cow milk do very well with goat milk. Anyone who has an allergy problem or catarrhal problems of any kind will do better on raw, fresh goat milk. Because goat milk is deficient in folic acid, a 100 microgram supplement should be taken per quart of milk or per day."[425]

Some doctors have found that people ingesting dairy products have too much calcium in their bodies, which would seem to indicate unusual calcium absorption. However, testing for minerals in the body is difficult and very deceiving. In tests, one can find elevated potassium, calcium, sodium, etc. and the truth can be the exact opposite. First of all, as I have said in a previous chapter, allopathic medicine does not recognize the difference between minerals that are usable (organic minerals from plants) and unusable minerals (inorganic minerals from rocks). **Tests usually indicate excess minerals when almost every patient shows evidence of such severe mineral depletion that he or she is falling apart at the seams.** How can this be? This is probably true with nearly all critically ill persons in America. The tests indicate the presence of the **unusable** minerals and not the usable minerals. Another factor that is not well understood by many doctors is that there are many kinds, types, or even groups of various minerals. This is especially true of sodium and calcium. Tests seldom, if ever, show the types that we need to know about. In his book *Biologic Ionization*, on page 67, Doctor Beddoe talks about giving the right kind of calcium to those who had shown excess calcium. After giving an abundance of the right kind of calcium, the high levels of unusable calcium dropped. I have found this to be true many times.[426]

Pasteurized cow's milk is dangerous to all animals' health, including calves.[427] Those who must use dairy products, should use those made with raw goat's milk since it is nearer to human milk, much less mucus-forming and easier to digest.

---

[425] Bernard Jensen, Ph.D, *Food Healing for Man*, (Escondido, CA: Bernard Jensen, Publisher, 1983), pg. 293.

[426] Dr. Alexander F. Beddoe, D.D.S., *Biological Ionization*, (Grass Valley, CA: Agro-Bio Systems, 1990), pg. 67.

[427] Morter, pg. 167.

# Avoid Meat - Two Lives Depend on It[428]

**The digestive system of the meat-eating animal is only 12 feet long and is very different from man's.** When meat has to travel through 30 feet of the human being's digestive tract before it is eliminated, it causes excess fermentation and putrefaction. It's no wonder that the fecal matter and gas have a foul odor, especially when compared to a cleaned-out vegetarian. The meat-eating animal has ten times more hydrochloric acid than can be provided by the human body and most people tend to be deficient in hydrochloric acid as it is.

An important factor that few people seem to consider is that with a normal meat-eating diet, huge quantities of protein are consumed. In the process of protein assimilation, massive quantities of proteins are stored in the intestines, kidneys, and the liver. This is one of the main reasons why these important organs become weak. Consider this: the more protein (acid-forming foods) we eat, the more ammonia is produced. Ammonia is supposed to be converted into urea and released from the body. When we have too much protein stored in the liver, the liver cannot function properly and urea is not released from the body. **Now get this**. When the liver cannot synthesize ammonia into urea, then ammonia accumulates in the blood. This is extremely toxic, especially to the brain. This condition can cause hepatic coma.[429] This condition is called alkalosis, in other words - over-alkalinity. **The number one cause of ammonia in the blood[430] (alkalosis) is acidosis.**[431] This helps explain why I say that we cannot become over-alkaline by eating too much alkaline food. Becoming over-alkaline is caused by consistently eating too much acid food.[432]

---

[428] Study after study reveals that meat eaters have much more osteoporosis, arthritis, bone disease, diabetes, asthma, liver and kidney problems, as well as cancer, AIDS, and heart disease, etc. So, eating meat may endanger your life, not to mention the life of the animal you are eating!

[429] Guyton, pg. 833 - 837.

[430] The pH of ammonia is 10.25

[431] Ibid., pg. 847.

[432] It is fairly well known among doctors who are aware of nutrition, that if a patient is over-acid, they can give the person alkaline-forming foods and they become normal. Is the reverse true; can we give a patient who is over-alkaline, acid-forming foods to become normal? No! They will become even more alkalotic, because it is acid that causes alkalosis.

A hepatic coma is an extreme situation, caused by consuming large amounts of acid-forming foods, as well as by other stressors. Many people are slowly moving towards this extreme imbalance in pH levels. My point is, that most people have a sluggish liver, most people eat too much animal protein (which is the worst kind of protein), most people are either too over-acid or too over-alkaline, and both those conditions are caused by too much protein.

I have always wondered why it was that advanced spiritual societies would not allow their members to eat meat. I used to think that it was simply the animal vibration that interfered with the higher levels of spiritual awareness. But, it may be that meat-eating, due to the toxicity of excess ammonia levels, interferes with brain function. I doubt if the old priests knew about ammonia in the blood. **They just knew as long as a meat diet was consumed, that those individuals could not acquire the deeper spiritual awareness**. Both history and my observation have proven this to be true, with very few exceptions.

I associate with many people who are on intense spiritual paths. Many of these people have traveled all over the world, seeking. Most of them have studied deeply. About 99% of them are vegetarian and most of these people agree, that after they became vegetarian, that they were able to think much more clearly and at much deeper levels. For myself, I can say that I noticed a slight increase in mental awareness after one year of being a vegetarian. Now, 26 years later, I can look back and see that mentally, emotionally, and in terms of spiritual awareness, there is no comparison. I am convinced that **the ability to love at higher levels, is also inhibited by the brutality associated with flesh-eating**.

Early Greeks, Egyptians, Hebrews, and Buddhists were all vegetarians. These are only some of the societies I was referring to. St. Paul also said, "**It is good not to eat flesh**." (Romans 14:21). In *The Essene Gospel of Peace* of Jesus Christ by the disciple John from which I quote frequently in this book, Jesus says, "**And the flesh of slain beasts in a person's body will become his own tomb. For I tell you truly, he who kills, kills himself and whoever eats the flesh of slain beasts eats the body of death**."

It's a mystery to me that those who read and study the Bible continue to order the death of innocent animals by buying their carcasses from their local supermarkets and restaurants. In Genesis, the Bible is clear on this issue, but in other parts of the Bible it gets confusing to many. Yet with a little thought it becomes clear to those 'who have ears to hear'. Have we not all read, "Thou shalt not kill."? Are we so ignorant we do not understand that when one buys animal flesh from the supermarket, he is placing a purchase order for someone to kill an animal? Maybe people just don't comprehend the word "kill". Isn't it interesting that the subject of eating animals is one area of the Bible that contradicts itself? *The Essene Gospel of Peace* explains this contradiction.[433]

---

[433] "Kill not, neither eat the flesh of your innocent prey, lest you become the slaves of Satan... " Then another said: "Moses, the greatest in Israel, suffered our forefathers to eat the flesh of clean beasts and forbade only the flesh of unclean beasts. Why, therefore, do you forbid us the flesh of all beasts? Which law comes from God? That of Moses, or your law?"

And Jesus answered: "God gave, by Moses, ten commandments to your forefathers. 'These commandments are hard,' said your forefathers, and they could not keep them. When Moses saw this, he had compassion on his people, and would not that they perish. And then he gave them ten times ten commandments, less hard that they might follow them. I tell you truly, if your forefathers had been able to keep the ten commandments of God, Moses would never have had need of his ten times ten commandments. For he whose feet are strong as the mountain of Zion, needs no crutches; but he whose limbs do shake, gets further having crutches, than without them. And Moses said to the Lord: 'My heart is filled with sorrow, for my people will be lost. For they are without knowledge, and are not able to understand thy commandments. They are as little children who cannot yet understand their father's words. Suffer, Lord, that I give them other laws, that they may not perish. If they may not be with thee, Lord, let them not be against thee; that they may sustain themselves, and when the time has come and they are ripe for thy words, reveal to them thy laws.' For that did Moses break the two tablets of stone whereon were written the ten commandments, and he gave them ten times ten in their stead. And of these ten times ten the Scribes and Pharisees have made a hundred times ten commandments. And they have laid unbearable burdens on your shoulders, that they themselves do not carry. For the more nigh are the commandments to God, the less do we need. Wherefore are the laws of the Pharisees and Scribes innumerable; the laws of the Son of Man seven; of the angels three; and of God one.

"Therefore, I teach you only those laws which you can understand, that you may become men, and follow the seven laws of the Son of Man. **Then will the unknown angels of the heavenly Father also reveal their laws to you**, that God's holy spirit may descend upon you, and lead you to his law." And all were astonished at his wisdom, and asked him: "Continue, Master, and teach us all the laws which we can receive." And Jesus continued: "God commanded your forefathers: 'Thou shalt not kill.' But their hearts were hardened and they killed. Then Moses desired that at least they should not kill men, and he suffered them to kill beasts. And then the heart of your forefathers was hardened yet more, and they killed men and beasts likewise. But I do say to you : **Kill neither men, nor beasts, nor yet the food which goes into your mouth**. For if you eat living food, the same will quicken you, but **if you kill your food, the dead food will kill you also**. For life comes only from life, and from death comes always death. **For everything which kills your food, kills your bodies also**. And everything which kills your bodies kills your souls also. And your bodies become what your foods

If one has a desire for truth and a love for all life, he will show kindness for those over which he has dominion and will care what happens to them; but if the love is for self, for gluttony, and if wisdom is canceled by rationalization, then when that one goes into the supermarket, he or she will continue to place the death sentence on completely innocent and helpless fellow creatures. Forgive me. I know the truth hurts; I have been shocked by it many, many times. Perhaps it would help to know, that I started out a totally dedicated hunter and meat-eater. I did not believe that anything could change that, because I was so determined to continue.

In my early years I ate a lot of meat, but I observed that whenever I was doing strenuous exercise, my body wanted less protein. Later, when I gave up meat, I noticed that I had more stamina, especially when I ate very little. Now when I am climbing or backpacking with a heavy pack and really pushing myself to the limit, I never want to eat much. When I do my week-long trips in the mountains, I eat very little and I rarely take any protein foods with me. At these times I feel the absolute best; and after a week of really hard exercise, I feel incredible for a month at least, even if I later pig out on things I know are not good.

In John Robbins' book, *Diet For A New America,* he disclosed, "Study after study has found that protein combustion is no higher during heavy exercise than under resting conditions." He also pointed out that the National Academy of Science made this statement: **"There is little evidence that muscular activity increases the need for protein."**[434]

In John's book, on page 201, he explained some other very interesting studies that everyone should know about. "Early experiments which found that rats grew faster when fed animal protein led to the hypothesis that animal protein was superior. Further research has validated that rats so fed do indeed grow faster, but the 'bigger is better' mentality has

---

are, even as your spirits, likewise, become what your thoughts are. **Therefore, eat not anything which fire, or frost, or water has destroyed**. For burned, frozen, and rotted foods will burn, freeze, and rot your body also. Be not like the foolish husbandman who sowed in his ground cooked, and frozen, and rotten seeds. And the autumn came, and his fields bore nothing. And great was his distress. But be like that husbandman who sowed in his field living seed, and whose field bore living ears of wheat, paying a hundredfold for the seeds which he planted. For I tell you truly, live only by the fire of life, and prepare not your foods with the fire of death, which kills your foods, your bodies and your souls also." From: The Essene Gospel of Peace.

[434] John Robbins, pg. 187, 188.

been dealt quite a blow by other discoveries. **It has been found that rats fed animal protein also die sooner, plus suffer from a multitude of diseases vegetarian rats do not."**

Another report John found went like this: "A report aptly titled, 'Rapid Growth - Shorter Life,' appeared in the journal of the American Medical Association. It showed that high animal-protein diets measurably shortened the life spans of a number of different animals. These findings corroborate the World Health statistics that show **human meat-eating populations *do not*, as a rule, live as long as vegetarian populations**. It has also been discovered that meat-eaters have a much higher rates of cancer than do vegetarians."[435]

**Study after study reveals that meat eaters have much more osteoporosis, arthritis, bone disease, diabetes, heart disease, asthma, liver and kidney problems, as well as cancer, AIDS, etc.** A group of top scientists in the field of heart disease and nutrition met in Tucson during the first week of October 1991. Their goal was to stop heart disease, cancer and many of the other diseases of the Western World. Published in the headlines of the Tucson Citizen, Friday, October 4, 1991, were the comments of these scientists. Their conclusion was: **"Throw all animal products out of our diet. We don't need them. They harm us. That's it. That's all. Period. End of story."** The paper continued: "These are experts who have conducted some of the longest, largest and most scientifically acclaimed studies of the diseases that most plague people living in developed countries such as ours. In brief, these are people who know what they are talking about. And what are they talking about? **In near unison, they are saying that all the advice from the American Heart Association and the federal government about how to live more healthful lives is largely wrong." People need to be vegetarians if they want to be healthy.**

This article points out that **if people with heart disease follow the recommendations of the American Heart Association and the federal government, that they will get worse. "We don't need animal products. They are the main culprit in what is killing us. We can absolutely live better lives without them." "Even small amounts of additions of animal protein to the diet is going to elevate the blood**

---

[435] "Protein, Calories and Life Expectancy," *Federation Proceedings,* 1959; 18, pg. 1190-1207. A. Exton-Smith, "Physiological Aspects of Aging: Relationship to Nutrition," *American Journal of Clinical Nutrition,* 1972; 25, pg. 853-59. P. Krohn, "Rapid Growth, Short Life," *Journal of the American Medical Association,* 1959; 171, pg. 461. H. Sherman, *Chemistry of Food and Nutrition,* (New York, NY: H. MacMillian Co., 1952), pg. 208. H. Sherman, *The Science of Nutrition,* (New York: Columbia Univ. Press, 1943), pg. 177-198.

**cholesterol."** These quotes are from T. Colin Campbell, nationally known nutritional biochemist and national adviser on food safety. He continues, **"To make matters worse, studies also show that a diet rich in animal protein enhances the growth of tumors in animals that have been exposed to cancer-causing agents. However, such tumors stop growing when plant protein, such as soy protein, is substituted."** Campbell also pointed out that the **Chinese who eat almost no animal products, also suffer very little heart disease or cancer**. And those diseases are the main killers of animal-fed Americans. **But as animal foods begin to appear in China, they begin to get our diseases. He states emphatically, "People can raise their children and live as healthy adults with no animal protein whatsoever. There's just nothing in animal foods that we need."**[436]

Dr. William P. Castelli, one of the top experts at the National Heart, Lung and Blood Institute, said: **"I can save your life if I can get you down to 15 grams of fat in your diet a day."** Average Americans consume 50 grams daily. **"Fifteen grams is what 4 billion out of 5 billion people on this planet eat, and they don't get these diseases** (cancer and heart disease). But to do that will force you to eliminate most of the animal products you eat and not many Americans can take that." And therein lies the deadly rub. **Americans have been raised, educated, brainwashed and literally hooked on eating animals, these experts pointed out.** The meat and dairy industries have high commercial stakes in making sure we keep consuming their deadly products.

More startling news from Tucson. The Arizona Daily Star, Tuesday, April 9, 1991, published: **Doctors Urge Dropping Meat, Dairy Products from Diet.** The Physicians Committee for Responsible Medicine proposed a "new four food groups" of grains, legumes, vegetables and fruits. **"Animal foods are simply not necessary in the human diet. At best they are options,"** said Virginia Messina, a nutritionist with the Physicians Committee and editor of its bimonthly magazine, "Guide to Healthy Eating." The Physicians Committee is "essentially proposing a vegetarian diet". **"Based on the knowledge we have today, we cannot go on recommending a diet based on the old four food groups."** Said Dr. Neal Barnard president of the Physicians Committee. "What we need is an entirely new food guide, and that is what we have developed."

**"Humans are natural vegetarians,"** Cornell Dietary research suggests, and further, **"Meat, dairy found to raise disease risk."** A seven-year Cornell University study involving 6,500 Chinese revealed shocking data. "Chinese consume one third less protein than Americans and only 7 percent of their protein comes from animal sources, compared

---

[436] From: *The Tucson Citizen*, Friday, October 4, 1991, a front page headline.

with 70 percent for Americans. The Chinese consume 20 percent more calories than Americans do, but Americans are 25 percent fatter. The Chinese diet contains three times the dietary fiber of Americans. **The average vegetarian Chinese adult consumes twice as much iron as an American meat-eating adult.** The study showed that people need less calcium than previously thought and that the Chinese received enough from vegetables.[437]

It is a proven fact, as many scientific studies have shown, that **diets consumed in areas with a high incidence of bowel cancer are high in fat and animal protein content.** High-fat diets result in a high fecal concentration of bile acids, thus providing more substrate for conversion to carcinogens.[438]

# Scientific Facts About Meat

At one time science supported the consumption of meat. It no longer does, for it cannot. The facts are overwhelming that indicate that the eating of animal flesh is the cause of the massive epidemics of cancer, heart disease and many other diseases. One day, mankind will look back in horror at the carnivorous habits of its predecessors. The eating of animals and other living creatures will seem as barbaric and disgusting to future man as the eating of human meat now seems to the average American. Animal-eating is only one step below cannibalism. Consider these facts:

* In 1961, the "Journal of the American Medical Association" reported that a vegetarian diet can prevent 90-97% of all heart diseases. Imagine that! The number one cause of death in the United States is heart disease.

* Studies reveal 59% less cancer among people who eat small amounts of meat, compared to average meat-eaters. (Imagine how much better those figures would be when compared to vegetarians.)

* Scotland has the highest rate of bowel cancer in the world and they eat 20% more meat than the English.

---

[437] *The Arizona Daily Star*, Tucson, Arizona, Wednesday, May 9th , 1990, pg.14 - Section A.

[438] Sydney M. Finegold, Howard R. Attenbery and Vera L. Sutter, "Effect of Diet on Human Fecal Flora: Comparison of Japanese and American Diets," *The American Journal of Clinical Nutrition* 1974; 27: Dec. pg. 1456-1469.

* The kidneys of the meat-eater must work three times harder than the kidneys of the vegetarian.

* Although meat needs to pass through the digestive tract quickly, it takes four times longer than grains or vegetables.

* During World War I, Norway and Denmark could not get meat. The death rate dropped 17% and then returned to normal when they returned to their meat diets.

* The American National Institute of Health, in a study of 50,000 vegetarians, found that they live longer, have far less heart disease, and a much lower cancer rate compared to meat-eaters.[439]

* In England, vegetarians pay less for life insurance.

* Studies show that **vegetarians are stronger, more agile, have greater endurance, and recover from fatigue faster than meat-eaters.**

* A Yale University study revealed that **vegetarians have nearly twice the stamina of meat-eaters.**[440]

* Cornell University announced through major newspapers in May of 1990, that "Humans are natural vegetarians." The report said: "Animal foods, in general, are not really helpful and we need to get away from eating them." "In addition to reducing the risk of heart disease, low cholesterol also protects against colon cancer, the most common life-threatening cancer among Americans."

* World starvation is well-connected to meat-eating habits. If Americans stopped feeding grain to cattle, the excess grain could feed 500 million people (not to mention the land that could be used to grow food instead of being used for grazing cattle). When people see those programs on TV

---

[439] Note: Most American vegetarians were once meat-eaters and even after many years on a vegetarian diet, they still carry old, dead meat or its toxins in their intestinal tracts. It takes serious cleansing to get rid of it. Lifelong vegetarians have a tremendous advantage, even if they eat poorly, as many do. When this study was made, most of the vegetarians ate large amounts of meat substitutes, the highly processed soy products, which are detrimental to the human body.

[440] In this study, they used athletic meat-eaters, and put them against vegetarians who did not participate in sport activities. Would you call that a fair study? Yet the vegetarians still won out.

about all the starving children, they should consider that their diets are a contributing factor.

* The protein brainwashing was done by the meat and dairy industries. Their facts were based upon unreliable data. The medical suggestions for the amounts of protein needed for human consumption is based upon rats, not humans. A baby rat doubles its weight in just a few days drinking rat mother's milk which is about 15% protein. Human babies double their weight in about 180 days, drinking human mother's milk which has about 2% protein. Yet the suggested daily protein is based upon rats. Make cents? No, it makes dollars.

* The essential and non-essential amino acids suggestions were also based upon a study of rats, not humans. Really, someone should tell some of these researchers that there is a vast difference in rats and humans, at least most humans.[441] But then again, maybe these researchers were rats.

I was flying from L.A. to Seattle one day and was seated next to a pretty young lady from Germany. We had struck up a lively conversation when a stewardess asked on the intercom for Rich Anderson to identify himself, so I pushed the button. The lady asked me what it was about and I explained that it was for my vegetarian meal. She said she ate meat and asked why I didn't. I answered, "I like animals." (Lots easier than going into the mucoid-fecal-matter explanation and besides, it's true.) "So do I!" she exclaimed. I looked at her in disbelief and said, "You do?" She got the message and just sat there, looking stunned, for several minutes. I suppose people love animals in different ways - some love to eat them; others just love them as friends with a desire to help them.

## How to Eat Meat

**If people are going to eat meat, they should eat it raw, because:**

1. Enzymes are destroyed by the cooking.
2. Eating meat raw causes less drainage of our alkaline reserve. (Notice that no animal in its right mind would ever cook its food. They are just too smart for that.)
3. More life force is retained.
4. In the process of cooking meat, the high heat changes the ionic bonds of the fats. The tighter the ionic bonds become, the more stress imposed upon the liver and the greater the drain of the alkaline and electrolyte minerals.

---

[441] Shils and Young, *Modern Nutrition in Health and Disease*, 7th Edition, (Philadelphia, PA: Lea & Febiger, 1988), pg. 5, 29.

Man is the only species on earth that cooks his food and is the only species that destroys himself. We are capable of being god-like, but often we choose to be lower than the animals. We need to raise our consciousness to a higher level and stop destroying ourselves and defenseless animals.

# Two Deer Stories

## The Doe and Her Fawn

I was raised to be a rough and tough independent man who knew how to survive in the mountains. In my family it was great glory to go out and kill something and bring it home to eat. I have not forgotten the first time I killed a deer, although I wish I could.

Our whole family, which included my mother, father, brother, grandfather and his brother, and several friends of the family, would go hunting each year in the Okanogen country in northern Washington.

In October of 1955 our camp had been set for several days and I had roamed the hills each day looking for those beautiful creatures called deer. One day as I was returning to camp after a long day scouting the hills, I spotted a doe. I had a doe permit and was programmed that it was OK to shoot doe since that helps to control the deer herds. The truth was, they did not want so many deer in the forest because they competed with cattle and there was only a limited amount of food to eat. Anyway, when I saw the doe I got excited. My heart was beating hard and fast as I took my 9 mm French Labelle off my shoulder and slowly aimed at her. Suddenly something in me began to say, "This is wrong, this is wrong," but my training had been effective. I pulled the trigger and down she went.

As she fell, a fawn ran from behind her in terror. The feeling that I had done a great wrong came over me. I wished that I had not done it. I walked sadly over to the fallen doe to find that she was not dead, but lay there looking up at me with suffering in her eyes. I felt so sorry and thought the best thing to do was put her out of her misery. I shot her again and that ended it.

As I stood there, part of me wanted to cry and another part of me was glowing with false pride for being a victorious hunter. As I struggled with the thoughts of whether I was a hero or a villain, everyone from camp came up to the place of the murder. My dad shook my hand, my grandfather said he was proud of me, my mother smiled and said that she would give me an anatomy lesson, and my brother just looked jealous and said nothing. Soon my little chest swelled and I felt the pride and glory of it all. I was feeling good about myself and thought maybe I had done the right thing. After all, I was responsible for putting meat on the table. I had assisted my father in bringing food to the family. I was doing my share.

All went well until we began dressing out the deer, which is a gentle way of saying, cutting her throat and draining her blood, then splitting her belly open and pulling out all her organs. We soon found that she had milk and had been feeding her baby. The guilt quickly came over me again. I felt a connection to both the doe I had killed and her fawn, now standing about 70 yards away, watching us dissecting her mother. Soon the guilt and sadness vanished as the conversation continued to glorify the little hunter.

## Animals are Smarter Than We Think

It was now 1963. I was full grown and was very at ease in the mountains. It was November and there were only a few days left of the hunting season. About 4 to 6 inches of snow was on the ground and by 9:00 in the morning, I was high on the Etiat mountains. I had just come over a rocky ridge when I spotted the largest buck I had ever seen. His neck was swollen from being in the rutting season. He was with several doe and was enjoying every minute of it. I got into position and fired. It was a long shot and the 30-06 Remmington pump was a very poor rifle. I missed. The buck bounced around trying to figure which way the shot had come from. He was downhill from me and I thought maybe I shot over him. I aimed lower and pulled the trigger. I missed again. The doe ran and the buck was trying to see me. I could see him straining to find something moving. I kept still and shot again. The shot hit his massive antlers; it swung him to one side. He was very confused and still afraid to run because he didn't know which way was safe. I was normally a crack shot, but this rifle was practically useless. I silently cussed at my rifle. The next shot hit his shoulder. It dropped him, but he got right back up. From this shot, he somehow was able to figure out which way to go. As he headed down towards the thickets, he could barely walk. His left front leg was badly broken; it just hung on him. Having only one shot left, I ran full speed to head him off and get closer.

I got within 50 feet of him, but the trees were too thick to try a shot. After he was covered by the trees he turned and instead of going down, he headed out on level ground at a fast run. I ran after him as fast as I could. He left me in the snow. I realized that he could not go downhill very well, but had no trouble going either up or on level ground. He was bleeding, but not badly. I decided to stop and let him think that I had given up. Impatiently, I waited for about 20 minutes, thinking that he would quickly tire and lie down. Maybe he would get stiff or just bleed to death. Soon I was on his trail. In less that a mile I spotted some more deer, all does, then I saw him. He was lying near the top of a ridge. I thought, "a perfect get-away position." None of the deer had spotted me and I was careful to move in quietly. I went from one tree to another very slowly. I was almost ready for a shot. I planned to get to one more large tree and I would go for it. I was crawling on my stomach and couldn't see the deer until I got to the tree. I got into position, put the rifle off safety, and slowly moved around the tree for a shot. The doe were gone and so was the buck.

I went to where he had been lying and saw that he had bled when he first got up. I sat down to think and decided to try it one more time. If I couldn't get close the next time, then I would push him really hard. In about 20 minutes I was off again on the hunt. I had no trouble following his tracks because he was much bigger than any of the other deer and a drop of blood fell about every 30 feet. I came up to where he had been lying down again. I realized that he was being more cautious. This was the second indication that he was thinking, not just reacting.

Now I was on the run. I would either get him or wear myself out. It was a contest and I liked contests, especially in the mountains. Competition with an animal that was supreme in his own element was appealing to me, but I had no idea that I was about to learn something from this animal that would have a powerful influence over the rest of my life.

As I trotted through the forest as fast as my endurance allowed, I had little trouble following his tracks until he suddenly turned and went downhill. I wondered about this because I knew that he would be in great pain going downhill and it was extremely difficult for him to do so. I checked to see if I were really following him rather than another deer, and sure enough, the blood was there. Soon the trail went into a very thick grove of trees. No snow and no noticeable tracks. I searched hard for his signs. I tried to follow the same line of direction, but when I got to the other side of the grove, still no tracks. I considered that he may still be in the grove and I ran from one end to the other — nothing. So I finally went out of the grove and walked all the way around in the snow until I found his tracks again. Sure enough he had gone in the grove at one angle and then changed directions. I thought, "That is exactly what an Apache would have done. It was a great defensive maneuver - no coincidence."

After about 20 minutes delay, I was on his trail again. The next thing I noticed was that he seemed to always walk in the trail of other deer and this made it harder to follow him. Then he began to go off the easy open areas and walk right into very thick brush. He seemed to always go out of his way to do this. This really surprised me as I realized that it had to be very difficult and painful to do this with such a badly broken leg. About then he entered another large grove of trees that had no snow. I took a peek inside and thought to myself, "Oh no you don't, I'm not going to waste my time doing that again." I walked around the grove until I found where he had come out, and then with all my might, I pushed on. Sometimes I would run until I was out of breath. Then I just walked fast. I was pushing him hard. Many times he would lie down and each time he got up he lost more blood. As I followed him, he continued to do his little maneuvers whenever it was appropriate. I began to have serious talks with myself, "Could he really be planning and thinking about what he was doing? I thought animals were dumb and could not really think like a human." More and more I saw evidence that he was indeed an intelligent being.

Hours went by. On and on I pushed. Finally we ran out of level ground. We were getting into the high country now and there was no way but up or down. I knew he could not go down without great pain and difficulty, and without slowing down. Soon we were going up very steep ground. Now after lying down and getting up, the blood spills were increasing. We climbed up about three thousand feet in elevation. He could easily go around and keep level without going up or down. Why was he not doing so? He would soon be getting to the top, and then he would have no other way to go but down. Then I thought, "Could it be that he knows the other side of this mountain is an extremely dense, wooded area and that he could easily lose me?" I thought about it and came the conclusion that if I were being chased, I too would stand a better chance of hiding on the east side of the Etiat Ridge than anywhere else in that country. But the snow would be deeper. How could he expect to hide his tracks? What he was about to do was the biggest shock of all.

I pushed faster and faster, to my maximum speed. I thought about trying to beat him to the top, but that did not seem possible. I tried anyway. It was getting late; the sun would soon be going down. Finally, I was at the top. The snow became deeper and deeper as I walked to the northeast side. The trees were smaller. Thousands had fallen over each other, and snow was piled high on the logs. The buck's trail hooked up to an old manmade trail and went into the tangled woods. Without the trail, it would have been really hard going. Drops of blood were still on the trail, but it became less as the way was now level. He was apparently with two other very large deer and I could not tell the difference between his tracks and the others. I was looking for tricks. I thought that he had a purpose for coming here and I was certain that the trail would go down very soon and then I would get him, unless he pulled some kind of trick. I could not imagine what that would be, but I was soon to find out.

I kept following the tracks until the trail did indeed go down and rather steeply. I looked for blood, but none was there. Now I was the one confused. I had been following very carefully, looking here and there, trying not to miss a thing. But something was wrong. He had gotten off the trail; I was sure of it. I followed for another 100 yards to be sure. No blood, I turned back and followed my own trail back. "Darn", I said to myself, "I broke my own rules; never step in the tracks I'm following." Following the deer tracks, I walked right in the middle of them and messed them up. I went all the way back to where I saw the last blood. Then I followed it all over again. I must have looked like Sherlock Homes. I looked at each track — at the direction of each track. All seemed in perfect order. Now it is a difficult thing trying to tell just how many animals are following the same path, but there came a time when it seemed that there were less tracks than before. However, I couldn't tell for sure. I looked carefully for a track moving in another direction. There was no such thing. Every print held the exact same direction. Then I thought that if I were right and he had gotten off the trail, maybe I could see his tracks if I got up in the logs next to the trail.

It was slippery and rough going, but I traveled about 10 to 15 feet off the trail and sure enough, I spotted his hoof prints. I followed them back to where he first got off the trail, and I couldn't believe my eyes. Here is what happened: he had gone along with the other deer. Now, without changing direction, and even though he had a broken leg, he made one mighty leap over a pile of logs that was at least 5 feet high (including about 14 inches of snow), and landed on the other side where it was impossible to see where he landed. For me that was the clincher. I was absolutely certain that he had planned it. From this point on, he walked or jumped between logs and snow in such a way that his tracks always remained at the lowest possible point, making it very difficult to see them.

I followed them for about 100 yards and there he stood. I walked up within about 35 feet from him, and he just stood there looking at me. He was the biggest deer I had ever seen. I knew that he must be close to 400 pounds and his antlers would make the Boon Crocket Record Club (which they did). I also knew that he knew I had won the contest. A contest which if he lost, he died. But if I lost, I lost nothing. As I stood there watching him, I felt a connection that I have never forgotten. I felt deep respect and love for him. I wished that we were together under totally different circumstances. I wanted to be his friend, rather that his dreaded enemy. I involuntarily started talking to him. I told him how sorry I was that I had done this to him, and that I wished I had the power to heal him and undo the wrong I had done. I also knew that he was in great pain and would die before morning. So I slowly took the safety off my rifle and with terrible mixed emotions, I aimed at his neck, for I could not bear to shoot him in the head.

When the shot went off, he fell very hard, as the power of a 30-06 is extremely impressive. I had hoped that the bullet would enter the front of the neck and then hit his vertebrae which would have instantly killed him. Instead, the bullet went through his juggler vein and slightly changed direction, missing the deadly point. Sadly, I walked closer to him. With the last bit of energy he had left, he looked up at me with his big brown eyes. They looked kind, as though he was forgiving me. He choked upon his own blood, his eyes began to dilate, and in a few moments he stopped breathing.

As I stood there with tears running down my face, I said a prayer from the bottom of my heart. "Oh, God, sometime, in some way, let me make it up to this beautiful being that I have just killed, and forgive me for doing this terrible thing."

I was feeling the goodness within me, the real me, the awareness which I really was. I felt great love and appreciation for that animal. I fully knew that I had done a great wrong and that I would also be made responsible for this selfish act; but I also knew that I would someday have the chance to clear the record. Somehow, I would be his friend.

A few minutes later, the unaware self, the human ego took over. I began to feel proud that I had shot such an incredible animal. What a victory! I had provided more meat for the table. How proud everyone would be of me. Today, as I write this, I can say that there is not much of the animal self left in me now. I would rather heal than kill, and I will not kill indirectly by buying meat from the supermarket or restaurant, which is worse in a way, for at least the hunter doesn't deny that he is a murderer.

When one reaches deep within, they find truth that cannot be denied. There is no excuse to kill animals for our food. No excuse but habit, lust, ignorance, and human ego. Perhaps, in some way, I am making it up to my friend whom I killed, by helping others see the truth of what they are doing.

# The Truth About Vegetarians

Sometimes we hear rumors that a vegetarian diet is harmful, that doctors cannot nutritionally balance vegetarians, or that vegetarians cannot get enough Vitamin B-12. Nothing could be further from the truth. **First of all**, any doctor or practitioner who cannot nutritionally balance a vegetarian just hasn't learned how. Few doctors know anything about nutrition, and medical doctors are not trained in nutrition. If a practitioner is not a vegetarian, then he generally does not understand what is needed.

**Secondly**, I am amazed when someone tells me she is a vegetarian but still eats birds and fish. I just don't understand how anyone can think that birds and fish are vegetables. If you plant a duck, will it grow another a new duck family? Every research report I have ever seen that came to negative conclusions about vegetarians did their research on macrobiotic vegetarians. Many of these people are really "grainarians," not vegetarians, and their diet usually consists of mostly cooked grains, soy products, some cooked vegetables and very little raw fruits and vegetables. This is a better diet than the standard American meat and dairy diet, but it is not a healthy diet as indicated by all the medical research that has been done. The macrobiotic diet is an acid diet; however, if it is not as acid-forming as the meat-eater's diet. Even though it is too acid-forming as far as I am concerned, and lacks enzymes, life force, and other important factors necessary for the highest level of health, such a person would have less cancer, heart disease, etc. than someone following a normal meat diet.

**Thirdly**, the last argument that meat-eaters have against vegetarians concerns vitamin B-12. That contention is going to crumble right now.

# Vitamin B-12

Vitamin B-12 is a very important vitamin. We only need very small amounts of this vitamin, for the liver stores enough B-12 to last for three to five years. However, the lack of this vitamin could cause glandular imbalance, lack of energy, brain damage, and pernicious[442] anemia which can result in death. Other symptomatic indications are anorexia,

---

[442] Pernicious: Destructive; harmful; denoting a disease of severe character and usually fatal without appropriate treatment. Pernicious anemia is caused because of a lack of B-12. Lack of B-12 is not usually caused by lack of B-12 in the diet, but in the failure to absorb this vitamin through the digestive tract. The number one cause is an atrophic gastric mucosa that fails to secrete the necessary gastric juices. Guyton, *Textbook of Medical Physiology*, 7th Edition, pg. 45.

intermittent constipation and diarrhea, abdominal pain, burning of the tongue, considerable weight loss, to name a few.

B-12 absorption requires the presence of an intrinsic factor, the secretion of the gastric mucosa by parietal cells , to transport the vitamin across the intestinal mucosa. **B-12 deficiency is really related to an intestinal problem, and not so much whether the food we eat has B-12**. However, keep in mind that it is the food we eat, or negative emotions, that in all probability cause the intestinal problems. To verify my statement, the Merck Manual claims that the cause of B-12 deficiency is chronic atrophic gastritis, achlorhydria (no hydrochloric acid secretion).

Critics of vegetarianism say that vegetarians do not get enough vitamin B-12 because a usable form cannot be found anywhere in the food kingdom except in animal flesh. That is not true. **We get B-12 from raw vegetables, algae, legumes, and most importantly, from our own intestinal flora**. Nearly all of the studies on B-12 deficiencies, which I have read, have been done with meat-eaters, not vegetarians. In addition, it is interesting to note that the majority of the people in the world are either entirely or primarily vegetarian.

I have in my files several research projects involving patients with pernicious anemia (the most serious B-12 deficiency). All these studies done with meat-eaters concluded that these people had no secretion of hydrochloric acid (achlorhydria) and had other severe digestive problems. Some of these patients developed stomach cancer and some died of other causes unrelated to pernicious anemia. Of course, with serious digestive problems, one can expect anything in our bodies to go wrong. Remember, all these people lost their sodium reserve,[443] and you can be sure that they had acquired mucoid plaque in the guts.

## Latest Research About B-12

**We don't need to eat food containing vitamin B-12 to obtain B-12**. The real trouble most people have is that they can't absorb the B-12, either from the food they eat or from the bacteria which is supposed to manufacture this vitamin in their small intestines, because their digestive system is on the blink.

Research has been performed involving vitamin B-12 growth and absorption in the digestive tract. In one study, it was found that **huge**

---

[443] Sheila Callender & G.H. Spray, *Latent Pernicious Anaemia*, (Oxford, England: Nuffield Dept. of Clinical Medicine, The Radcliffe Infirmary, Oxford, Br. ) *Journal of Haematology*, 1962; 8, pg. 230-240.

**amounts of Vitamin B-12 were produced in the colon when the correct type of bacteria was present**. Another study found that colon bacteria of vegan vegetarians (no animal products such as cheese or eggs) make enough vitamin B-12, but the B-12 was not being absorbed through the colon wall (probably due to an old buildup of mucoid plaque). **When they fed the bacteria from their own B-12 rich colon feces to some of these people orally, the B-12 deficiency diminished**. This would indicate impaired colon absorption. They should have first tried intestinal cleansing and rebuilding the bowel.

We know perfectly well that in a healthy body, all the necessary vitamin B-12 is produced in the intestines; this vitamin mixes with the bile and is easily absorbed by the small intestine. The only requirement is a healthy digestive system.

There were some studies done indicating that vegans all eventually have slowed DNA synthesis, which is corrected by vitamin B-12. In one study, several hundred vegans showed that they all eventually got vitamin B-12 deficiency diseases with anemia, pancytopenia, low white counts, low red counts, and low platelet counts.[444]

My response to this study is that vegans, as well as everyone else, should cleanse their bowels, rebuild their digestive organs, make certain that they have the right bacteria implants, and alkalize their bodies. Another thing they can do is take vitamin B-12 supplements, which are almost always included in any B-complex formula (but this should be unnecessary if the above steps are taken).

When we read medical research reports, we must do so with an open mind. Almost every report I have yet read is strongly one-sided. What I mean is this: each report reflects only a small fragment of the whole picture, and even that fragment may be wrong. For example, I have a report that states that vitamin B-12 is in milk or milk products. Then later in the same report, it says that boiling milk before drinking may destroy much of the vitamin B-12. As you probably know, it is difficult to find raw milk anywhere in the United States. It's all pasteurized. It is boiled at temperatures that are sometimes extremely hot. If that doesn't kill the B-12, nothing will.

Remember, medical researchers are usually paid by those who want certain information. If they don't get the facts they want from the research, some people could lose their jobs. I know of cases where this has

---

[444] Victor Herbert, M.D., J.D., "Vitamin B-12: Plant Sources, Requirements, and Assay," *American Journal of Clinical Nutrition*, 1988; 48, pg. 852-858.

happened. In 1942 a study was done on a breakfast food that is still one of the more popular cereals on the market today. Four sets of rats were given special diets.

### 1942 Breakfast Food Study

| Group | Received | Results |
|-------|----------|---------|
| 1 | Plain whole wheat, water, vitamins, and minerals | Lived over 1 year |
| 2 | Nothing but water and chemical nutrients | Lived 8 weeks |
| 3 | Water and white sugar | Lived 4 weeks |
| 4 | XX cereal, water, and chemical nutrients | Lived only 2 weeks |

Don't you think that group 4 should have at least lived as long as group 2? What this report is saying, is that sugar is not good for you, right? Wrong. What it is really saying is that **the XX cereal is not only lacking in nutrients, but is also toxic.** This 1942 report was rediscovered in 1978. The researcher went directly to the president of this well-known cereal manufacturer and showed him the report. The response from the president was, "I know people should throw it on brides and grooms at weddings, but if they insist on sticking it in their mouths, can I help it? Besides, we made $9 million on the stuff last year." Next, this company did all it could to discredit the researcher and intimidate members of the media interested in his message. This company no longer does animal-feeding studies on most of its products, because too often the tests show its foods are incapable of sustaining life.[445]

### One Last Note About Vitamin B-12

Research conducted among vegetarians in southern India found that healthy subjects had normal vitamin B-12 absorption, but those who had a stagnant bowel syndrome (constipation) did have a deficiency. It was also found that healthy Indians with normal B-12 levels developed deficiencies

---

[445] Paul Stitt, *Fighting The Food Giants*, (Manitowoc, WI: Natural Press, 1981), pg. 62-64.

after they immigrated to England, which probably involved a significant change in their diet.[446]

The point that we need to remember is that **there is no B-12 deficiency among vegetarians or vegan vegetarians who have a healthy digestive system**; but if we have a lack of hydrochloric acid, lack of organic sodium, lack of friendly bacteria, or indications of constipation, it could mean that we are moving in the direction of a B-12 deficiency. Keep in mind that this deficiency occurs much more often among the eaters of flesh, for when meat and dairy products are cooked, this vitamin is usually destroyed.

# What To Expect As Your Intestinal Tract Becomes Purer

Pure, clear, clean, calm water reflects the sun perfectly. Put a drop of black dye in it and observe the contrast. Then try red, brown, yellow, etc. At first, each drop makes a significant difference, but later it makes very little change. Keep doing this for some time and two things will happen: the sun will not be reflected, and any further drops will cause little or no contrast. There are two points here: 1) Purity is required to reflect the light; and 2) When the body is filled with filth from eating "non-foods" (anything other than raw fruits, raw vegetables, and sprouted seeds, nuts, and grains), there is little noticeable effect when we eat dead foods, but when our bodies become more purified, we begin to notice the effects of the dead foods much more keenly.

## Cooked-Food Experiment

Years ago, Barbara, my wife at the time, and I decided to experiment with that contrast. After a great deal of intestinal cleansing and a couple of months on raw foods (mostly fruit), we went back to eating the average American diet, minus meat, for four days. Each morning it became more and more difficult to get out of bed, let alone feel good. We each began to develop the world's worst case of baggy eyes until by the fourth morning we had pouches instead of bags. The wrinkles in our faces became decidedly more pronounced. My vision became increasingly fuzzy (but taking my herbal formula for the eyes cleared it) and tiny little bumps developed on our skin as our bodies made a desperate attempt to eliminate the toxic overload. Our complexions became dull and lifeless. We noticed

---

[446] M.J. Albert, V.I. Mathan & S.J. Baker, "Vitamin B-12 Synthesis by Human Small Intestinal Bacteria," *Nature*, 1980; 283, pg. 781-782.

that our love for each other lessened. Our sleep was interrupted by weird dreams. Our whole bodies became puffy, but it was especially noticeable in our faces. Our energy levels became lower and lower and for the first time in years, we found ourselves getting sleepy during the day. I felt some pain in my kidneys, and we both experienced inflammation in various joints. We felt congested in our sinuses and throats, as well as having various aches and pains throughout our bodies. My memory became less effective, and we both found it difficult to turn our attention to God. Our appetites for food became almost uncontrollable, we were hungry when we shouldn't be, and work became an effort instead of the joy it usually was for us. We experienced feelings of low self-esteem and a lack of confidence. We had puffy stomachs. Our mental efficiency lessened and we became more and more prone to negative feelings. We were easily irritated and rather short-tempered. Our bodies developed foul odors that had been absent for a long time. Being neither TV-watchers nor movie-goers, we were amazed when we actually had the desire for such amusements. We found it difficult to entertain ourselves and began to search for outside diversions. All these things really did occur, for this was another research project and we took notes.

Believe me, we were so happy to get back on our cleanse that we marveled at our enthusiasm. Our baggy eyes disappeared in three days. We looked and felt good again. Our energy returned, along with our increasing love and gratitude for each other and for God. In fact, almost every one of the symptoms we had developed disappeared within three days of cleansing.

A few days later we experimented again and ate cooked foods for another four days. This time we even had chocolates and pizza (we still did not eat meat), and the same symptoms of ill-health and lifelessness gradually returned. After those four days, we truly embraced the raw foods diet with the fervor of religious converts. We have developed such appreciation for God's fresh foods that they bring us joy just to look at them in their lovely, pure simplicity. Eating God's unadulterated, wholesome foods brings greater life and energy into us instead of depleting us. It makes us feel good, the breath is fresher, the mental capacity is increased and uplifted, and our love and joy toward all life is accelerated in its expansion. Blessed is the life that grows and provides real foods and blessed are those who eat them in their raw, fresh state!

My earnestness and zeal to conquer all desire for non-foods still remain. For once you have cleansed your body and lived on raw food for even a few days, you cannot deny the power of it.[447] Then, if you choose to

---

[447] **See Chapter 14: Secrets of Super Health, "Why Raw Foods are the Perfect Foods," and "Raw Food is Quickening."**

go back to cooked food, you begin to understand what cooked food does to you; to your consciousness. You'll know beyond a shadow of a doubt that it weakens you mentally, physically, emotionally, and spiritually. And again, you may wonder why these things are not taught in school, why more people do not do this, why churches do not suggest it, and you may suspect that there are forces that deliberately try to keep mankind limited for purposes of control and manipulation. Yet, we all know, so help us God, that all lower desires will one day be mere faded memories, as we go forward on the path to complete purification of the mental, emotional, and physical structure.

# The Vital Energy That Heals

Disease can only exist in a de-vitalized body. The higher our vitality, the less disease we can have. When we have enough vitality, disease is impossible.

There is an energetic force that actually repels disease very similar to magnetic repulsion; it is like a light bulb that repels darkness. This force is not derived from the physical level. This energy, measured at the physical level, comes from the energetic or etheric levels. Only a few scientists are aware of this force field. Albert Einstein and Nikola Tesla were both very interested in this force as are most acupuncturists and homeopaths. This force can actually be seen by clairvoyants for it is semi-physical. I believe it is only the gross density of mankind, mentally, physically, and spiritually, that prevents more people from activating the glandular and etheric vortexes that open the awareness to see into these higher levels. With a small amount of training, people who are inclined to know more about themselves, can open their inner awareness and see these etheric levels. I believe that the creators of acupuncture developed this science by the use of clairvoyant sight. They could actually see energy meridians and the blockages along those energy currents. After careful study they were able to map out the energy meridians and determine what physical organs were connected to them by clairvoyance. They learned that sticking a needle into the blocked area actually attracted energy, like an antenna, into the blockage and that would release the blocked energy at that point and then the cells and organs could heal themselves. It works very well as long as the acupuncturist is able to connect to main "chi" meridians. If there were no blockages in the etheric field, disease would be unlikely to develop. For these blockages actually short circuit the energy our cells need.

As Albert Einstein pointed out, the earth is surrounded by an etheric energy field. Many scientists, not medical scientists unfortunately, have worked for years to tap the tremendous energy of the etheric fields.

Apparently, Tesla had figured out how to do this and had constructed an huge antenna system at Colorado Springs to draw the energy into one focal point. His intent was to harness the etheric energy, and power all automobiles, airplanes, boats, and all appliances worldwide from this one central focal point. When his financial backers learned what he was doing, they cut him off and this incredible invention was never initiated. Consider how much money was made because this one invention was blocked.

The point is that this energy field does exist and all our bodies live off it to some degree or another. The great secret of many of the Yogis is that they have learned how to tap into it. If it is not accomplished just right, however, it can be dangerous. Instantaneous combustion is an example of one of its dangers. This topic was covered on the science fiction television program "Outer Limits," many years ago. One story went something like this. The lady who experienced instantaneous combustion was feeling a little strange one evening and went to bed rather early. A slight concern arose with the rest of the family. After a few minutes they heard her scream. They all ran upstairs to her bedroom. There was nothing left of her but carbon and ashes. The heat was so tremendous that even her bones and all fluids had been carbonized. Authorities concluded that the heat had come from within her own body in one mighty flash, for the bed covers were not even burned.

The yogi spends a whole lifetime preparing the body to handle this immense energy and this is why so many of them have such healing powers and can perform such incredible feats, such as maintaining warmth in freezing cold temperatures as the Lamas have demonstrated. This energy can be directed to feed our own energy fields and cells of our body. It is the great secret of living hundreds of years or overcoming death. There are critical necessities to safely using this energy: purity and a strong healthy body. For impurity creates congestion and blockage. Purity of thought, feelings, and everything else within our beings is essential. For once this energy begins to increase, it amplifies everything with which it comes in contact. If we have anger, that anger is amplified many times; if we have Love, the Love is amplified many times. This is why when we experience the love of a Divine being, we are all so overwhelmed, usually to the point of uncontrolled tears.

When we understand these things, then we begin to view that which is called Divine from a more scientific and practical viewpoint. This does not take away the reverence and respect of spiritual things, but actually creates new concepts that place the previously unknown and the unbelievable into a realm which we can understand and believe. Mankind, primarily through religious dogmas, has placed that which we call 'spiritual' on such a pedestal that it is viewed by many as nonsense. **The truth is that which is called spiritual is really very scientific, but beyond our present means of measurement or perception.** I have always viewed the spiritual in a very scientific framework. Yes, there is a very good scientific reason why it is beneficial to follow spiritual exercises. The great Masters were incredible scientists. They knew about these energy fields and used them wisely to better themselves and all they contacted. They knew that the law of cause and effect was a reality at all levels of existence, including thoughts and feelings. That is why they warned their disciples, "whatsoever you do unto another, it shall be done unto you." There teachings were designed to help their students to align with the forces of the universe. Most people don't listen; most people who worship a great Master, don't follow the teachings. Millions of people have died horrible deaths at the hands of those who kill in the name of their Master, which is the opposite of what their Master taught.

The healing force within our bodies is this vitality. Some have called it the "life element", and some even call it God's energy. It's nature is electrical. A little comes from food, but it's everywhere throughout the entire Universe. When we raise our consciousness and have purified and strengthened our bodies to a certain degree, we can become receptive to this universal energy. To conquer "the last enemy," death, we must arrive at a very high level of purity. Until then, we must get the life element through the air we breathe, the food we eat, and the liquids we drink. The more vitality we bring into our bodies, the more life, energy, and freedom from disease we have. When we deplete this vitality, we move toward disease and death. One of the main reasons I have developed my cleansing program is to help people prepare for this increased vitality. Many, after cleansing, access it to some degree.[448] How do we deplete this "vital energy"?

* Negative thoughts and emotions (stress, worry, fear etc.)
* Alcohol and drugs
* Eating cooked foods
* Misuse of the sex energy

## How Do We Replace This Vital Energy?

* Purification of our bodies (allows the nerves and vital energies to flow)
* Gradually eating more and more raw foods
* Drinking pure water that has oxygen in it but with no short-circuiting inorganic minerals in it, or poisons such as chlorine and sodium fluoride
* Drinking fresh, organic, fruit and vegetable juices and eating fresh, organic produce
* Breathing deeply of fresh clean air

---

[448] **See Chapter 14: Secrets of Super Health, and Chapter 15: The Experience in Teeshi Lumbo** for more on this subject.

* Exercising enough to get our hearts beating faster and our lungs breathing more
* Having happy, joyous, and loving thoughts and feelings
* Being outdoors and in the sunshine
* Spiritual exercises

An important goal: eat and drink *only* foods that have vitality in them. This means fresh, raw fruits and vegetables. However, I have seen some people force themselves to eat nothing but raw foods because they believed that they should. Yes, we should, but many can't, as yet. After thousands of years of eating unnaturally, our bodies have deteriorated to the point where disease is probably within every human being on this planet. Disease is far more normal than having good health. True health is an almost unheard of phenomenon.

Hardly anyone today can live a long life without getting some disease, and few live long lives. If someone survives to the age of 120, we think that is exceptional. Those that do live that long look like they've already died but haven't been buried yet, and they can hardly function. Do you call this healthy? I don't. There are people alive today that have reached ages well past 100 and are more vital than you and I put together. We don't hear much about these people, but they do exist. We may meet them on the street and think nothing of it because they just look like healthy young people. We would have no idea how old they really are.

When the World Health Organization reported that we are in the greatest epidemic the world has ever known, it was in relation to chronic and degenerative disease. The U.S. Department of Health said that six out of ten deaths are caused by bad diet (the truth is more like nine out of ten). Our digestive systems have degenerated to the point where very few people can digest and assimilate raw foods healthfully. Many generations of cooked food and meat-eating have caused an imbalance of bacteria and enzymes. When we lack hydrochloric acid, have an over-acid body, lack enzymes, have acid bile, have Candida or other fungal diseases, or lack friendly bacteria in the intestines, we cannot handle raw foods or protein foods very well. We must cleanse and rebuild. I would like to again state that the most important cleansing we can do is for us to cleanse and rebuild our minds and emotional processes, as well as our bodies. We should not expect too much success with anything until we do. Our attitudes, our points of view, have brought us to where we are now; we must change them if we want a better life.

Another problem with going on a raw-food diet without cleansing is that when the average person eats raw foods, even for just a few days, he begins to cleanse the cell structure (not the intestinal tract). That doesn't clean out the mucoid plaque, but raw foods will do serious cleansing. What's wrong with that? Well, one must be very careful. **The average** person is so full of toxic waste that without serious preparation, such as complete intestinal cleansing and then deep tissue cleansing, a total raw-food diet could stir up more problems than he or she could handle. I know of people who did this and it took about two years before they felt good again.

Fruits are the most cleansing of all foods. Vegetables do not cleanse us nearly as rapidly. It is ironic that because of severe cleansing reactions, it would sometimes appear that eating fresh, raw foods makes a person sick, while eating cooked or junk foods makes a person feel better and appear well. This is an illusion. Please do not forget this: in these cases, all that has happened is that **the eating of junk foods has stopped the cleansing process.**

I read about the death of a person who was exceptionally toxic and ate only raw fruit for a long period of time. Cleansing reactions on a raw food diet, without cleansing the digestive tract first, can be extremely severe for the average person; and lack of energy, spaciness, eruptions of the skin, overloaded kidneys, liver, and other organs can weaken the body to the point of ineffectiveness. This is, unfortunately, why many who have studied health have became discouraged when experimenting with the raw food diet and even concluded that raw foods were unhealthy. We need to be careful and use wisdom in all this, never going to extremes.

Thus, I recommend that we first cleanse the intestines, then work on the liver, gallbladder, kidneys, and then the glands. Once the digestive system is repaired, we will be strong enough to cleanse the rest of the body. Cleansing should be done gradually and carefully. This is why I occasionally suggest that a person who is having extreme cleansing reactions to my program, eat a baked potato or switch to a lighter phase of cleansing. It instantly slows the internal cleansing and he feels better immediately. He is also giving his liver a breather. Whenever possible, however, I would still prefer that a person suffering those reactions first try an enema.

One time I was in the kitchen at a resort. The lady in charge of the kitchen was about 70 years old, strong, and full of energy. Many of her helpers had been on the "Fit for Life" program, which is mainly raw foods. Many of them were going through cleansing reactions and she was disturbed about it. I heard her make this comment, "You kids should just stop all this crazy dieting and eat what normal folks eat." Well, she got into some arguments and I was determined to keep quiet. Finally she made the following comment, "I would like someone to tell me why it is that I have twice as much energy and can outwork everyone of you who are on this raw food diet."

Well, that did it, so I went up to her and told her that I would like to answer the question for her. So I said: "Please understand that people of your generation come from a far more healthy stock than the younger people of today, who are getting weaker and sicker with each generation. One of the main reasons for this is the way their parents have been eating, which is exactly what you are promoting. Now these employees of yours are intelligent enough to recognize all this and are trying to do something about it. If their parents had lived properly, they wouldn't have even considered doing extreme diets to get back in control. The truth is, raw food is not an extreme diet: it is the natural one. Had these 'kids' been raised properly on a raw food diet, they wouldn't be going through those symptoms now. To answer your question, the reason these people feel tired from eating raw food, is simply because the raw food is stirring up all the toxins and poisons the cooked food produced. Now when these poisons enter the blood, which they must do to get out of the body, they feel bad. Too bad isn't it, that we have to pay a price for eating naturally, by feeling bad?" By the way, this lady was having problems and didn't tell anyone. Later, she did do my cleanse program.

I spent 20 years trying to cleanse the cell structure of my body first. Besides eating raw foods, another way to initiate this is through water fasting. I fasted a great deal. I did not always eat the way I should have between the fasts, which was one of the main reasons I was not successful. However, I did quite well until an accident kept me from exercising (which helps get rid of toxins). Then it was downhill, with occasional ups during my fasts. Of course, I was dealing with a weak heart, weak liver, and sluggish kidneys from poor eating as a child. Eventually I learned to cleanse the intestinal tract and my health greatly improved.

# A Problem Vegetarians and Raw-Fooders Can Have

For unknown generations, western people have consumed meat and cooked food. What a crying shame! Most of our bodies have adapted to this unnatural diet by reconditioning the enzyme and bacteria production to synchronize with the dead foods. When we have finally gained the wisdom to switch over to the harmonious way of eating and living and become a vegetarian, we often have problems digesting raw foods and cooked carbohydrates. What our bodies need to do is switch back over to its natural enzyme production and synchronize with the much improved and natural way of eating. This seldom happens naturally. Over a period of decades or generations, it undoubtedly would, but many people have trouble digesting and assimilating enough of the carbohydrates and raw foods. Even so, vegetarians who have these problems are still far healthier than those who eat flesh, but why settle for "just better"?  Why not go for incredible energy and vibrant health?

# Digestive Enzymes

There are many different kinds of digestive enzymes on the market. My research indicates that what is commonly found in health food stores (at this time) are not necessarily the most effective.  I am interested in enzymes that are similar to what the body itself produces, and have developed some key formulas to provide these.  Most of us have come from a genetic line of meat-eaters, which is unnatural for the human body; but over the many decades of this kind of eating, our bodies were forced to modify the enzyme and bacterial production.  So, at least for a time, it can be critical to use enzymes to match the foods you are eating, especially if you make changes in your diet.  In addition, as we age and the mucoid plaque builds up, the ability of the body to provide critical digestive enzymes declines.  This condition should improve as the body is cleansed and freed from the destructive influence of old mucoid plaque. Digestive enzymes may also be critical anytime one indulges in cooked food, which is enzyme poor, since cooking destroys enzymes.[449]

# How to Combat the Effects of the Occasional "Pig-Out"

When people have been working on cleansing their bodies but have the occasional splurge or "pig-out" (as the popular and accurate saying goes), they may be apprehensive about what their body is going to have to go through, and may want to eliminate the effects of the "pig-out" as rapidly as possible. Here is what can be done:

### If You Overate...
### or the Food was Poor Quality
### and Needs to be Removed Quickly:

1. Take one heaping teaspoon of papaya powder (also good to sprinkle on meals, except on fruit because fruit already has plenty of digestive enzymes).
2. About 2-1/2 to 3 hours later, take enough herbal laxatives to produce a semi-watery stool.
3. Drink lots of water.

---

[449] **See Chapter 14:  Secrets of Super Health, under "Enzymes,"** for more information.

4. Take as much cayenne as you can stand.
5. Take an enema before bed and one in the morning.
6. Take a psyllium shake when you get up in the morning.
7. Take the two herbal cleansing formulas[450] again, 1-1/2 hours after the shake.

## Quick Way to Get Rid of Food Poisoning:

1. Take about 4 to 8 tablespoons of **extra thick "Hydrated Bentonite"** with a psyllium shake using only one teaspoon of psyllium.
2. Two hours later take enough herbal laxatives to produce a semi-watery stool (usually 4 or more)
3. 30 minutes later take about 2 or 3 bacteria containing large amounts of *Lactobacillus acidophilus*
4. 1-1/2 hours later, take a normal psyllium shake. (If it is late at night and you want to sleep, then wait until morning.)
5. 1-1/2 hours after the shake, take the two herbal formulas.
6. If you're feeling bad, take an enema.

Sometimes it is better to prevent the contamination from going through the system. Using lobelia tincture, about two dropper's full in a four ounce glass of water will help you achieve this. It's easier than sticking your fingers down your throat to force vomiting.

Once, during our four-day experiment, we ate in what appeared to be one of the nicest restaurants in Klamath Falls, Oregon. We had good ole' pancakes and omelets (which we hadn't had in ages). The pancakes tasted so bad that I could only eat one of them. The omelet had a piece of ham on it (which to me ranks the highest in levels of repulsiveness), and some chili. I picked out the animal parts as best I could and ate the rest of it. YUK! It was the worst omelet ever. This was the ideal eating experience, for we were attempting to destroy all desire for cooked foods. We laughed all the way through breakfast. About a half-hour later I felt the full effects of such low vibration and decided that this so-called food was too bad to keep in my body; it had to go. (I rarely do this.) We stopped the car. I put about four squirts of super-powerful lobelia extract into some water (that's two-and-a-half times the dose required to induce vomiting) and drank it down. Then I thought about what I had just eaten and took two more eye dropper shots, undiluted, straight into the mouth. Nothing happened. I couldn't believe it. I did it all over again. I used almost half

---

[450] See Appendix II: Essential Elements for Effective Cleansing and Rebuilding, #1 and #2. Note: the Appendix offers simply a list of ingredients, not the proportions required to create the actual formula.

an ounce of the lobelia extract. Believe me, that's enough to make a rhinoceros upchuck his cookies. Either it was just plain karma, or else we can assume that the cleaner the body becomes, the less effective lobelia is in its emetic effects. Even though I never did vomit, the lobelia did make me feel enormously better.[451] A half-hour later I took the psyllium shake, using a good fluid ounce of hydrated bentonite, and felt good the rest of the day.[452]

# Giving Up Desires For Poor Food

When people have a strong desire for perfect health, they will eventually lose the desires for non-foods when their bodies are ready to let go of them. I do not mean to imply that we should not set goals or give our human desires a good nudge in the right direction once in a while;   but I don't think we should impose too lofty a goal and set ourselves up for failure and disappointment, just because we were not ready. The greatest assistance may be found when we ask God to help. The human ego and all its puny desires are nothing. Our real self, our God-self, is what will empower us to make these sorts of changes. It also helps to read inspiring books about raw food diets.

One thing that will be a great help is to visualize the good food we are going to eat, while cleansing (but for some, it is best to not even think about food while cleansing). **We should never allow ourselves to think about the garbage food we may want after cleansing. That sets us up for poor control later.**

Here is what worked for me, better than any other thing. I stopped criticizing myself, for my many pig-outs and other food desires.  When I had my pig-outs, I did my very best to enjoy them, not to criticize myself, eliminate all guilt, and stop telling myself how bad it was for me. It wasn't long, and I lost all my really bad food desires.

You see, before that, I was doing the complete opposite.  I would really rip into my-self. **What we criticize, we become. Anything we run from, chases us. But to admit our weaknesses, face them square on, takes away all the power of our desire monsters.** There are some who

---

[451] Lobelia is one of the most out-standing herbs grown.  It is often referred to as "the intelligent herb", because it always seems to know what to do.  Read Dr. John Christopher's book: *School of Natural Healing*, published by the School of Natural Healing.

[452] Anytime one uses bentonite, friendly bacteria should be replenished with a general use supplement.

apparently had never created these overwhelming desire entities, and they can just say, "Well I'm not going to have this anymore". Lucky them!

# Summary: Man's Natural Food

Seven years ago I said, "In a few more years, the scientific world will be forced to announce that a vegetarian diet is a far healthier way of eating, than flesh-eating." That has come true already. Sometime in the future it will be known that the natural food for man is raw fruits, raw vegetables, sprouted seeds, sprouted grains, sprouted nuts, and herbs. The Bible [453] in Genesis 1:29 makes it crystal clear, yet how many students of the Bible have the determination, the strength, the desire or the intelligence to overcome lustful habits of eating meat and other harmful substances? People love to rationalize. We all do it. It is not my intent to criticize those who rationalize their poor eating habits; in fact, I've thought about writing a book called, "1,001 Ways to Rationalize", because I thought that I was a true expert.

Can you see how difficult all this might be? Have you noticed how our society abundantly provides every energy draining, emotion degrading, and attention sucking mechanism to keep everyone down and under? Think of how our food, water, and air are all contaminated and devitalized. Consider the chemicals in our food and medicine. How about what you see on television, hear on the radio and see in movies; the violence, the programming of negativity. Look at education! Shocking. The world seems to want to sabotage itself just like many people. Can you see how society is moving towards the "Big Brother" society? A slave world - and the populations are too weak and dull to resist it. Do you think this is being done by accident or by design?

---

[453] *The Holy Bible*, Genesis 1:29 ..."And God said, Behold, I have given you every herb-bearing seed, which is upon the face of all the earth, and every tree, in which is the fruit of a tree yielding seed; to you it shall be for meat." ; & Ezekiel 47:12 ..."and the fruit thereof shall be for meat, and the leaf thereof for medicine."

# Chapter 14

# SECRETS OF SUPER HEALTH

*Feelings control our glands. Glands control DNA.
Anything less than feelings of love depresses all body
functions, propelling us towards death. Calm,
vibrant joyful love vitalizes all body functions,
propelling us towards unending life and health.*

-Dr. Richard Anderson

## The Basics

I am convinced that fresh, raw, ripe fruit is the natural food for a clean, healthy body.[454] Intuitively, it is obvious to me that it has the highest vibratory frequency of all foods. What I mean by this is that fruit is like condensed sunshine: it is jam-packed full of life, yielding an abundance of life force when consumed. Once your body is cleansed, you will notice the obvious difference in how much energy you receive when eating fruit as opposed to other foods. It is this higher level of life force that allows man to tune in to his true nature and his relationship with the rest of the Universe. But don't kid yourself; though the spirit is willing, the flesh is weak. No one can function effectively on an all fruit diet until they are pure. The purity I am talking about is more than just physical; it is mental, emotional and spiritual, as well. It has been said that God works for man, through man, as man, **when man is pure**. The Bible announces that, "Only the pure shall see God." But few have the ears to hear this message, and even fewer know what it means to be pure.

**The greatest secret of perfect health is to eliminate every thought and feeling that is less than unconditional love for everybody and everything**. We must cleanse and purify our minds, emotions, and actions - these, in fact, are more important to cleanse than the body, because it is through impure thoughts and emotions that we contaminate our

---

[454] All my research indicates that man must be very healthy mentally, physically, and emotionally, before he can handle an all-fruit diet. Most people are not ready for a total fruit diet. They need to cleanse, rebuild their digestive organs, and eliminate their negative emotions first.

bodies. Yet it is also true that cleansing the body is one of the most effective methods of cleansing our minds and emotions. **Many will find that in order to successfully clean out those old mental and emotional impurities, that they must first cleanse the physical structure, for it is in the cell tissues that a great amount of our negative consciousness is stored.** Our physical condition affects the mind and the emotions (and vice versa). At the risk of being redundant, I will now repeat the following, which explains the state of man and his ability to raise himself. Please heed this carefully:

* The cell structure, and in fact everything within our bodies including the mucoid fecal plaque, constantly radiates some form of consciousness, just as everything does, to some degree. It emits a vibratory frequency which reflects the thoughts and feelings we were experiencing at the time we ingested the substance which contributed to the creation of those cells.

* When the mucoid plaque breaks up and is pulled from the intestinal wall, associated thoughts and feelings surface and can exert a great influence upon a person. When that substance is evacuated, it and its inherent consciousness no longer have an effect upon us.

* Therefore, as we remove mucoid layers, it becomes increasingly easier to control desires, appetites, and bad habits, as well as negative thoughts and emotions. Cleansing the digestive tract is an important first step to mental and emotional transformation.

* The next step is to begin cleansing our entire cell structure through juice fasts, consistent clean diets and water fasting. When we arrive at this level, we will know that we are making impressive progress. But, it is not likely to be easy. No one who achieves this level should still eat meat.

* Certain foods - those which yield the greatest life force - should be eaten to maintain that purity of mind and body. Other foods, which give less life force and which may carry associated emotions experienced by animals before and during slaughter or when confined inhumanely (such as meat and dairy), should be avoided in order to assist ourselves in overcoming unwanted feelings (such as hate, fear, and anger). Sticking to foods which yield high life force with the least amount of digestive effort and toxins supports our cell structure in much more effectively eliminating negative thought, feeling, habit, and attitude.

One secret to super health is to **cleanse and rebuild the entire intestinal tract and then the rest of the body,** so that one can live an energetic, happy life sustained by raw fruit alone - this may include sprouted seeds and a few nuts. Before attaining that goal, we need to eat mostly raw fruits and vegetables and occasionally, lightly steamed or cooked foods to control cleansing reactions. During this stage, a baked potato or some steamed vegetables now and then are fine.  One should cleanse or fast periodically, but especially during this period.

The eating of raw fruits only is a very high level of achievement. It can only be obtained after great advancements have been made in eliminating almost all negative thoughts, feelings, and patterns from the deepest core of our beings.  There can be practically no ego (selfishness) left.  At this point we will have the attitude that we are working for all life, not just ourselves.  We will be in conscious contact with our Higher Self or our spirit guide and will demonstrate proof of this.  Beware of imitators.

Before achieving the ideal diet, all of the above mentioned foods are appropriate, as well as occasional grains and squash.   Dr. Jensen advocates the use of these four grains only: millet, rye, yellow cornmeal, and brown rice.[455]  We know that millet is the best of the four in terms of alkalinity. And we add the ancient grain quinoa to this list.  They should be whole and natural.    Sprouted grains and seeds[456] are considered vegetables and are both good, live foods. Others than those just mentioned will actually undermine our efforts and lead us backward to some degree; however, they can sometimes prove useful when controlling cleansing reactions, or when being used to trigger unconscious emotions to come to the surface. The key is to be in touch with our deeper knowing, and allow that to be our guide.

# Raw Food is Quickening

As important as a raw food diet is,  I believe that less than ten percent of the people can adequately handle a total raw food diet without preparation. The main reasons for this are: suppressed negative emotions, lack of control of thoughts and feelings, weak digestive system, and a weak liver. The last two are obvious, but the first two are no less important, **for when we eat raw foods, there is a "quickening of consciousness".**

**This quickening often occurs during or after fasting and cleansing.**  This is one of the reasons fasting has always been utilized among various spiritual orders, and is strongly discouraged among the religious groups that seek to control, limit and manipulate their members. During the accelerated cleansing process, the body takes advantage of the

---

[455] Jensen, *Iridology, The Science and Practice in the Healing Arts*, pg. 426-427.

[456] One needs to eat sprouts in moderation.  They are not all complete foods and can cause imbalances; however, they are very high in life force and enzymes. See:  Dr. Edward Howell, *Enzyme Nutrition*, (Wayne, NJ: Avery Publishing Group, Inc., 1985), pg. 26.

lack of food and opened elimination channels and dumps its overloads of mucus and toxins. After a certain amount has been released, the energy of the body and mind is increased. **The body and mind "lighten up" and perception and awareness are increased and sometimes increased by quantum leaps.**

In our society, people who experience this releasing activity are considered sick. It is common to drug these people, sedate them, get them out of the way. Again, the influence of the dark side. For when we fully realize just how we all are suffering and live such short lives because of the pent-up, stored, and suppressed emotional sludge, we want to do everything we can to get rid of it. In other words, Cleanse and Purify Ourselves at every level of our being. When you fully realize the importance of this, especially at the spiritual level, you will want to know why churches do not teach this, for until one becomes completely pure within, his or her relationship with God, the Creator, Christ, Buddha, whatever term you use, is greatly limited.[457,458]

Over the last 34 years, I have had a deep interest in this quickening, expansion, or acceleration of consciousness. The very first Christians, who were known as the Essenes, were masters of this process. Some of their members included Jesus Christ, Joseph, Mary, John the Baptist, and most of the apostles. These incredible individuals were all advocates of fasting and raw food. It was only after the Roman Empire took over the Christian movement (or I should say, the Essene movement which later faded into the present Christianity) that all this began to change, for they wanted control, and it was impossible to control those who knew how to expand their awareness in these ways.

Anyway, as I said, there is a problem with this quickening. It brings up unsettled issues which the average person is unprepared to handle. As these old suppressed feelings, thoughts and habits surface, we have to deal with them once again. Forgotten memories often surface, bringing all sorts of fluctuations in consciousness. Sometimes, they affect our bodies, feelings, and affairs. Sometimes these memories cannot be identified with this life and we begin to suspect, as Jesus taught, that we have lived before.[459]

---

[457] "Blessed are the pure in heart: for they shall see God." *The Holy Bible*, Matthew 5:8. Are there people who are pure enough to see God? Yes. Are they condemned by those who call themselves authorities? Of course. One of the problems is that people do not understand what it means to be 'pure' - a word our society applies to anything but a person!

**[458] See Chapter 15: The Experience in Teeshi Lumbo.**

# Why Raw Foods are the Perfect Foods

Raw foods are the perfect foods for man and can bring him exceptional health. They keep the body clean and congestion-free. Only raw foods have life force and enzymes, and they are more important to our health than taking vitamins, minerals, and amino acids. It's the life force and enzymes that keep us vibrantly alive and internally clean. We can eat foods without life force or enzymes and still get minerals and proteins, but we cannot get vitamins, enzymes or life force from those foods.

Alexis Carrel of the Rockefeller Institute and recipient of the Nobel Prize was able **to keep tissue cells alive indefinitely**, by nutritious feedings and by washing away tissue excretions. These cells grew and thrived as long as evacuations were removed. Unsanitary conditions resulted in lower vitality, deterioration, and death. He kept a chicken heart alive for 29 years until someone failed to cleanse its excretions!

The same thing holds true in the human body. If it is not kept clean inside, congestion occurs, the blood becomes impure, and the result is lowered vitality, disease, and a depleted immune system which eventually leads to so-called death. How many times have we marveled at the seemingly endless energy of a young child? When the body is in its pure state, before it is congested, it is wonderfully alive, vibrant, and bursting with energy. We should not have to deteriorate from that state, but on the contrary, improve upon it. Raw foods maintain internal purity; cooked foods create mucus and congestion. **Negative thoughts also cause congestion in our physical bodies; I estimate that they actually have a greater impact upon our health than the food we eat**.

On an emotional level, it is the impure emotions and desires that cause a conflict between our outer and inner selves, and this leads to congestion. Physical congestion, which generally begins in the intestines, is really the number-one killer in the world. Without congestion, the cells easily repair themselves. Carrel believed that the cell was, therefore, immortal. I believe that this is only possible in humans, when mind and emotion have been purified.

Congestion starves the cells of needed nutrients and oxygen. The body is not only capable of repairing itself, but what's more, it never stops trying! All we have to do is get the congestion out of the way and then

---

[459] Read the *Gospel of the Holy Twelve*. In my estimation, this is a pure "New Testament" uncontaminated by those who seek to control. For more information about this book and the Essenes, contact Brother David Owen, PO Box 1113, Creswell, Oregon 97426. This book reveals that Jesus Christ does indeed teach reincarnation, vegetarianism, and equality of men and women.

give our bodies what they need, and nothing else. Most people know that if you put sugar into the gas tank of your car, it clogs up the engine and the car stops running. Eating cooked and processed foods is like putting slime and glue into the body. No wonder the body wears out - it's been forced to work a few too many overtime hours! Cooked food leaves residue, eventually causing congestion. Raw food, properly digested, leaves no residue.

So, the key is to eat foods that keep the body congestion-free, and that means raw fruits, raw vegetables, raw sprouted grains, and small amounts of sprouted nuts and seeds. Moses lived 600 years. Melchizedek lived over 900 years. Who knows how long we would live if we cleansed ourselves, ate raw foods, and harmonized with the laws of Nature.

# Simplified Eating

One key to outstanding health is to **not eat any more than what we need**. After our bodies are clean and the digestion is working the way it should, one small meal per day might be enough. People would be surprised how much energy is wasted in digesting food. If we eat more than we need, even if it is perfect food, then we place unnecessary stress on our bodies and dilute our digestive fluids.

Another secret that will surprise the gourmet cook, is to **limit the variety of the food eaten at any one time**. Eating only 1 - 3 different foods at one meal is best. For example, if it's fruit, eat only nectarines, or another fruit that is compatible. Don't have the normal fruit salad, especially with whipped cream. If it's vegetables, just have one to three vegetables and no more. We should not make all these multi-combo salads everyone likes to have. We need to stop mixing everything and stop using salad dressings, oils, and seasonings, in hopes that we can make something taste good. We need to try to develop the natural taste buds again and enjoy the individual fruits and vegetables. I wonder how may people have ever tried to eat only some butter lettuce, a bell pepper, a cabbage, or some watercress, all by themselves? This is a very advanced way of eating — the healthy way.[460]

---

[460] Study the *Essene Gospel of Peace,* the entire book. This offers the very best advice ever given about how, when, how much, and what to eat.

# Life Force

Life force is the potency of Innate Intelligence that gives life to everything that lives. It is the only healing force there is or ever will be, and is *the* most powerful and effective contributor towards good health. It is the source of energy and nerve vitality. It is what gives the spinal fluid its life and power. It gives life to every cell in our bodies. It is even the life in the electron of the atom. It is what gives enzymes the ability to function. Without life force no one can exist, and the amount of life force you have determines your health, energy, happiness, and how long you will live.

Every atom of the body is filled with electricity or life force, to some degree. These atoms are composed of electrons and protons, which are negatively and positively charged particles. The greater the voltage, charge or force of each cell, the more power it can generate to be healthy. The cell itself can be so charged with life force that it can become radiant light. It is this light that repels disease. It is energy in its purest form. The greater the power flowing, the more one is able to think clearly and accurately. When this energy flows in full force through the nerve channels and the emotional body, it is easier to remain positive in the feelings. Charismatic qualities of happiness and joy surface more readily. The mind and heart are naturally drawn to higher things. One is inclined to express love and kindness more freely and seldom tires at work or play. When this life force flows through every cell of the body, we ward off disease, handle stress effectively, stay healthy longer, and our aging is slowed. When we have purified ourselves completely and have strengthened our bodies with the necessary substances, we can become transformers of massive focal points of life force or energy. In comparing the vibrancy of a young, healthy child to an elderly, diseased person, we all know that there is a great difference in life force. What we often fail to realize is that we can continue to increase that life force within us to unlimited degrees. It is in this way that we can go beyond perfect health and beyond the ultimate disease called death.

The life force of the body is not dissipated or destroyed by over-exertion, for exercise helps to eliminate toxins, deep breathing helps eliminate acids and helps draw part of the life force back in, and the joy of exercise draws etheric energy in through our energy vortexes. It is dissipated or destroyed by drugs, misuse of sex, negative emotions, and dead foods. Foods that have been cooked, frozen, canned, or processed have had the life force removed. Each time these dead or devitalized foods are consumed we are, in effect, "killing off" our energy, our alertness, our health and the process of aging speeds up.

Following is a good illustration. When one fully-charged, 12-volt battery is hooked up to a dead 12-volt battery, the dead battery will draw from the charged battery until the median level is reached. The fully-charged battery becomes considerably drained - in fact, it is drained to half its original force - while the dead battery takes on some of the energy from the charged battery.

So it goes when eating dead foods. A portion of our life force is drained from our electrical reserves (located in the spine and in each atom) to feed the devitalized foods. On the other hand, eating raw foods helps build the life force, adding zest and energy while keeping the body free from congestion. Eating raw foods is like eating fully-charged battery cells.

Once we have eliminated congestion from the body, along with the obstruction of negative thoughts and feelings, the life force connection with God and the solar system may flow in unlimited power through the other centers (which are now sealed) in the body. Who knows the potential of this? Only those who have attained this exalted state, and they are the legends of mankind's history. Ponder the words of Jesus: "...the works that I do, shall ye do also and even greater works than these shall ye do." When do we start?

# Sunshine

Almost everyone has experienced a noticeable increase in energy, strength, mental alertness, health and happiness during and after spending time in the sun. Yet there are forces that are trying to keep people from spending much time in the sun.

We are told that the sun can cause skin cancer. I can hardly believe that anyone would fall for such nonsense. Millions of people soak in the sun every day and never get skin cancer. I am convinced that it is not the sun that causes skin cancer; it is the impurities - the toxins in the skin that cause this condition. Those who are prone towards skin cancer need only cleanse themselves and they will find the sun to be rejuvenating and healthy. I believe that many suntan lotions can cause skin cancer and damage internal organs such as the liver and kidneys.

We need the sun to assimilate minerals, especially calcium. Calcium is used for many things besides bones. It is needed for strength, healing, emotional stability, pH, and more. Over a period of 20 years I have observed myself and others becoming stronger, more rejuvenated and whole when we spend time in the sun. Ideally, we should spend at least an hour every day in the sun. The more skin we expose to the sun, the better. I believe that the most important part of the body for the sun to kiss is the solar plexus. Exposing this area for just a few minutes can make wonderful changes.

# Enzymes

Enzymes are essential in maintaining internal cleanliness, not to mention health, youth, and strength. Our breathing, sleeping, eating, working, and thinking are dependent upon enzymes. Enzymes are substances that make life possible. They are far more important than any other nutrient. Proteins cannot be utilized without enzymes, nor can vitamins and minerals. Enzymes are destroyed after use and must be constantly replaced. Like the battery analogy, cooked foods draw from the enzyme reserves, depleting the body's precious "labor-force." Life force is the central core of each enzyme. Enzymes are the vehicles through which life force works to make things happen. Vitamins, minerals, proteins, and body chemicals depend on enzymes to do all the work. Enzymes, however, also depend upon vitamins, minerals, and proteins in order to function — one depends upon the other.

Raw foods are full of enzymes. Cooked and processed foods have none. Enzymes play a vital part in the digestion of our foods, in fighting disease, and in breaking down foreign matter. With a decrease in enzymes, a process of internal decay rapidly develops, creating mounting problems in the body which can even be transmitted, through DNA, to one's future children.

According to Dr. Edward Howell (who was probably the world's authority on enzymes) each person is given a limited supply of body enzymes at birth. The faster we use up our enzyme supply, the shorter our life span, the weaker our immune system, and the more dis-eased the body. As he puts it, "Both the habit of cooking our foods and eating them processed with chemicals, and the use of alcohol, drugs, and junk food, draw out tremendous quantities of enzymes from our limited supply." He also says that colds, flu, and other sicknesses deplete the supply.

Dr. Howell exposed the unsuccessful attempts of modern medicine to heal disease and its failure to attack the root of the problem. He said that many, if not all, degenerative diseases from which humans suffer and die are caused by excessive use of enzyme-deficient cooked and processed foods.[461] This is one of the many reasons that herbs cure, and drugs stimulate but do not heal. **Drugs have no life force, no nutrition, and no enzymes, but herbs have them all.**

By 1968 science had identified 1300 enzymes. There are three classes of enzymes:
1. Digestive enzymes, which digest our foods.
2. Food enzymes, which are abundant in raw foods.

---

[461] Howell, pg. 26.

3. Metabolic enzymes, which run our bodies.

Raw food supplies food enzymes which provide many of the digestive enzymes that the body would otherwise have to come up with from its limited reserves if one ate cooked food. When we have lived for many years on cooked foods we can easily have depleted our abundance of enzymes. When this happens, our digestive systems will withdraw from our metabolic enzyme reserves to aid in digestion. **When metabolic enzymes are depleted to a certain point, the body begins to deteriorate at an ever increasing rate.** If this depletion goes far enough, the body dies.

Science does not know how to replenish these enzymes. A few digestive enzyme supplements are now available, but not metabolic enzymes. The only way we know to create additional metabolic enzymes is to increase the flow of life-force through the body. This activates the energy at the base of the spine that gives the yogi his powers; this is known as the kundalini energy. I have discussed the importance of this life-force to a small degree throughout this book.

Heating food over 116-120 degrees F. destroys all food enzymes (and most vitamins) and forces the body to deplete itself. This causes enlargement of the digestive organs, especially the pancreas. **Foods and drinks which are at too high a temperature will also injure the enzymes in the stomach.** In addition, eating high protein foods, forces the bowels to become acid, thereby destroying enzyme function in the bowel, for enzymes in the intestines can only function to their maximum degree at a pH between 7 - 8.[462]

Enzymes are the active ingredients that cure disease. They are the central core of the immune system and necessary for the maintenance of health.[463] It is the enzymatic activity that makes the brain function, the memory work, and keeps the body alive. So, for a longer, healthier, and happier life, one should eat less and eat only raw foods. Consider the words of Jesus the Christ from the *Essene Gospel of Peace*:

---

[462] Guyton, pg. 780.

[463] How do you think the immune system destroys our enemies? The white cells release enzymes that kill pathogens. For example, eosinophils release histaminase and aryl sulphatase. These enzymes are needed to help reduce inflammation and destroy parasites. Neutrophils secrete hydrolases, myeloperoxidase, and muramidase which can kill a variety of microorganisms. Ivan Roitt, Jonathan Brosoff, David Male, *Immunology*, (Philadelphia, PA: J.B. Lippincott Co., 1989), pg. 2.11, 2.14, 2.16.

(**Note**: Whether you believe that these are the words of Jesus, should not matter, but let us listen and learn from the deep wisdom they contain.)

"So eat always from the table of God: the fruits of the trees, the grain and grasses of the field, the milk of beasts (raw milk), and the honey of bees. For everything beyond these is of Satan, and leads by the way of sins and of diseases unto death. But the foods which you eat from the abundant table of God give strength and youth to your body, **and you will never see disease**. For the table of God fed Methuselah of old, and I tell you truly, if you live even as he lived, then will the God of the living give you also long life upon the earth as was his.

For I tell you truly, the God of the living is richer than all the rich of the earth, and his abundant table is richer than the richest table of feasting of all the rich upon the earth. **Eat, therefore, all your life at the table of our Earthly Mother, and you will never see want**. And when you eat at her table, eat all things even **as they are found** on the table of the Earthly Mother. **Cook not, neither mix all things one with another, lest your bowels become as steaming bogs**. For I tell you truly, this is abominable in the eyes of the Lord.

And be not like the greedy servant, who always ate up, at the table of his lord, the portions of others. And he devoured everything himself, and mixed all together in his gluttony. And seeing that, his lord was wroth with him, and drove him from the table. And when all had ended their meal, he mixed together all that remained upon the table, and called the greedy servant to him and said: 'Take and eat all this with the swine, for your place is with them, and not at my table.'

Take heed, therefore, and defile not with all kinds of abominations the temple of your bodies. **Be content with two or three sorts of food**, which you will find always upon the table of our Earthly Mother. And desire not to devour all things which you see around you. For I tell you truly, **if you mix together all sorts of food in your body, then the peace of your body will cease, and endless war will rage in you**. And it will be blotted out even as homes and kingdoms divided against themselves work their own destruction. For your God is the God of peace, and does never help division.

*Arouse not, therefore, against you the wrath of God, lest He drive you from his table, and lest you be compelled to go to the table of Satan, where the fire of sins, diseases, and death will corrupt your body.*

*And when you eat, **never eat unto fullness**. Flee the temptations of Satan, and listen to the voice of God's angels. For Satan and his power tempt you always to eat more and more. But live by the spirit, and resist the desires of the body. And your **fasting is always pleasing in the eyes of the angels of God**. So give heed to how much you have eaten when your body is sated, and always eat less by a third.*

*Let the weight of your daily foods be not less than a mina,[464] but mark that it go not beyond two. Then will the angels of God serve you always, and you will never fall into the bondage of Satan and of his diseases. Trouble not the work of the angels in your body by eating often. For I tell you truly, **he who eats more than twice in the day does in him the work of Satan**. And the angels of God leave his body, and soon Satan will take possession of it. **Eat only when the sun is highest in the heavens, and again when it is set**. And you will never see disease, for such finds favor in the eyes of the Lord. **And if you will that the angels of God rejoice in your body, and that Satan shun you afar, then sit but once in the day at the table of God**. And then your days will be long upon the earth, for this is pleasing in the eyes of the Lord. Eat always when the table of God is served before you, and eat always of that which you find upon the table of God. For I tell you truly, God knows well what your body needs, and when it needs."[465]*

---

[464] Greek unit of measurement.

[465] An interesting thought: when reading Biblical or Essene works, try replacing the word Lord with "law" and see if this gives new insight.

# Exercise

Vigorous exercise offers many important benefits. One is: removing toxins everywhere that the blood and lymph circulate. Vigorous exercise flushes our pipe system (circulatory and lymphatic). It not only helps to keep our systems clear, but it allows oxygen and other nutrients to enter areas of the body that have a tendency to remain stagnant. It prevents our bodies from becoming swamps!

When we exercise hard, we also create or maintain maximum mitochondria levels. Mitochondria are the energy factories in our cells. They convert glucose into ATP (Adenosine Triphosphate), or pure energy. The less mitochondria in our bodies, the less energy, strength and endurance. When we fail to exercise on a regular basis, the number of mitochondria gradually decreases. When we exercise vigorously, we can increase the mitochondria and our bodies will have an increase of energy. This increased energy will improve all areas of our beings: physical performance, mental ability, and emotional well-being, too. Even our immune systems and overall health will improve; thus our resistance to disease becomes much more effective.

Vigorous exercise means to me: moving our bodies in such a way that we breathe hard: lungs pump, our hearts beat fast and we sweat. We should gradually build ourselves up to at least one hour of exercise, three times a week.

# Reversing the Aging Process

"**The cell is immortal**. It is merely the fluid in which it floats which degenerates. Renew this fluid at intervals, give the cell something upon which to feed, and as far as we know, the pulsation of life may go on forever." - Alexis Carrel

**Alexis Carrel won the Nobel Prize for proving that the cell is immortal**. His chicken heart experiment was the key to this conclusion. So the question is: if our cells can continue their existence indefinitely, how is it that they die so early? Is there something that we can do to prevent their early death?

Basically that is what this book is all about. However, there is an important consideration that I wish to discuss at this time. Science has found that one thing that damages our cells, hence causing pre-mature aging, is the free radical, which is imbalanced on a molecular level.

While we have come to expect that we will undergo the aging process and all of the disorders that we associate with it, there is a general consensus within the scientific community that free radicals play an enormous role not only in how we age, but also in how fast we age. Aging, by the way, is currently defined in medicine as an increase in the risk of death. In other words, the more free radicals, the faster we age and the shorter our life span. Take a look at a person with sun damaged skin. The "age" or "liver" spots on the back of the hands or face of a person with sun damaged skin are a perfect example of free radical damage. Well, the same thing is happening to the other organs of the body, including the heart, the brain and other internal organs. Sounds pretty dismal doesn't it? It doesn't have to be. The most effective way to *decrease the amount of free radicals* and oxidative stress is to cleanse our bodies of the toxins that are the source of free radical activity, and to defend ourselves from the continual onslaught of toxins in our environment as well as from those we choose to ingest, by choosing to eat purer foods. If, however, we are unable to cleanse effectively, and/or to eat pure foods, we should take antioxidant supplements.

# Free Radicals

Actually, free radicals are a normal byproduct of cellular metabolism, the everyday task of our bodies in the creation of energy, cellular repair, and fueling ourselves with nutrients. We need oxygen during these processes, and more importantly, we need it to live. The free radicals produced during our usual metabolic functions are not a problem and can even be beneficial. How is it then that free radicals are blamed for cellular damage, aging and even death? It is when oxidation caused by free radicals gets out of hand that we get into trouble. When we bombard our bodies with the toxins contained within meats loaded with nitrates, as well as with herbicides, mucus producing foods, cigarettes, drugs, smog, ultraviolet radiation, artificial colorings, physical trauma, and emotional stress we drastically increase the amount of oxidative stress and the formation of free radicals. Even exercise, which increases our intake of oxygen, increases oxidation. The results can be devastating for those who are deficient in antioxidants. Excess levels of free radicals damage the cell membrane structures (organelles) within the cell, particularly mitochondria (the powerhouse or energy source within our cells) and even our DNA which carries the code for reproduction. When you have massive cell damage, it affects tissue, and eventually the organs and health. These cell damaging processes are primarily determined by the course of mitochondrial respiration and the rate of damage to the mitochondria. The cellular damage associated with the increase of free radicals has been correlated to the prevalence of cancer, heart disease, neurodegenerative disorders such as Huntington's disease, Parkinson's disease, Alzheimer's, inflammatory disorders such as rheumatoid arthritis, amyotrophic lateral sclerosis (more commonly known as Lou Gehrig's disease), and the acceleration of the aging process.

## Causes of Excess Free Radicals

* poor diet
* excess stress (worry, fear, anger)
* unhealthy water (containing chlorine, sodium fluoride, inorganic minerals)
* radiation (coming from computers, fluorescent lights, microwaves, power lines)
* pesticides, herbicides, inorganic fertilizers, and other chemical residues in our food and environment
* air pollution
* too much exercise (over exertion)
* colds, flu, inflammations, disease
* chronic and degenerative diseases
* any toxin

Excess free radicals present a major threat to the immune system and to the entire metabolic function. As we age, or whenever our cells cannot receive adequate nutrients due to either congestion at the cell level or lack of needed nutrients, our natural body production of antioxidant enzymes decreases. These enzymes are a major part of the immune system.

So what is a free radical and what are these "free radical chompers" called antioxidants? A free radical is a molecule that has lost one of its electrons and becomes hungry for another one. It is like someone who was bit by a vampire and became a vampire. Quite simply, a free radical is an incomplete, unstable molecule, often in the form of oxygen, that reacts with other molecules in a destructive manner. How does this happen? Molecules, which are one of the basic units in nature, are usually balanced and have paired electrons around their nucleus. When a molecule loses one of it's electrons, it becomes unbalanced. That is a free radical. In an effort to regain it's balance, it will rob an electron from a second molecule. In doing so, it creates a free radical of that molecule. Needing an electron, that molecule will do the same, and so on, creating a chain reaction or a cascade effect. This theft of electrons is called oxidation. And each time an electron is stolen from a molecule, that molecule is damaged, causing a malfunction of one type or another in the body. It is exactly the same process that causes metal to rust! That's oxidation, and it is even more damaging to the human body. It is the "free radical chompers" (often referred to as scavengers or antioxidants) which stop this terrible destruction.

The "free radical chompers" are called "antioxidant enzymes". However, the problem arises when there are far too many free radicals and not enough antioxidant enzymes. In other words, when the levels of free radicals are greater than the supply of antioxidant enzymes, our cells are being damaged beyond the capacity to repair them.

## Types of Free Radicals

**Peroxide free radicals** tend to damage the fats in our bodies. Rancid fats are high in peroxide free radicals and too many of these can damage our livers, injure the heart function, and cause premature aging. Other problems also occur such as skin diseases, pre-mature wrinkling, age spots, dermatitis, eczema, and psoriasis. The solution to these free radicals is stopping the causes, of course, but also important is glutathione peroxidase. This enzyme eats peroxide free radicals. How important is glutathione? Our bodies can only live three days without it.[466]

**Hydroxyl free radicals** are usually formed from a response to radiation, too much exercise, or heavy metals in our bodies. This includes mercury in our fillings, lead from gas fumes, aluminum from cooking with aluminum pots, and other heavy metals we get from the environment, as well as pesticides from commercially grown foods. This free radical has the ability to damage any type of cell tissue and is considered to be the most dangerous free radical. Removing amalgam fillings would be a wise move. **We should not jog or exercise near heavy traffic** where exhaust fumes are abundant, nor in closed rooms where oxygen is limited. We should never breathe exhaust fumes or eat commercially grown produce, frozen or canned. Methionine reductase is the enzyme that reduces the hydroxyl free radical.

**Superoxide free radicals** are the most common free radicals. They are a by-product of oxidation. We all know that we cannot live without oxygen, the most important physical element. Yet

---

[466] When people have a serious illness or receive chemotherapy and lose muscle mass, it is because the body broke down muscle to gather glutamine, and then glutamic acid to make glutathione to save the life of the body.

few of us realize that there are unbalanced oxygen atoms and they do cause serious problems in our bodies. The superoxide free radicals activate the break down of synovial fluid, the lubricating element. This can affect the joints, causing inflammation. This radical can cause many other problems as well. When the body is well nourished, it creates its own antioxidants to combat these free radicals.

# Antioxidants

Antioxidant molecules and enzymes protect our cells from the damage of oxidation by either neutralizing the free radicals or by interrupting the cascade of oxidative damage. There are a number of antioxidants available from the food we eat, including vitamins A, C, and E as well as some of the trace minerals such as selenium, copper, zinc, magnesium and much more. Theoretically, given that we were designed to live in perfect balance, the foods we eat should provide us with ample amounts of antioxidants to combat the effects of free radical damage. I'm sure that was true before we introduced the vast array of poisons that we ingest and use to destroy ourselves and the earth. (Ever wonder why the people in biblical times lived to be hundreds of years old?) **The amount of antioxidants in our food doesn't cut it anymore, folks - unless we eat from our own perfect garden grown in rich, undepleted soil.** We need to supplement our diets with antioxidants to fight the effects of oxidation caused by pollution, bad food, preservatives, too much ultra-violet radiation (the result of an ozone depleted atmosphere) and emotional and physical stress.

# Uses of Specific Antioxidants

Until recently, the major antioxidant players were believed to be vitamins A, C, and E. And they are effective, especially in the treatment and prevention of certain types of cancer and degenerative disorders of the eyes (our mothers were right on when they said to eat our carrots to keep our eyes strong). However, we now recognize that there are a number of even more potent antioxidants. **Many of them are synergistic with each other**, working to spare or recycle one another or sharing nutrients as needed when scavenging free radicals.

Vitamin E and Selenium interact to provide strong protection against oxidative damage to the liver. Vitamins C and E work as a team to produce an antioxidant effect that is far greater than any one individual antioxidant, and they help protect each other from the onslaught of free radicals. Both Vitamin C and Co-enzyme Q10 interact with Vitamin E to regenerate E's antioxidant form. When there are enough of the other antioxidants, such as Vitamin E, Selenium and Beta-carotene, CoQ10 can significantly reduce free-radical damage in the liver, kidney and heart cells. It has also been shown to eliminate breast cancer in some people. Selenium and Vitamin A work together to help prevent cancer.[467] The amino acid L-Cysteine works in tandem with Vitamin C (ascorbic acid) to create a reciprocal relationship with Glutathione: ascorbate spares Glutathione and increases mitochondrial Glutathione in Glutathione deficient animals.[468] Vitamin C and Glutathione also work together in protecting mitochondria from oxidative damage.[469] Selenium also interacts with Glutathione (GSH), which is a vital component in the production of Glutathione Peroxidase - an enzyme which is essential for life.[470]

The liver can only survive for about three days without the action of GSH, hence, support for all the essential aspects of GSH activity should be found in an ideal antioxidant formula: this would include Selenium, GSH, L-Cysteine, Co-enzyme Q10, and Beta-carotene. In a recent study on GSH and aging, it was found that GSH concentrations are positively correlated with age and good health. In fact, those individuals with higher GSH levels experienced less disease, and better health overall than age-matched subjects with lower GSH levels.[471]

Some antioxidants are known to target particular disease states or organs; or, they may act to prevent a myriad of disease states, including cancer. Co-enzyme Q10, Quercitin (a bioflavonoid), an all-natural grape seed extract rich in biologically active flavonoids), and pine bark extract are all known for their anti-inflammatory effects and are, therefore, extremely effective in the treatment of allergies, asthma and certain inflammatory disorders such as lupus, rheumatoid arthritis and in some cases, cancer.[472,473,474] Chromium seems to have a regulatory role in glucose and

---

[467] Maryce M. Jacobs, *Vitamins and Minerals in the Prevention and Treatment of Cancer*, (Boca Raton, FL: CRC Press, 1991), pg. 105.

[468] B. S. Winkler, S. M. Orselli, T. S. Rex, "The Redox Couple Between Glutathione and Ascorbic Acid: A Chemical and Physiological Approach," *Free Radical Biology and Medicine*, 1994; Vol. 17(4), pg. 333-349.

[469] Ibid.

[470] T. M. Bray, C. G. Taylor, "Tissue Glutathione, Nutrition, and Oxidative Stress," *Canadian Journal of Physiology and Pharmacology*, 1993; Vol. 71, pg. 746-751.

[471] M. Julius, C.A. Lang, L. Gleiberman, W. DiFranceisco, and A. Schork, "Glutathione and Morbidity in a Community-based Sample of Elderly," *Journal of Clinical Epidemiology*, 1994; Vol. 47, pg. 1021-1026.

insulin metabolism. Without glucose balance, we become vulnerable to all sorts of diseases, including Candidiasis, as well as target for a substantial increase of free radical activity. Therefore, adequate supplies of chromium assist all other antioxidants by reducing levels of free radicals created in the body. Zinc (Zinc L-monomethionine) is an essential trace element that is vital to protein synthesis, nucleic acid production, and healthy immune system function. This type of zinc supplement has also been shown to help reduce excess levels of superoxide free radicals and to detoxify cellular membranes by displacing heavy metals and toxins from body tissues.

As regards the effects of antioxidants on specific organs, the liver is a most important organ to address. Without a good strong liver, the brain, the heart, lungs, kidneys and all of the glands become vulnerable to various toxins, drugs, chemicals and poisons. I believe a number of antioxidants are essential for the liver: Silymarin, Curcumin, Lipoic acid, Glutathione, Selenium and L-Cysteine all help detoxify, strengthen and protect the liver[475] Very few diseases can be established in the body as long as the liver is able to perform its full function.

In my opinion, an ideal antioxidant formula would also address brain function. Ginkgo Biloba is well known to strengthen the walls of even the tiniest blood vessels and capillaries. It is also known as the most effective nutrient for improving blood circulation to the brain. Ginkgo is effective in relieving migraine headaches and has become famous for improving the memory.[476] **Another important antioxidant for the brain is lipoic (thioctic) acid. In addition to it's importance in the production of cellular metabolism, energy production, and it's ability to detoxify tissue of heavy metals, lipoic acid is particularly important in**

---

[472] R. M. Facino, et. al., "Free Radicals Scavenging Action and Anti-enzyme Activities of Procyanidines from Vitis Vinifera. A Mechanism for Their Capillary Protective Action," *Arzneim-Forsch*, 1994; Vol. 44, pg. 592-601.

[473] A.K. Verma, et. al., "Inhibition of 7, 12-Dimethylbenz(A)anthracene - and N-Nitrosomethylurea - Induced Rat Mammary Cancer by Dietary Flavonol Quercitin," *Cancer Research*, 1989; Vol. 48, pg. 5754.

[474] K. Lockwood, et. al., "Partial and Complete Regression of Breast Cancer in Relation to Dosage of Co-enzyme Q-10," *Biochemical and Biophysical Research Communications*, 1994; Vol. 100, pg. 1504-1508.

[475] J. Feher, et. al., "Hepaprotective Activity of Silymarin (Legalon) Therapy in Patients with Chronic Alcoholic Liver Disease," *Orvosi Hetilap* (Budapest, Hungary), 1989; Vol. 130, pg. 2723.

[476] Carolyn Rueben, *Antioxidants - Your Complete Guide*, (Rockland, CA: Prima Publishing, 1995), pg. 186

**protecting the integrity of neural (brain) tissue.**[477] Generous amounts of these antioxidants should be included. And only the highest quality ginkgo biloba extract and lipoic acid should be used, to do the job right.

Other benefits of an outstanding antioxidant formula would include the following. In addition to **reducing the risk and incidence of cancer**, antioxidants have also been shown to diminish tumor size once cancer has been established. What else? How about **slowing down the aging process, reducing the risk of heart disease, maintaining strong bones, teeth, beautiful hair and skin, sparing the eyes from the effects of free radical damage and reducing the risk of diabetic retinopathy, reducing respiratory infections, and protecting against heart disease? In other words, the regular use of an excellent antioxidant formula can protect and maintain your body in optimal health.**

As you can see, a supplement containing a *combination* of antioxidants would be highly beneficial for the prevention and elimination of the detrimental effects of free radicals. I believe that I have created the most advanced antioxidant formula available today. It is so effective that people have reported a difference in their well-being in just a few days of using it. It also seems to effectively enhance athletic performance.

## Very Quick Glance List of Important Antioxidants

**Vitamin A** - helps to prevent the formation of cataracts.
**Vitamin C** - slows down glutathione loss and vice versa.
**Vitamin E** - gamma-tocopherol can quench peroxynitrite, a highly destructive nitric oxide radical.
**Proanthocynidin and Pycnogenol**-extract from grape seed or pine bark - weapons against premature aging and disease.
**Curcumin** - an extract from turmeric with anticancer properties, purifies and strengthens the liver.
**Alpha lipoic acid** - a sulfur containing antioxidant that protects the nervous system from the damages of free radicals, protects the liver, and helps to detoxify the body of heavy metal pollutants.
**Coenzyme Q-10** - free radical scavenger, protects the body from cardiovascular disease.
**L-Cysteine** - an effective precursor of glutathione synthesis, L-cysteine helps to prevent oxidative cell death by supplying the cell with glutathione, and by scavenging free radicals.

---

[477] L. Packer, H.J. Tritshchler, K. Wessel, "Neuroprotection by the Metabolic Antioxidant Alpha-lipoic Acid," *Free Radical Biology and Medicine,* 1997; Vol. 22(1-2), pg. 359-378.

**Glutathione** - works as a chelator of toxins to carry them out of the body, and as a cofactor in the production of essential enzymes.

**Selenium** - activates the production of the enzyme, glutathione peroxidase. Destroys fat soluble oxidants in the cell.

**Silymarin** - detoxifies and protects the liver.

**Vitamin B-6** - essential for the production of antibodies, red blood cells and absorption of vitamin B-12.

**L-Monomethionine** - vital element in protein synthesis and a healthy immune system function.

**Ginkgo Biloba** - strengthens the walls of blood vessels and capillaries and improves blood circulation in the brain.

**Chromium** - aids in the metabolism of fat, protein and carbohydrates. Works with insulin to facilitate the uptake of glucose into the cell.

**Quercitin** - helpful for all inflammatory and allergic conditions.

# "Friendly" Bacteria

**The proper bacteria in our gut are essential for health.** Few people realize just how important they are. In a healthy body, the total number of bacteria outnumbers man's own cells! Their total weight is comparable to the liver and includes close to 500 different strains.[478] A perfect combination is required for health. **The lack of certain bacteria can cause severe imbalances and an overabundance of other strains can also cause severe metabolic disturbances**. This may include a chain reaction of digestive disturbances, assimilation problems, liver weakness, and deficiencies which can contribute towards a gradual and consistent decline of health. Due to unnatural diet and lifestyle, most people have drastically altered their normal intestinal bacterial flora.

**Many people have used various** *acidophilus* **products with temporary success only to later find that they had merely exchanged one set of problems for another.** Few, however, have realized this because it is so difficult to trace symptoms back to the cause. Most bacteria formulas (probiotics) contain a predominance of acid-producing bacteria (*Lactobacillus acidophilus* etc.) which are highly beneficial under various pathogenic conditions. However, when used consistently, these bacteria contribute towards abnormal bowel acidity, which may be very challenging to the electrolyte balance as well as to a healthy bowel environment. Some studies have shown that patients suffering from metabolic acidosis may have triggered this potential death-causing extreme by consuming *lactobacillus* tablets and/or milk and yogurt.[479,480] **What are we doing to future**

---

[478] B. E. Gustafsson, "The Physiological Importance of the Colonic Microflora," *Scandinavian Journal of Gastroenterology*, Supplements, 1982; 77, pg. 117-121.

metabolic functions when we saturate our bowels with acid-forming bacteria which produce large amounts of unnatural lactic acids consisting of a pH of 3.9 to 4.5?[481] Doesn't this tend to reverse what the bowel is attempting to accomplish when it secretes fluids of 7.5 to 8.9 pH?[482] And what does this do to the digestive enzymes of the small and large intestine, **which can only function optimally in a pH of 7 or above?**[483] Some doctors and scientists believe that this poses a potential futuristic problem.

Is *L. acidophilus* even natural to the human gut? I do not think so. Studies show that approximately 25% of the human population do not have *lactobacillus* in their guts.[484] It appears that *L. acidophilus* is found in humans that drink dairy products or take probiotics containing *L. acidophilus*. Even those who take probiotics and consume large amounts of dairy products have only small amounts of *lactobacillus*.[485] This indicates that *Lactobacillus acidophilus* is not natural in the human bowel and tends to die off rather quickly if a constant source is not used. I do not believe that man was intended to rob animals of their milk or take probiotics. It is only after the "fall of man" so to speak that that these unnatural activities developed. And here we are, the fall continues. What do we do to restore ourselves to the natural healthy position that is our birth right? I believe that ***Lactobacillus* probiotics have a place in the treatment against pathogens, however, they need to be used with intelligence and caution and not as the main bacterial implant.**

---

[479] Joseph T. Thurn, Gordon L. Pierpont, Carl W. Ludvigsen, John H. Eckfeldt, "D-Lactate Encephalopathy," *The American Journal of Medicine*, 1985; Dec.; Vol. 79, pg. 720.

[480] Lawrence Stolberg, Rial Rolfe, Norman Gitlin, Jeffrey Merritt, Lewis Mann, Jr., Jean Linder, Sydney Finegold, "D-lactic Acidosis Due To Abnormal Gut Flora," *The New England Journal Of Medicine*, 1982; June 3; pg. 1347.

[481] Noel R. Krieg, ed., *Bergey's Manual Of Systematic Bacteriology*, Volume 2, (Baltimore, MD: Williams & Wilkins, 1984), pg. 1210-1212. According to Dr. Khem Shahani, some strains of acidophilus create a lactic acid pH as low as 3.9.

[482] Guyton, pg 772.

[483] Ibid., pg 780.

[484] Glen R. Gibson and George T. Macfarlane, ed., *Human Colonic Bacteria - Role in Nutrition, Physiology, and Pathology*, (Boca Raton, FL: CRC Press, 1995), pg. 260.

[485] Ibid.

Studies indicate that ***Bifidobacterium infantis* is the predominant bacteria in breast-fed infant feces**. This is the first bacteria that young healthy infants receive from breast milk, and may be the most essential and basic bacteria for the human gut.[486] Other *bifidobacterium*, such as *B. longum* (which is closely related to *B. infantis* and is found in both healthy children and adults),[487] and *Bifidobacterium bifidum, (*which is found in healthy adults),[488] are probably the most natural and essential bacteria for man. **These bacteria generate a pH between 6.5 to 7.0,[489] which is much more beneficial for a healthy human bowel than the lactic acid producing *lactobacillus***. Beneficial bacteria begin to die off at a pH near 4.5, the pH normally produced by *Lactobacillus acidophilus*. **This indicates that *L. acidophilus* may actually destroy the natural health offering bacteria**. *Bifidobacterium* are also resistant to a wide spectrum of harmful medical drugs, including some antibiotics.[490] *Bifidobacterium* species are also known to produce large amounts of amino acids[491] and other nutritious elements including vitamins. Clinical studies have shown that out of all the other *bifidobacteria* strains tested, both ***B. infantis* and *B. breve* were most effective in repelling *E. coli* and *Salmonella* and their toxins.**[492]

This is not to say that *lactobacillus* do not have a place in the alimentary canal. On the contrary, I believe that they can have a constructive place and serve an important role in the proper balance of the gut. However, *lactobacillus* should not be the predominant specie. Some strains of *Lactobacillus acidophilus* create lactase, which may assist lactose intolerant people. It has been shown to help reduce serum cholesterol and create a wide spectrum anti-microbial activity (antibiotic). Some strains have shown anti-carcinogenic activity against particular cancer cells, especially those found in the esophagus, stomach, colon, prostate, breast and pancreas. It has also been shown to modify and inhibit the growth of

---

[486] Krieg, pg. 1424.

[487] Ibid., pg. 1424.

[488] Ibid., pg. 1424.

[489] Ibid., pg. 1418.

[490] Ibid., pg. 1422.

[491] Gibson, and Macfarlane, pg. 88.

[492] M. F. Bernet, D. Brassart, J. R. Nesser, A. I. Servin, "Adhesion of Human Bifidobacterial Strains to Cultured Human Intestinal Epithelial Cells and Inhibition of Enteropathogen-cell Interactions," *Applied Environmental Microbiology*, 1993; Dec.; 59 (12), pg. 4121-4128.

*Candida Albicans.*[493]   Again I would like to point out that using *lactobacillus* for longer than a few months may be detrimental, especially if it is not replaced with the more natural and more alkaline *bifidobacteria* such as *B. infantis, B. breve*, etc.

Note:   Some doctors have recognized that various disorders have been associated with alkaline-forming bacteria. From this point of view, they have reasoned that the bowel should be strongly acid, for the acid-producing bacteria are effective in destroying the over-alkaline producing bacteria which cause disease. This is all true, but an important point has been missed. The nearly alkaline-producing bacteria of the *Bifidobacterium* species (pH 6.5), are not pathogenic and the bowel does not have to be over-acid to prevent pathogenic bacteria. It is not the more alkaline environment produced by health-producing bacteria that causes infections. It is the overall weakened state of the bowel and its impaired immune function that allows *any* infection to develop. This weakness is initially a direct result of mineral deficiency which has created an over-acid environment. When certain pathogenic bacteria begin to thrive in this depleted environment, the pH then becomes overly alkaline due to the build-up of waste products of those bacteria. *Either* extreme pH condition is a sign of disease. Infections of any type are more likely to occur in a bowel that has first become deficient as a result of an overly acid environment.

A similar reasoning has occurred with theories on urinary infections. There is an alkaline-producing bacteria that can cause urinary infections - hot burning urine. Using cranberry juice or distilled vinegar will kill off this bacteria usually within three days. Some doctors reason, that the urine should be acid to prevent alkaline pathogens. However, nothing could be further from the truth. When we have a full reserve of alkaline producing electrolytes and we eat alkaline-forming foods, it is natural, soothing and healthful for our urine to be alkaline, for it is simply removing the excess electrolytes from the body. This is a sign of good health and urinary infections are less likely to occur during this normal activity. However, when the urine is consistently acid, because we are deficient in electrolytes, we are more vulnerable to infections from any pathogens, including alkaline-producing ones.

Friendly intestinal bacteria are essential to good health. **Most raw foods, especially those with chlorophyll, feed the friendly bacteria. Cooked and processed foods feed the harmful bacteria. Undigested foods also feed pathogenic bacteria**. The whole body must be in balance in order to have good health. When the bowel is out of balance, it becomes essential to take supplements of friendly

---

[493] From the files of Dr. Khem Shahani with the University of Nebraska.

bacteria.  It is critical, especially after the use of antibiotics.  The friendly
bacteria are needed to:

* reduce cholesterol in the blood
* produce certain digestive enzymes necessary to digest proteins,
  carbohydrates and fats
* help control the pH factor (acid-alkaline levels) in the intestines
* reduce unhealthy bacteria in the intestinal tract
* reduce high blood pressure
* detoxify poisonous material in the diet
* strengthen the immune system
* assist in elimination of ailments such as colon irritation,
  constipation, diarrhea, acne and liver and kidney problems
* manufacture and assimilate B-complex (which includes niacin,
  biotin, folic acid, riboflavin, and B-12)
* produce natural anti-bacterial agents (antibiotics) which inhibit 23
  known pathogens
* produce cancer-suppressing or tumor-suppressing compounds
* detoxify hazardous chemicals added to foods, such as nitrates
* increase calcium assimilation
* help eliminate bad breath and gas
* retard yeast infections
* help alleviate anxiety and stress.
* retard proliferation of vaginitis, flu and herpes

# The Most Dangerous Enemies of the Friendly Bacteria, In Order of Importance

* drugs - especially antibiotics, since one dose can
  eliminate it all [494]
* alcohol - it destroys enzymes and friendly bacteria, not
  to mention actual cells (particularly brain cells)
* cooked meat - it feeds the bacillus E. coli (harmful
  bacteria) which in turn destroys the good bacteria
* bread - especially white flour or any wheat bread that
  was baked in an oven (wheat is only good in its raw,
  sprouted state; then it's excellent)
* sugar - yes, that includes most breakfast cereals,
  chocolate, cakes, pies, cookies, ice cream, pop, etc.
* fried foods - *e.g.* potato chips, French fries, anything fried in oil

---

[494] Yamada, pg. 2063.

* acid-forming foods, when overused (these include all processed/cooked foods - all foods not in the natural state in which mother nature made them.

# More About *acidophilus*

We have all heard so many good reports about *Lactobacillus acidophilus*, but as I have said, I think it is not beneficial except under certain conditions. The more I learn about it the more I tend to think that it can do more harm than good. A man called the other day and gave me a list of all the problems he has acquired in the last two years, and they all pertained to the digestive tract. They included constipation, diverticulitis, fatigue, depression, and many other conditions which he summarized as "falling apart". I began asking questions to try to find out what he had changed in his life. After all, he was in his 60's and had pretty good health up until one year ago. Why the sudden problems? The only thing he had done differently was that two years previous to our phone conversation, he began to take *acidolphilus*. When he said this, I remembered other people making similar statements. This was another confirmation pertaining to what I was learning about *acidophilus*.

Here are a few facts I have found in medical and microbiology textbooks:

*Lactobacillus acidophilus* **requires a great deal of nutrition to survive**. It may actually compete with us in terms of the food we eat. After all, when you stop to think that 25 to 35% of the fecal matter is composed of bacteria, it becomes plain that there is a great deal of substance that must be fed. It is hungry stuff. It needs folic acid, niacin, and riboflavin, to name a few of the vitamins. It uses calcium, and who doesn't have calcium problems these days? It also uses amino acids.[495]

*Lactobacillus acidophilus* creates a pH of 4.5. That's too acid! Its optimal growth pH range is between 5.5 - 6.2. Any intestinal fluids above that pH, begin to weaken and kill *acidophilus*.

### The pH that *acidophilus* Creates, Presents Four Serious Problems for our Bodies.

1. Enzymes of the small intestine cannot efficiently function at the pH that *acidophilus*

---

[495] Krieg, pg. 1212.

creates and which it must live in if it is to survive.

2. The acids that *acidolphilus* produces, are too acid for our bodies and force the body to use more organic sodium and calcium to buffer these acids.[496] These minerals are the electrolytes. Those who have electrolyte problems are likely to have bacterial problems. The more *acidolphilus* we take, the harder our bodies must work to compensate for the increased acids. As already explained, the optimum pH range for most of the digestive enzymes in the bowel is about 7.5.

3. For the body to have to deal with this kind of situation causes an energy drain as well as a mineral loss.

4. Unnecessary fermentation may occur because the alkaline fluids from the Crypts of Lieberkuhn will be killing off the *acidophilus*.[497]

The reason that *acidolphilus* does not thrive in the human gut, is because sodium bicarbonates and electrolytes are secreted by the pancreas, gall bladder, and also secreted by the crypts of Lieberkuhn, to reduce the intestinal acidity that acid-producing bacteria manufacture. This alkalinity kills off the *acidolphilus*. If we have lost our alkaline minerals to a certain level, then *acidolphilus* is not being controlled by our alkaline reserve and we could develop more serious acid conditions of the bowel and potential acidosis. It makes sense that this could this trigger more serious bowel diseases to develop.

## A Quantum Leap

Even though I recommended a very useful probiotic formula for many years, I always kept looking for improvements. Maybe I enjoy watching the little critters through my microscope; I continued

---

[496] Ibid., pg. 1210.

[497] The Crypts of Lieberkuhn secrete alkaline fluids of 7.8 to 8.6, all the way from the duodenum to the anus. It does this to maintain healthy bowel pH. In these fluids are the electrolyte or alkaline minerals. Guyton, Hall, pg. 830.

experimenting with other bacteria formulas. In conjunction with Khem Shahani, Ph.D., of the University of Nebraska, I have subsequently developed an even more refined formula, which includes *Bacillus subtilis*, the most beneficial strains of *Bifidobacteria*, the proper percentage of the best *acidophilus*, plus the new addition of bacteria cultured from human colostrum: *Bifidobacterium infantis*. I suspect that this new bacteria may very well be the foundational bacteria of the human race. It certainly is designed and capable to 'kick start' the human digestive system from 'scratch.' This new formula again represents a quantum leap forward in terms of its overall effectiveness and in terms of its regenerative as well as protective applications.

# The Perfect Bacteria

So what is the perfect bacteria? The perfect bacteria may well be a combination of the natural bacteria given to us by healthy mothers (B. infantis), and the bacteria found on fruits and vegetables that have not been sprayed or irradiated and are fresh and raw. For this is what is natural for man, if man lived by the natural laws of his own species. However, for most people this is not practical. For those who cannot eat fresh, raw, unwashed fruits and vegetables may need to take bacteria products. I have been researching this subject for quite some time. At this period in time, the better bacteria seem to be those which will support the body to maintain a pH between 6.5 - 7.5, the ideal for digestive enzyme function. These bacteria should contribute nutritionally, rather than deplete the body.

Perhaps the best bacteria for the colon are *Bifidobacteria*. They can function between 4.5 - 8.5 pH. These bacteria create amino acids and other nutritional products including the B vitamins.[498]

It is evident that a healthy body needs several kinds of bacteria. **I believe that the environment in our digestive tract has the ability to change bacteria into various forms**. It may be necessary to use implants of the correct bacteria for a period of several months to be sure that the correct bacteria is holding, but there comes a time to stop putting in so much bacteria and allow the body to adjust it to the way it knows best. Let us hope that our bowels are in a condition in which they can successfully adjust the ingredients of bowel substance for optimum health. In my opinion, it is necessary to cleanse our bowels first, in order to effectively adjust intestinal flora.

*Bifidobacterium infantis* and other *bifidobacteria* appear to be the most beneficial.

---

[498] Krieg, pg. 1418 - 1426.

The bacteria found in the general use probiotic formula, which I recommend, offer a combination which actually creates amino acids, many vitamins, including vitamin B-12, and even antibiotics. They are critical players on the digestive team which allows us to receive the nutrients we need from our foods. In terms of defense, a good bacterial activity is a major part of our immune system.

## Comparison of *Lactobacillus acidophilus* with an Ideal Probiotic Formula for General Use

| *acidophilus* | An Ideal Probiotic Formula |
|---|---|
| Fragile and unstable in the human gut | Very durable and stable in the gut |
| Unnatural to human species | Natural to human species |
| Imbalances human bowel | Balances human bowel |
| Produces 4.5 pH lactic acid or less | Produces a pH of 6.5 |
| Contributes to serum ammonia levels | Reduces serum ammonia levels |
| Has little effect breaking down carbohydrates | Effective in breaking down carbohydrates |
| Has little effect on *Candida* | Effective against *Candida*, when used with a second probiotic formula specific for eliminating unwanted pathogenic organisms |
| Contributes to bowel irritation | Reduces bowel irritation |
| Improves digestion in upper stomach only | Effectively improves digestion in the small intestine & colon |
| Requires complex nutrition to survive | Manufactures abundant nutrients |
| Originally animal-derived, not natural to humans | Naturally found in healthy breast-fed infants, children, and adults |

# Water Fasting

## The World's Greatest Tool for Removing Toxins and Harmful Emotions

After completing a cleanse program as many times as it takes to remove all mucoid plaque, some cleansers have an interest in exploring water fasting. **Unless working under the care of an experienced health practitioner, we do not recommend water fasting until the body is already strengthened and healed as much as possible.** However, when the body is ready, **water fasting can be one of the greatest tools to make our dreams come true, to eliminate the causes behind cause, to eliminate the sources of sorrow and pain, to strengthen and purify our spirits, and open the flood gates for love to flow through us**. Yet, most find it very difficult, and only the brave and the strong can accomplish it.

Almost all the great spiritual leaders such as Gautama Buddha and His disciples, Jesus and His disciples, all the great Essene adepts, and millions of others who followed high spiritual paths fasted. **Contrary to what many people think, I believe they fasted to release toxins from the body, mind, and spirit, not as a test of will**. Legends state that certain groups of the Essenes would not allow anyone to enter their secret sects unless they passed certain stringent tests. There is one written record of a man who had to fast, living only on water for 40 days and 40 nights. He stated that he had originally thought the fast was a test of will and endurance. But he found out that **the fast had so cleared his mind that then and only then, would he be able to comprehend the instruction that was later given**. He admitted that previous to the fast, he had no idea that the fast could improve his mental faculties as it did.

Water fasting is indeed, an incredibly powerful and rapid method to release the sludge, mucus, and toxins from the body's thousands of miles of pipelines, trillions of cells, and all the fluids. **When one is ready and well prepared, there is no physical activity that can bring such rapid relief and balance as water fasting**. And even more important, it can be used to help dig out the negative emotions that ruin so many people's lives.

Water fasting, more rapidly than any other tool, clears the mind and feelings in such a way that we can see far beyond our previous limits. **It increases our awareness, improves our eyesight and hearing**. It even opens us to **levels of understanding and comprehension that had been beyond us before**. It helps to put us in touch with the who we truly are.

If water fasting is so incredibly effective, why, you may ask, has it been so condemned in the Christian and the Western World? For many reasons. **Those who know how to fast properly and practice it, arise to a greater awareness and cannot be controlled and manipulated as easily as the masses**. Potentially, they can become a threat to the dogmas and creeds of world orders, governments, church theocracies, and others who impose their selfish scenarios upon others.

Now when we talk about water fasting, we mean that we do not eat or drink anything except water. Juice fasting is really a juice diet. This is a very beneficial method to detox gradually and build our reserves at the same time. I believe that a juice diet is a powerful way to prepare for a water fast.

It is important to know that there is nothing that works like a water fast. When we stop feeding our bodies with food, juice etc., a metabolic activity takes place that happens only when we are water fasting. Basically, **the body begins to digest everything within that is not a part of a healthy cell structure. It literally eats up the excess proteins, fats, sugars, pathogenic microorganisms and then takes on the weak and dying cells.** There is nothing physical that can work this miracle. However, it must be done properly and with great care.

A few decades ago, when the average person was not filled full with toxins, chemicals, preservatives, pesticides, heavy metals, processed foods, sugar, etc.; when people where stronger and healthier, almost anyone could accomplish a long water fast. But today, the constitutional strength of most people is terribly compromised. They are chuck full of potentially harmful material and not only does this make it more difficult to fast, but for some it can be harmful and dangerous. And yet, even though this is true, it is all the more reason to work towards fasting. We need it more than any other time in history, but we need to do it with great care.

## Situations Where Water Fasting Can Be Dangerous

Heavy metals stored in the body.
Drugs (medicinal and otherwise) stored in the body.
Poisonous chemicals stored in the body.
Having certain diseases such as some cancers, tuberculosis, diabetes.
Having severe liver, kidney, heart disease or some other severe disease.
Having an exceptionally toxic, weak and debilitated body.

Although at least 90% of the people who practice water fasting have no dangerous situation to deal with, the above factors still need to be addressed. People need to be alert to the above toxins and conditions, and do what is needed to proceed with safety in each case. There may be people who are confronted with serious situations because of by-products of modern society. In the past, out of ignorance, many water fasters have been inclined to "tough it out" when difficulties related to the above situations arise. This is *not* recommended!

Does this mean that if we run into difficulty that we should never fast again? No, it does not mean this at all. It means that we need to change course and proceed with intelligence, knowledge, and caution. It means that we really need to get to work on our bodies and minds. We need to learn what to do and do it. We must never allow ourselves to become weak. We must use the necessary tools that will remove these toxins. We must repair any organs that were damaged by these poisons. Once they are removed, we can go back to cleansing or fasting. We should never give up.

Of the list above, heavy metals, and especially lead, are my greatest concern. Lead has a half life of twenty-five years. It can cause the greatest damage. However, if it is already in our bodies, you can be sure that it already has caused damage. How are your liver, kidneys, heart, and bowels? Are they perfect? If not, there is a good chance that lead has already done damage to you. It is better to remove these toxins now, when you have the strength, rather than later, when you don't have the strength and ability required to handle them.

Notice how the older people get, the thinner many become. I believe that it is possible that as many as half of the deaths in America may be related to heavy metals. I don't mean that half the people wouldn't eventually die, but that they may be dying prematurely. Yes, heavy metals are that serious.

## Benefits of Fasting

Eliminate harmful undigested proteins and fats.
Eliminate excessive proteins, fats, sugars, cholesterol, acids.
Strengthen and improve functions of all organs and glands.
Remove harmful negative emotions stored at cell level.
Release congestion in lymph, blood, organs, and cells.
Purify the lungs so that greater amounts of oxygen can enter the system.
Tune and tone all tissues, especially the skin and muscles.
Improve digestion.
Improve all senses - and mental abilities. Expand awareness and inner knowing.

## Guidelines for Water Fasting Safely

Cleanse the bowels first. Do several full intestinal cleansing programs.
Do juice diets for a week or longer.

Take pH test prior to water fasting. Have a full supply of electrolytes before fasting.[499]

Start with short water fasts, such as 36 hours. When you can do this and feel good, then increase the time. For most people there is almost nothing that can go wrong when doing short water fasts. It is the longer ones which require caution.

Drink plenty of water, preferably distilled. Never drink water with chlorine or fluoride in it.

Take enemas once or more a day.

Take coffee enemas when feeling headaches, nausea.

Be outside as much as possible and in the sunshine.[500]

Take bacteria supplements after each enema.

# Water Fasting, Enzyme Therapy and Heavy Metals

Again, the effects of heavy metals are my greatest concern. I experienced them in my own body. After many years of cleansing, mostly the alimentary canal, I finally ran out of mucoid plaque. At that time, my body made it clear that bowel cleansing had come to an end for me. I was excited, for I had never felt so wonderful in all my life. I began to do a few short water fasts with miraculous results. My mind soared like an eagle. My awareness expanded beyond anything I had yet experienced. I looked forward to a 40 day water fast and I gradually prepared myself for this special event. It was about that time that I began to experiment with enzyme therapy.

It happened during a trip I made to Pasadena, California to speak at the National Health Federation. Suddenly, for the first time in many years, I felt unusually tired and my mind was dull. I had to go up to my room and lie down. I felt so weak, that I was afraid that I would not be able to give a good performance at the conference. I gave my talk, and then, I went back to my room and laid down again. When I got back home, I became progressively worse. I did everything I could to figure out what was wrong with me. Over a period of several years, my mind and memory deteriorated. There were three times that I really thought I was at the edge of death. And every time I fasted, my health would get worse. One time I forced myself to water fast for 7 days. That was a serious mistake. It took

---

[499] **See Chapter 2, under "Minerals - Important Key to Health," and Appendix I: How to Do the pH Test.**

[500] I believe that skin cancer from the sun occurs not because of the sun but because of the toxins in the skin. Otherwise, I and many people I know, would be chuck full of skin cancer, yes every inch.

three weeks to recover. However, I would not give up, for I knew that even though I was going through hell, there were deep memories of terrible thoughts and feelings that were in the process of being released through my traumas. Although I studied less, worked less, produced less, I learned more. For I learned from a very deep, spiritual level that all disease is primarily a natural by-product of our own negativity of the past. I also knew that if I persevered, I would get through this and would be far better and healthier as a result. During this time, I still did not know that I was dealing with heavy metals.

Finally, after years of research and experimentation, I determined that my problem was related to lead poisoning. Once in the bloodstream, lead is distributed and deposited in soft tissue and mineralized tissue such as bone. My research revealed that lead is accumulated in the body over a lifetime and normally, is released very slowly. However, when we experience undue physiological or emotional stress, lead may be released from its many hiding places and this can significantly increase the amount of lead in the blood. Even after complete removal of the source of lead exposure. It's removal can take decades. In fact, while the half life of lead in the blood is only 25 days, the half life of lead in bone tissue is 25 years. So, even small amounts, over time, can cause long term problems with lead poisoning.

Apparently, as a result of my water fasting and perhaps, more importantly, the enzymes I was taking, I unlocked old stores of lead deposits that I had **gradually accumulated since childhood**. When I realized that most of my symptoms were related to lead poisoning, I began to research everything I could about methods of extracting lead out of our bodies. I also found that this is a very serious problem in our society and that our government and conventional medical system has covered up this important issue. We have all been exposed to toxic levels of lead, particularly those of us who grew up in the 50's, 60's and 70's, through lead gasoline, paint, the solder used to seal food cans, lead dust from ceramic glazes, lead in the soil and vegetables grown in contaminated soil. That doesn't even include the atmospheric lead from glass manufacturers, printers, smelters and all of the other sources of industrial lead. We've all heard of how bad mercury is and how the American Dental Association has covered up the mercury facts, but I say that the problems associated with lead toxicity are even more serious.

Once I recognized that I was suffering from heavy metal toxicity, I began to experiment with different methods of removing lead, which, by the way, is not an easy thing to do. However, within three days of using a program I developed to detoxify the body of heavy metals, new hope spread throughout my being. I actually awoke one morning feeling good. I began to experience, more and more, days of feeling stronger and more mentally alert. I began gaining weight. My strength gradually came back. I could once again hike up Mt. Shasta. Finally I decided to give fasting another try. I did a 36-hour water fast. I recovered quickly with more energy and mental alertness. My memory began to come back to me. So I did another and then another. The third time, my energy level and alertness went back down. I had uncovered another storehouse of poisonous lead. Immediately I went back on my heavy metal detox program. In a few days I was better, but I found that every time the lead surfaced that my kidneys and liver went haywire.

One day I found that I could not eat fruit without the body becoming incapacitated. A few days later, I could eat all the fruit I wanted. Basically, it has been an up and down battle and that is the way it is when you are eliminating heavy metals from your body. Perseverance in detoxifying and cleansing are the keys to ridding your body of these unwanted toxins. While it has been a long process, I am finally getting rid of the heavy metals in my body. And I am feeling much better. I am actually excited and have no regrets. The years of suffering purified many suppressed emotions and memories, and greatly strengthened me emotionally and spiritually.

In addition to the acute effects of lead poisoning which, in severe cases, can include convulsions, coma and death, there are a number of **long-term effects including increased incidence of cardiovascular disease and cerebrovascular deaths** in those who had been exposed to lead as children.

## Long-Term Lead Poisoning Effects Include

| | | |
|---|---|---|
| Anemia | Anorexia | Anxiety |
| Attention deficits | Bone pain | Chronic fatigue |
| Concentration difficulty | Constipation | Depression |
| Eye problems | Gout | Headaches |
| Hearing problems | High blood pressure | Hyper and hypoactivity |
| Indigestion | Insomnia | Irritability |
| Kidney problems | Lack of appetite | Malaise |
| Memory poor | Metallic taste | Muscle pains |
| Numbness or tingling | Personality changes | Poor coordination |
| in extremities | Poor memory | Reading/learning |
| Reduced IQ | Restlessness | disabilities |
| Symptoms of dementia, Alzheimer's-like | | |

Note: Lead is such a severe toxin, that symptoms may recur over and over and often many chronic conditions are considered irreversible. Nothing is irreversible.

## Severe Acute Toxicity In Children

Paralysis
Attention deficit and reduced IQ
Encephalopathy
Aggressive behavior disorders
Coma and death
Development regression
Convulsions
Hyperactivity
Severe abdominal
Linked to sudden infant death syndrome
Forceful and persistent vomiting
Mental retardation
Diarrhea
Seizure disorders
CNS symptoms (Central Nervous System)
Unusual thirst
Ataxia
Mania
Seizures and coma
Brain abscess, brain tumor
Acute encephalitis, and meningitis

When lead damages such organs as the liver, gallbladder, kidneys, heart, brain, etc., then one can experience specific symptoms related to those organs. I wouldn't be at all surprised to find that many diseases, even cancer, liver disease, heart disease and more, are actually related to heavy metal toxicity.

Cadmium is another heavy metal toxicant, which is commonly found today and can be extremely damaging. Cadmium toxicity may be taken in from exposure to residue or run-off from phosphate fertilizers, exposure to sewage sludge, the burning of fossil fuels, gases released from zinc, lead and copper smelters, the smoking of tobacco, and the breathing of second-hand cigarette smoke. The body's main avenue for intake of cadmium is through inhalation.[501]

---

[501] This information is from the website of the Center for Disease Control's *Agency for Toxic Substances and Disease Registry.* See: http:\\atsdr1.atsdr.cdc.gov:8080\hazdat.html

# Cadmium Is Sometimes a More Serious Toxic Pollutant Than Lead

| | | |
|---|---|---|
| Decreased appetite | Sore joints | Mouth lesions |
| Dry & scaly skin | Loss of hair | Loss of body weight |
| Lung damage | Shortened life span | Hypertension |
| Kidney problems | Sodium retention | Edema |
| Liver problems | Poor zinc metabolism | Zinc deficiencies |
| Low body temperature | Decreased growth | Hemoglobin |
| Depressed immune function | Impotence | problems |
| Anemia | Sugar problems | Poor milk production |
| Poor absorption of iron, copper and manganese | Loss of smell | |

# Teeth

## Mercury - Heavy metal in "Silver" Fillings

I began to investigate silver fillings, properly called amalgam fillings, because after all the cleansing I had done, things still were not right in my body, although my health had improved immensely. **These amalgams should really be called "mercury fillings" because they contain over 50% mercury and only 35% silver**. Symptoms caused by mercury and other metals include many of those indicated for lead and cadmium. Because of mercury amalgam fillings, most people probably have mercury residues which have very negative effects upon their bodies.

The American Dental Association (ADA) and the FDA say that mercury in the mouth is perfectly all right. Nothing could be further from the truth[502] and the fact that they make this statement seems to show a decided lack of concern, responsibility, integrity and love. It is another fact implying a conspiratorial action about our health.

**Mercury is a deadly poison**. It is a medically proven fact that it can damage the brain, and digestive tract, and can be passed into a fetus from the mother.[503] Mercury is one of the most poisonous substances on

---

[502] Dr. Hal Huggins, D.D.S., *It's All in Your Head*, (New York, NY: Avery Press, 1993). For more information you can contact Dr. Huggins office at (719) 522-0566 in Colorado Springs, CO.

the planet. Some claim it's the most lethal. In terms of lethal potential, it even beats out sodium fluoride and chlorine. Please understand that it is an extremely virulent poison. Even in minute concentrations it is very *very* toxic.

A friend of mine, Dr. Gardaphe, DDS, in Tucson, told me why he quit using mercury filings in 1960. He was having dinner with his father-in-law, who was a medical doctor. He saw that the doctor was troubled about something that evening and inquired as to the cause. Here is what the doctor said. "Some friends of mine went out to dinner the other night, and they left their nine-year-old boy alone. While his parents were gone, the boy began to experiment with some mercury that he had taken out of a broken thermometer. He put the mercury into a frying pan to heat it up. The mercury turned into a vapor, the boy breathed the mercury vapor and died instantaneously."

Dr. Gardaphe was shocked. He said to the doctor, "Is mercury that poisonous?" The doctor nodded his head, and said, "Yes". Then Gardaphe said, "I have been putting mercury in people's mouths for years and that can't be doing them any good."

Well, Dr. Gardaphe had the good sense to never use mercury in his work again. The trouble is that mercury in the mouth creates a mercury vapor which is released from the amalgam by enzyme and bacterial action. This gets into our bodies and accumulates so slowly that as disease develops, we cannot trace the cause. Many, many people find their problems disappearing after having their amalgams removed. I have listened to many people with multiple sclerosis claim that within a few months after mercury removal, they were walking again. Some people who could not get rid of their Candidiasis after trying various other treatments without success, did experience improvement after amalgam removal. It is known that these toxic fillings damage the kidneys in test animals, and you can be sure they do plenty of damage in people's kidneys. The mercury fillings are known to severely suppress the immune system and anything can happen after that. Mercury fillings may be a contributing factor to cancer and AIDS, as I have heard a doctor say that **everyone who has AIDS also has mercury amalgams too.**

---

[503] Lars Friberg, Gunnar F. Nordberg and Velimir B. Vouk, *Handbook on the Toxicology of Metals*, (Amsterdam and New York, NY: Elsevier/N. Holland Biomedical Press, 1979), pg. 510-516.

# Dr. Huggins' Experiences

There is no doubt that amalgam fillings are causing many horrible diseases in many people. Here are a few examples of how bad it really can be. The following stories are from Dr. Hal Huggins' book, *It's All In Your Head*.

### Leukemia Gone in a Few Days

"The physician had arrived in our office on a Wednesday, certain that he would die of chronic myelogenous leukemia (CML) in three months. He returned to his home four days later, certain that he would live. Was he qualified to make this decision? Yes, he is a physician.

"What was his dental condition when he came to us for diagnosis and treatment planning? He had a nickel crown and 21 amalgam fillings. Twelve of them showed negative current with one as high as -40. Though he was extremely skeptical until the follow-up CBC (complete blood count), we knew that we had a good chance of helping him."

Continued: "... It was 235,000 white blood cells. It was leukemia. Normal is 5,000-10,000. Within less than 48 hours after amalgam removal his white count was down to 176,000, a drop of nearly 60,000 cells from Thursday afternoon till Saturday morning. That's okay, but the lymph was the big story. Lymphocytes are good fighters against chronic myelogenous leukemia (CML). He was a CML'er. On Thursday he had 1 Percent lymph. The highest he had had since onset of CML was 9 percent and that was due to an intravenous injection of a powerful drug for that purpose. His lymph in the absence of amalgam had skyrocketed to 21 percent. The dignified, terminal MD before me melted into tears. He cried for half an hour. I cried with him."

**I cannot help wondering how many thousands of innocent people including children have died from leukemia due to amalgam fillings.**

### 11 Years Young

"How often does she have seizures like this?" "Every 15 minutes." "How long have they been going on?" "Since October...two months. But we could see it coming on in August." "What happened in August?" "She had two tiny fillings placed. That's why we're here. She's had $8,000 worth of testing at the finest hospital in Denver under one of the best neurologists." "What do they suggest?" "That she be put in an institution and both her mother and I undergo psychotherapy."

"This child couldn't stand by herself. Couldn't walk. She could just barely think. She had been a straight A student and now this eleven-year-old girl would take an average of 90 seconds to answer the simplest addition problems."

"We had 15 minutes between seizures to give anesthetics on both sides, place the rubber dam, get the amalgam out and place new mercury-free fillings. We did it in 14 minutes. Then it hit. She had a violent seizure right in the dental chair. This chair had metal parts. Sharon put her hands on the child's forehead to hold her head in the headrest. Her father sat on her right leg and I sat on the left. Another assistant draped herself across the waist. All of us were thrown up and down like we were on a bucking bronco. We were a combined weight of over 650 pounds and yet we were tossed into the air like rag dolls. I wonder what the American Dental Association would think about this one, I remember thinking."

"On December 25th she woke up. The numbness in her body was gone. Her brain was clear. She got out of bed and walked downstairs by herself! There were no more seizures. The next spring we videotaped her running the 100 yard dash in 14.8 seconds. I later had a chance to hear a reaction to her improvement from the American Dental Association (ADA). Their official comment to a Florida newspaper was, 'We are not impressed.' Later they were reported to say that we faked the videotape."

## How Many Suffer with Amalgam Fillings?

I wonder how many people have seizures, brain disorders, and muscle problems because of amalgam fillings. I wonder how may children suffer because of this.

Dr. Huggins said in his book, "The largest part of our practice involves MS (multiple sclerosis) patients. The next largest is patients with suicidal tendencies followed closely by those suffering fatigue."

But those are not the only diseases that have gone away when the amalgam fillings have been removed. Allergies, arthritis, lupus, chest pains, cardiovascular, immunological, and digestive problems, depression and suicidal tendencies, blood problems, etc. etc. etc.

I suggest we all read Dr. Huggins' book.[504] I also suggest that we all start making phone calls and write letters to dentists and the American

---

[504] Dr. Huggins says one thing in his book, *It's All in Your Head,* with which I disagree. He said something to the effect that he found it difficult to nutritionally balance vegetarians. One day in San Francisco,

Dental Association (ADA), telling them what we think. I suggest we tell them, **"Why chance it? Use something else that isn't a deadly poison."** I think that is reasonable, don't you?

Amalgam fillings should never be put into the mouth. If they are in the mouth they should be removed. If they are going to be removed, then they must not be yanked out by just any dentist. **It is very, very important that they be removed properly, and in the proper sequence by a dentist who has been educated in the correct procedures.** Many people who had their amalgams removed have experienced more health problems because they went to a dentist who did not know these procedures. For more information you can contact Dr. Hal Huggins at (719) 522-0566.

Dr. Hal Huggins has done research on these subjects. You may want to contact them so they can refer you to a good dentist in your area who knows the proper methods. Don't take any chances. Most dentists appear to be like most medical doctors, for they trust in the organizations that seem to care nothing about the people, except about taking their money. However, **when we can find a doctor or dentist who has an open mind, he or she is exceptional, and we should do all we can to support that individual.** "...for the powers of evil seek every means to place obstacles in the path of those who become a force for good." - Cyril Scott, Author of *The Initiate.*

# Root Canals

### The Miracle

Dr. Gardaphe saw me as I walked into his office. He rushed up to me and with an excited expression he said, "Rich, last week I pulled out a root canal from a lady who had lupus. 72 hours later she called me and

---

Hal Huggins and I were sitting together in a microscope class. It was Sunday, just after lunch. All the students had used the microscopes to see their own blood except me, for I have my own microscope and had seen my blood many times. So after lunch, I came back in early to look at my blood. Finally Hal came in and sat next to me. We were both watching my blood on the monitor and Hal says, "That is really good-looking blood." Then he asked, "How long has this blood been on the slide?" I looked at my watch and said, "One hour." Hal responded enthusiastically, "My gosh, that's the best blood I've ever seen. Who's blood is it?" I said, "That's my blood, and it's the blood of a strict vegetarian." He looked at me, stunned. His mouth dropped open. Then he looked again at the blood on the screen and shook his head.

said that all symptoms of lupus were gone." I said, "Get her testimony, I'll put it the book."

A few weeks later Dr. Gardaphe was putting the finishing touches on my root canal removals. After he was through and I was talking to his receptionist, the doctor came in and said, "Come in here, Rich. I want you to meet someone. Rich, meet Faith Snyder. Faith, Rich is writing a book about health and would like to hear your story about your lupus." The doc left the room and as Faith was lying in the dentist chair, I listened to her story.

She had the root canals and many mercury amalgam fillings placed in her mouth 12 -13 years ago. About 2 or 3 years ago things began to go terribly wrong. She developed systemic lupus, and pain arose in her joints, arms, and legs. The last year the pain became so intense that she could hardly get out of bed or walk. She had almost no energy. She had to be in bed more than out of bed. She couldn't open doors or take bottle caps off. She became more and more depressed, and her bright mind faded into a poor memory. She couldn't remember simple things. After talking to Dr. Gardaphe, she began to think that perhaps her problems were related to mercury and root canals. Last October and November, she was too ill to make it into the dentist office. Finally, in December, she started having the amalgams removed. After several fillings had been replaced, she still felt terrible. On January 13th, Dr. Gardaphe removed the root canal. The next morning she got out of bed for the first time in years with very little pain. The next day her mother-in-law called the doc. He said he heard screaming in the background - screams of happiness, of celebration. Most of the pain was gone. Her mind was also responding, her depression was gone, and her memory was returning. Her family rejoiced in gratitude for the miracle.

### At the University of Arizona

I was attending a lecture by Dr. Huggins, D.D.S., M.S., at the University Medical Center in Tucson. That was when I first met Hal. He explained that Dr. Weston Price, Director of Research for the American Dental Association for 14 years, spent 35 years of his professional career researching the systemic diseases of the heart, kidney, uterus, nervous system, and endocrine system, that resulted from toxins seeping out of root-canal-filled teeth. A certain percentage of people are sensitive to toxins that are manufactured within these dead teeth. He stirred up the dental community. Even with his vast experience, education, and thousands of controlled experiments, dentists were resistant to changing their thinking about the root canal procedures that they had been performing for decades. Here are a few of the facts that Dr. Price found that have been suppressed by the ADA.

If he removed root-filled teeth from people suffering from kidney and heart disease, in most cases those people would improve. In an effort to establish a relationship between the tooth and the disease, he inserted the root-filled teeth under the skin of rabbits. Rabbits have a similar immune system to that of humans. In fact, a normal, non-infected human tooth (as removed for orthodontic reasons) can be inserted under the skin of a rabbit for a year with practically no reaction. A thin film will form over it, but microscopically there are no infection cells present.

When a root-filled tooth was implanted under the skin of a rabbit, the rabbit died within less than two days, sometimes within 12 hours. If a very small fragment were used, within two weeks the rabbit would lose more than 20% of its body weight, and die of heart disease if that is what the human donor had, or of kidney disease if that is what the human donor had. To further challenge this observation, he removed the fragment and transferred it to another rabbit. In two weeks he observed a duplicate performance. In one case, he re-implanted the same tooth fragment in 100 rabbits, each, in succession, dying from the same exact disease that the human had had. In most experimental cases he transferred the fragment 30 times.

This is all that I'm going to say about silver fillings and root canals. I suggest that we all investigate.[505]

After the lecture at the medical center, I went upstairs to the medical library to look up Dr. Price's many writings. I checked the computer and lo and behold, everything that he had written seemed to have been pulled from the files. Nothing was there and it most certainly should have been, for after all, Dr. Price was head of the American Dental Association research lab for over 17 years. I also have records from *The Journal of the American Medical Association*, which prove that there had been a great deal of information published about his studies. But I could not find it on the computers. So, while I was there I decided to look up Dr. Koch. There was very little reference to all his works on cancer and other diseases. Then I searched for Dr. Kellogg of The Kellogg Institute. No information could be found. Need I say more?

Well yes, I should say one more thing. From "USA Today", Monday, Dec. 30, 1991: "Health Costs Soaring: Total U.S. health-care spending will rise 11% next year to $817 billion, the Commerce Department predicted Sunday. The growth rate, the same as this year's,

---

[505] Of course, all investigations should be free of cruelty to animals. Contact Dr. Hal Huggins office in Colorado Springs, CO, for more information about the root canals and all the studies done. (719) 522-0566.

will put health spending at 14% of gross national product. The report projects health-care spending will continue to grow 12% to 13% a year for the next five years, putting it at roughly $1.5 trillion by 1997." Sorry, I just had to say it one more time.

# Chapter 15

# THE EXPERIENCE IN TEESHI LUMBO

*When Magellan sailed around the tip of South America, he came to a certain island, anchored his ship, and with some of his men, rowed to shore. They were met by natives and were able to communicate with them. The natives were astounded, and wondered how they had come to the island.. The Captain pointed to the huge ships in the bay and said, "We sailed here in those great ships." The natives, who had good eyesight, looked long and hard, but they could never see those ships. Were those ships beyond the comprehension of the natives, and thus beyond their sight?*

## North Cascades

In August, 1987, White Crow and I hiked about eight miles over a high mountain pass into Teeshi Lumbo Valley of the North Cascades in the State of Washington. This is one of the most secluded and rugged mountain valleys in the continental United States. First we waded through the Chiwawa River. Then we hiked on an old, dilapidated trail which winds up through steep, rugged brush and rocks until it breaks into high, mountain meadows that stretch for miles on end. The first day we hiked until dark, which brought us past some rocky cliffs at the base of a meadow made by an avalanche, where the year before we had seen a bear and her cub. Then we broke into the high mountain meadows, which were filled with heather and blueberries. Here we ate a few peaches, nectarines, and *acidophilus* (a big mistake). This was to be our last meal for six days. The purpose of this trip was to fast, drinking only water.

The next morning we hiked over the pass and down into one of the most scenic mountain spots on Earth. By the time we came to the river in the bottom of the valley, we were feeling the effects of the fast. We had already been living on raw fruits with occasional salads for several months. We began to realize that our bodies were cleansing at a very rapid rate. We had just covered many rugged miles of exceptionally steep terrain, carrying fully-loaded backpacks, since we intended to stay as long as three weeks. The hot sweat rolled down our bodies. The combination of such a clean diet, the acids produced by strenuous exercise, the *acidophilus* we had taken, thinking it would help our fast, and then the water fast, put us into a maximum-cleansing mode which rapidly depleted our electrolytes.

As we set up our tent, we were feeling tired and weak.[506] We then took a plunge into the icy cold river, to wash off the sweat and dust, and to help regain our strength. White Crow had long ago taught me the therapeutic advantages of cold water, and how it could bring strength and healing. We had taken hundreds of icy cold plunges, and I was quite impressed with what Mother Nature can do for us through cold water. This river was indeed cold, as its source was only a few miles upstream and was fed by mighty glaciers. The water was, in fact, glacier-silt water. It was so clouded with silt that we couldn't even see our hands when submerged just inches below the surface. This plunge had marvelous effects on us and we immediately felt much better.

The air was crisp and clean in this valley. There were no other people, no noise, and no pollution or any sign of it. When the sun set, the temperature dropped quickly with a sharp edge to it that bit into our bare skin. That was how we began our water fast.

Three days passed, and we were saved by those cold baths. We both were feeling worse on this fast than on any other fast or cleanse we'd ever taken. We wanted to be rid of all toxins, poisons, the emotions, and anything else that interferes with our connection with the Great Spirit. The cleaner, the more pure we became, the more immaculate we wanted to be. We had developed a driving compulsion to be totally pure. These biblical words kept coming into my mind over and over, "Pluck out all things that are not of the Father", and my responding thoughts were always, "Yes, and what is left?" Not only had we been working on the physical structure, but we had been striving to purify every thought, feeling, appetite, and desire. Much progress had been made, but we had a long way to go and we hoped that a high level of purification would be attained with this fast.

# Angel of Light

The evening of the third day, I had just finished reading the book *The Gospel of Peace of Jesus Christ* by the disciple John.[507] I was deeply

---

[506] Usually on a water fast, we would start feeling good after three or four days. That is why we were willing to go so far into the mountains and fast; we were confident in this fact. We kept thinking that we should start feeling better any day, but it didn't happen like it would have, had we not taken the *acidophilus* bacteria. I did not find out for several years, that it really was the *acidophilus* that was causing most of our weakness during water fasts. This bacteria had a great time fermenting and creating acids inside our bodies. The strenuous hike also created massive lactic acids and water fasting is also an acid-producing experience; thus, we drained ourselves of electrolytes quickly.

[507] Also known as the *Essene Gospel of Peace*. See first chapter.

touched by the wise words in the little book, given to me by a friend. I wondered, did it really happen that way? Were those truly the words of Jesus himself? We crawled into our sleeping bags, hoping that we would sleep until noon of the next day, as our bodies were not feeling very well at all.

My thoughts turned to Barbara, my wife at that time. I let my thoughts drift with her. I soon entered the state between sleeping and waking, and I just let my imagination wander. We were walking through beautiful, landscaped gardens, up a walk-way to a pure, white temple, and we were dressed all in white. We were prepared to enter the temple when an elderly couple approached. I recognized them. They had just been on an ideal cleansing program. Their faces glowed with health, a light shining in their eyes, which were full of gratitude for the cleansing that had helped them so much. As I looked at their beaming faces, my love went forth with great intensity. I went up to them and put my arms around them and these words spoke through me - "Blessed are you for your willingness to purify yourselves." I was filled with a tremendous sense of appreciation for their willingness and efforts to purify themselves.

Tears of joy and love gathered in my eyes and increased, until I felt embarrassed to show them. I turned to Barbara, went to her, and another wave of even more intense love came. We walked to the trees as the love continued to flow through me, this time so powerfully that I awoke from my reverie. Then another wave of even more incredible love flooded through me so powerfully that I knew that I was having another intense Divine experience. I could feel an intense vibration all through my body. I placed my finger on my arms to see if I could feel and understand this powerful and unusual vibration. I realized that my body was simply not pure enough to handle so much power for very long. I sensed that if this vibration continued for a few hours, the body would begin the disintegrate - but, if that meant I could continue being in the presence of this much love - let it be so! As I enjoyed this immeasurable love and happiness, tears continued to pour and dampen my sleeping bag. I did not care if my body disintegrated. I just wanted the feeling to continue forever.

Suddenly, another even more potent wave of love shook my body and with it I heard the loving, sweet words, **"Blessed are you for your willingness to purify yourself; you shall be rewarded openly, if you persevere!"**[508] My eyes flew wide open and to my utter joy I saw right through the tent, where above it hovered a beautiful, glorious Being of intense and brilliant white light. Words cannot describe Her. She was surrounded with an aura of light so bright that I could see only brilliant

---

[508] It would be more than a decade later before I more fully understood what was meant by, "if you persevere..."

light. Instantly I had the desire to see into this light, to see the form of its source. I struggled to see and slowly Her form grew more and more vivid. She had long wavy golden hair which fell below her shoulders and large, bright eyes filled with energizing and potent love, infinite wisdom and knowing. Her Presence was potent, yet the feeling was calm and peaceful. I could clearly sense awesome energy and power - indeed, the eyes of a Master. No mortal's eyes could compare. She floated just a few feet above the tent. Millions of tiny, quarter-inch light rays rippled in various colors - blue, gold, pink, green, violet, purple, aqua, and white - and flowed gently, but intensely, in all directions. I studied those wonderful light rays, trying to take in everything. Truly I did not want to miss anything.

Instantly I was filled with information I had not had a few seconds before. With absolute certainty I understood her meaning. Anyone and everyone who willingly purified themselves - not only physically, but also mentally, emotionally, spiritually, and completely - would receive rewards beyond their fondest dreams. For it is through self-purification that we can become vehicles of immense love and intelligence. Mankind has no idea as to the power of love and what it can do. With enough love, there is no poverty, sickness, no death, no limitation, except what we consciously choose. Enough love solves every problem, every hurt, every limitation. All happiness is a product of love. The more love, the greater the happiness. Enough love dissolves selfishness, greed, hate, fear, limitations and struggle.

I then knew the truth of the biblical words, "only the pure shall see God." Not that I was totally pure — Ha! — not by a long shot. But certainly I had the desire and it was intense and sincere. I also realized that self-purification is a necessary ingredient for entrance into what is called Heaven, for only those may enter therein who have first purified themselves. And those who are willing to do so shall have the help of God's mightiest messengers and, if necessary, legions of angelic beings. All must someday do this and the sooner, the better. This must be accomplished before one can overcome the last enemy, death.[509]

This is one of the great secrets of life and explains why those great intellects - the spiritual leaders, priests, ministers, evangelists, writers, and teachers, etc. who claim that their way is the only way - have failed to win the great goal and achieve the fulfillment of the great work. I do not mean to criticize anyone for their endeavors, for this understanding was not made known in the past, but it is now coming to the attention of those who truly seek the Infinite One. Even though this knowledge has been available in writings for thousands of years, only a few were ready to grasp it; and only

---

[509] Jesus said, "Verily, verily, I say unto you, If a man keep my saying, he shall never see death." *The Holy Bible*, John 8:51.

a few have been strong enough to make use of it, for it is in direct conflict with man's lusts, appetites, and desires. Divine Love offers Divine benefits while man's lusts, desires, and appetites offer only temporal pleasure, well-mixed with pain and suffering.

I listened to Her words and was then allowed to ask questions. My first question: "Were the words written in the *Gospel of Peace of Jesus Christ*, by the disciple John, the actual words of Jesus?" Her answer: "With the exception of a few translation errors, those words are the words of Jesus, and are true."

About then, though I found it difficult to move, I finally managed to jab White Crow in the back with my elbow for I wanted him to see this. He awoke and rolled over. I found I couldn't talk, and he rolled back over on his side. I jabbed him harder, oops, a little too hard right on his back bone and he turned over and said, "Rich! Why did you do that?" I tried to talk, but the words barely came out. "Crow, look above the tent! What do you see?" To his surprise, he saw Her. Blessed were we both. I was really hoping that he would see Her. It is always more enjoyable to share these experiences. She then asked me to include this experience in the next publication of my book. For about 30 minutes more we talked and for those 30 minutes, we were filled with an essence of such love that made all things on earth seem small and insignificant in comparison. The only thing that seemed to matter on this level of existence was that which could assist us in reaching this state of transcendent love and peace, permanently. Later those feelings transformed into the desire to help others.

When our conversation was completed, She said that She would come again. She then began to arise and shine, straight up. As She did, She grew in size. The higher She rose, the larger and brighter She became. By the time She reached the top of the mountain peaks, She appeared to me as being well over a thousand feet tall. Her light lit up the entire valley almost like daytime, except Her light shed a deep golden essence.

It was made crystal clear to me that all the studies and learning we could do amounted to nothing when compared to the need to purify the mind, feelings, habits, and even our bodies, for our physical bodies are the extension of our consciousness. We must remove the filthiness of our consciousness - the greed, judgments, selfishness, hate, and fear. We must replace it with kindness, love, and the desire to give and help life everywhere. Knowledge without purification brings rewards to the human ego, but little for our spiritual selves — our real selves. The beautiful thing is that the very humble, weak, and ignorant, are just as capable as any other person, if they will purify themselves. It is only through purification that one may obtain divine wisdom, love, and power. It is only through purification that one can find entrance to the higher awareness known as Heaven and especially if obtained without passing through death. All these things are possible for mortal man when he purifies. The full power of Christ, the Higher Self, can only function in a pure temple. Through meditation, one can achieve great things, but the full power of Christ would disintegrate an impure body. Those millions — no, billions — of people, expecting to find heaven upon death, are in for a rude awakening. Jesus said, "Ye must be perfect before you enter the kingdom of heaven." Contrary to popular Christian belief, He meant exactly what He said, and the key to perfection is purification. For purification allows the Divine love, wisdom and power to act through us. It becomes the doer, we become the observer. For, by ourselves, we are nothing. We cannot even beat our own hearts.

Obtaining perfection is not brought forth by jamming our brains full of more human concepts, opinions, and knowledge, or by forming more limited beliefs. The key is removing the obstacles of human thought and emotion, and allowing Divinity, which is love, wisdom and intelligence to flow through us. Prayer, meditation, uttering mantras, cranking prayer wheels, staring at walls, going to church, and reading books are futile and impractical, unless they help eliminate our human opinions and beliefs, and purify our thoughts, feelings, and bodies. For obtaining, experiencing, or realizing that which is called heaven, cannot occur from human egoic consciousness, but only by accepting or allowing Divine consciousness to experience itself through us. It is a gift called grace. It happens only when we deserve it by becoming a pure instrument or vehicle for it to use. "Thy will be done" can only be achieved when we are no longer victims of habits, opinions, beliefs, judgments, hates, resentments, and fears. Only after we have cleared away this human created filth and become non-judgmental, non-opinionated, forgiving channels of Divine Love are we capable of living, "Thy will be done."

There are those who now walk physically on Earth and have become "heaven on Earth". They are masters of themselves, because they conquered the human ego and have become individualized focal points of the oneness of all life - love. They all teach that it is not the "I" (human ego) that accomplishes this exalted state. True freedom is obtained only at the point in which the human ego lets go. The crucifixion is a symbol in which man's ego dies, and then the Divine or Christ takes full control. My Angel friend was once like you and me, but through purification of Her Being, she became One with the One Life, the One Love.

It was made clear to me, that a cleanse program is a tool that all may use, regardless of their religious beliefs, to help achieve their greater potential, whether it be to accelerate their spiritual lives, heal their bodies and minds, or just to have more energy. Some will use such a program to heal their disease and pains, some will use it to sharpen their minds, and some will use it to achieve their full potential.

Do not misunderstand this experience in Teeshi Lumbo. It probably did not come about just because we had been physically cleansing our bodies. That was an important step, but even more important than that, was the fact that we had been trying to cleanse the mind and the feelings and consume every human condition that we had ever created since the beginning of our existence - every imperfect thought, feeling, habit, and negative experience of the past. It may also have been because we have an intense desire to know the truth, to be free, to help others, and the willingness to do anything and everything that's necessary to unify with all life.

Three more days went by, and it was the sixth day of our fast. We awoke and I felt that a shift had occurred. It no longer felt right to keep on fasting. I expressed my feeling to my white-bird friend, and he expressed his feelings too, "Rich, I wanted to quit on the second day and you talked me out of it. Now I want to keep going with this. I'm not stopping."

"Crow", I said, "it isn't that I want to break the fast. We have gone through the worst part and the best is just ahead, but something deep inside tells me that we must stop for reasons I don't understand. Let's go take a bath and maybe we can get some answer on this." We crawled into the icy river, floated downstream, hiked back up and did it again until we were so cold our bodies started to turn blue; but our energy increased and we could think better. Then we waded out to the island, sat on the sand just where the water met from both sides of the island and meditated. I called to my guide for help.

# My Guide Appears

The atmosphere began to change and a thrill of ecstatic joy penetrated our beings. A violet radiance formed right in front of us just above the swirling water, and the form of our instructor etherically materialized. This was His real self, not a projection and He was letting me know it. He hovered in His royal, majestic beauty, His eyes luminous, knowing, and loving. His love radiated through His voice and He said, "I want you both to know that your fasting has brought you three wonderful benefits. First, you were able to remove certain undesirable etheric accumulations (thought forms). Second, the physical benefits of fasting have purified and strengthened your bodies. And, **third, now We know just how far you are willing to go to purify yourself. That! will be your greatest benefit.**"

As He said this, the twinkle in his eyes made me know that He was serious; and He suggested that we break our fast, eat our mangoes, and be back at the car by the next day. "There is someone We want you to connect with on the way out," He said, then added, "The weather is going to change and you will not want to be here."

Then I asked if the experience we had on the third day of our fast was the surprise He had said we would have. He nodded, yes. And I continued, "She asked me to put that experience in my book. Did I get that right?" For some reason I felt very uneasy about doing it because I thought that I would be terribly criticized for doing so, and I had never intended to put spiritual things in my books.

When I asked the question, He suddenly became very still for about ten seconds, then reanimated Himself with that majesty that only He has, and with his majestic gestures said, "You are authorized." Sometimes I am so slow; it took me two days to get the point, "You are authorized." With a few parting words, saying that He would see us again soon, and with love, a smile, and joy in his incredible eyes, He disappeared.

We hiked out the next day with great difficulty. It was a very steep climb, and in some places the slope was almost vertical. When we were about three-quarters of the way up the mountain, we stopped to rest. Crow took off his pack and balanced it upright on the edge of the trail. It was sitting in a rather precarious position. We plopped into a patch of wild currants and blueberries. Our appetites were screaming. Suddenly, Crow's pack tilted and began to roll down the mountain. I thought, "Oh no, it will take hours to get it back and neither one of us has the energy." Crow quickly stood up and commanded his pack to stop. To my absolute surprise, it did. The slope was about a 70-degree angle. I always wondered how that happened.

We did meet someone on the way out who was deeply interested in the things that we know. The next day the weather changed for the worse, and we both agreed that we were glad to be out of there.

In obedience to the request of Her who came to me, and in the hopes that this story would indeed help and encourage others, I did place this in my book. As anticipated, I was criticized, I received strange letters, several friends completely avoided me, and I saw many weird looks and felt the judgments placed upon me. Several times I was accused of talking to Satan and told that I must be evil. But I also received many letters from grateful individuals whose intuition told them it was true, and who shared how this story gave encouragement when most needed.

So what did this experience do for me? Not only did it give me encouragement to aspire towards greater purification, but it produced an immense desire to love others, to stop judging, accept others as they are, and to be like our Angel friends. So I have dedicated my life and energy to assist life everywhere that I can, to help our Angel friends in bringing love and peace to this world, and to do it without force or violence, but with love. And with this attitude, I found more and more happiness and love flowing through me, and that is what this book is all about. To those who have read this, who believe it, who are encouraged by it, and who seek that ultimate purity: Though we may not have met, you are my brother or sister. We are friends and more, and I pray that you will also be rewarded along your path with experiences of love such as this story represents. *Ish konno say yam.*

# APPENDICES

# HOW TO DO THE pH TEST

## Before Starting Dr. Anderson's Cleanse Program,
### *Please Do a pH Test*

Vegetarians who consume large amounts of bread, pastas and grains are very apt to be too acid to do any rapid cleansing, fasting, or strenuous exercise. Most meat-eaters are even more over-acid. Being over-acid is the same as being electrolyte deficient. Doing a simple pH test is very useful, for it will help us decide if we are healthy enough to safely do the deeper phases of cleansing. However, even if we're slightly over-acid, we can still cleanse slowly by using the mildest phase. If we begin with an over-acid pH, we simply need to remember to continue providing abundant electrolytes (alkalizing organic minerals) for the body to use, since the body's reserves are low at the outset. When choosing an electrolyte supplement, make certain that it has plenty of organic sodium, such as is found in goat milk whey or celery. Make certain it contains natural electrolytes (organic minerals - minerals chelated to plant proteins) from vegetables. Fresh carrot/beet/celery juice, and a homemade vegetable mineral broth are also good sources of alkalizing organic minerals.

The pH test is the most important test to determine if it is safe to cleanse, fast, or perform strenuous exercise now, or whether we must alkalize our bodies first.

**The tools needed** are pH papers, pencil, and paper. I suggest pHydrion from Micro Essential Laboratory - with 4.5 to 8.5 pH range. It is important to have pH paper that can be read in two-tenths increments. (For example: 6.2, 6.4, 6.8 etc. instead of 6, 7, 8, etc.) You may be able to get these pH papers at your local drug store or maybe at the health food store. (At the drug store you can expect to pay about $25.00.) It should be less than half that amount at the health food stores that carry it. When testing, it is important to get the paper very wet with saliva. Spit on it. <u>Do not lick</u> the pH paper. You should read it between 10 and 30 seconds after first getting it wet. For the urine test, the paper can be placed into the mid-stream of urine, or one can fill a container with urine and test it by dipping the paper into the fluid. Use just enough to get a reading. I know one person who uses about a quarter of an inch and his papers last for a very long time. Some people use strips two inches long and that seems to be a waste. It's your choice.

# The pH Test (There are three parts. )

The normal pH in the mouth should be about 6.4 to 6.8. When we abruptly change the saliva pH with an acid lemon, the mouth should react quickly to this extremely acid condition by flushing alkalinity into the mouth. At first it will become very acid from the lemon, but within a few minutes after swallowing the lemon juice, we should have readings of 8 or above. If this does not occur, it indicates a lack of electrolyte minerals in the liver. This is fairly normal in this day and age of diseased America. Our supply of minerals is an important indicator of our health profile.

---

**Part 1:  Saliva**

We do all the pH tests after we have had no juice or food for at least two hours. Before picking up the lemon, before cutting the lemon, or even thinking about the lemon, take a pH reading by wetting a strip of pH paper with saliva, and then holding it up to the color chart which is provided with the papers. Compare the wet paper to the nearest color and, presto! you have the pH reading. Now record it.

**Interpreting Part 1:  Saliva:**

**6. or below** - Possibly in a seriously depleted condition and further testing is necessary. Indicates potentially life-threatening danger, when exercising or fasting.[510]

---

[510] When we exercise we create lactic acid. Though the body can easily remove the lactic acid created by exercise through the lungs, its ability to do so can be inhibited when our bodies are already over-acid due to a lack of buffering minerals. In other words, when our bodies have lost the ability to maintain its normal alkaline pH, the body's metabolic function is decreased. It can't function as quickly nor as effectively as it should. Therefore, under already over-acid conditions, if the body is creating

**6.1 - 6.3** - Indicates depletion, but not dangerous. Further testing needed.

**6.4 - 6.8** - You passed. Now proceed to Parts 2 and 3.

**6.9 or higher** - Something may have interfered with the reading. It may be the thoughts of the lemon, or it may indicate stress or excitement. Wait for about an hour and do the test again. Continued high readings indicate metabolic stress - cleansing is needed. An abundance of electrolyte minerals will **_not_** cause a high reading like this. Readings consistently above 6.9 reveal a serious digestive problem.

---

### Part 2: Saliva with Lemon

Cut and squeeze the juice of 1/2 lemon into 2-4 ounces of water, and drink. Swish in the mouth just a little bit as you drink all of it — no sweeteners. Drink the lemon water only once, at the start of the test. This test has five readings and lasts for six minutes. Check saliva pH two minutes after consuming the lemon water, then every 60 seconds, and record all six readings on paper.

### Interpreting Part 2: Saliva with Lemon

Within six minutes, (regardless of how low the reading was before touching the lemon) if the pH reading reaches **8 or higher**, then you passed the second part of the test and most likely will pass the third part, too. This would mean that **you have ready alkaline reserves in the liver, which is a very good indication that you are in good health**. However, test results could be misleading if your saliva reading _before_ the lemon test was 7 or above. _If this was the case, it is necessary to take the 3<sup>rd</sup> part of the test to see if you pass._

If your saliva reading _before_ the lemon test (Part 1: Saliva) was between 6.1 and 6.8, _and_ you pass this test (Part 2: Saliva with Lemon), then it is safe to do the full cleanse. However, if your readings are on the low side, you should do all in your power to increase your alkaline reserve. Read "Rebuilding the Alkaline Reserve" at the end of this appendix. By following these procedures during the mildest phase, a full alkaline reserve should be obtained before you begin any deeper phases of cleansing.

---

excess acids through exercise or stress, the body may not be capable of getting rid of the excess acids fast enough, and "boom" - the heart is flooded with excess acids and it stops. Many athletes and those who had a weak heart, have died for that reason. Saliva readings below 6.1 indicates this potential.

If readings were 7.5, you have *marginally* passed Part 2, but your electrolyte reserves are not fully charged. *Ideally it should be* **8 or above**.

If readings were **7 - 7.4,** you did not pass the test and **need to work on building up your electrolyte storehouse**. This result indicates that you have ready reserves of alkaline minerals, though not as much as you should. It means that you should stay away from acid-forming foods. It indicates that your body sometimes has to take minerals from body organs, bones, joints, muscles, etc., but not always. This means that you should do only the mildest phase of cleansing. To confirm this reading, it is necessary to take the third part of the test and it is not likely that you will pass it.

If readings are **below 7**, but higher than the reading taken before squeezing the lemon, it would mean that there is some alkaline reserve left, but not much. You must take the third part of the test to confirm your pH condition; and it is not likely that you will pass. **A reading below 7 is an indication that health may be in serious condition; it is a sign that chronic disease is developing**. However, if stress is unusually high, it could cause an uncharacteristically low reading here (in which case, you might pass Part 3); but even so, this level of stress will weaken all bodily functions very quickly. In any case, it is necessary to take the third part of the test.

If readings from Part 2 remain at or below the reading from Part 1 (before swallowing lemon), then this person is in **a seriously depleted condition. This is a sign that chronic or degenerative disease may have already developed**. Fasting, cleansing (other than the mildest phase), and **strenuous exercise should be avoided until the alkalinity is restored**.

---

**Part 3:  Urine - Test A** — *After Consuming Alkaline-Forming Foods*

Urine pH changes quickly. **If taken in the morning, it reveals how our bodies reacted to the food we ate the day before**. To complete this test you need to devote a day to eating only vegetables and their juices. No grains, no fruit, and nothing other than vegetables. The next morning, wet a strip of pH paper in a midstream of your first voiding of urine. Record the results.

**Interpreting Part 3:  Urine - Test A** (the next morning's urine test after eating *alkaline*-forming foods the day before):

**7.0 or above -**  You passed! A pH of 7.0 or above after eating only alkaline-forming foods (vegetables), indicates **your body has a good**

supply of electrolytes and is eliminating the excess through the urine — because it already has what it needs.

**6.5 - 6.9** - Depletion is indicated, but not serious. **Your body is retrieving electrolytes from the alkaline foods and hanging on to them.** However, it is releasing some, as well. You will want to replenish your electrolyte reserve *fully* before cleansing. These results are not bad, but not perfect.

**5.6 - 6.4** - Depletion is more serious. **Acid accumulation is greater than your electrolyte supply.** This means that your body may be digging into other body parts to retrieve electrolytes for normal metabolic function. It is a definite sign that **you are moving towards chronic and degenerative diseases. You must focus on replenishing your electrolyte storehouse before beginning a cleanse.**

**5.5 or below** - This indicates extreme depletion of electrolytes. **Some type of chronic or degenerative disease has probably already developed.** It is unlikely that you have passed the other tests. **You should not do any kind of cleansing beyond the very mildest phase. You should be eating only vegetables, vegetable juices, taking electrolyte supplements and doing all in your power to eliminate stress.**

---

## An Alternate Urine Test - Urine Test B

Following is another test that can be done, *but I do not recommend it* simply because it could be harmful for people who have extreme electrolyte depletion. The main reason that I am including this test is so that you can better understand how these pH tests work. There was a time when I recommended this test, but I found that we didn't need it and that for some people, it brought them to a lower pH level, and *that* they did *not* need. Here is the test, you may use it if you feel that your electrolytes are not too depleted.

**Part 3: Urine - Test B —** *After Consuming Acid-Forming Foods*
As noted in Test A, urine pH changes quickly. It reveals how our bodies reacted to the food we ate the day before. Choose a day when you can eat only acid-forming foods. (A list of acid foods is available following the Appendices. See Chart 1.) People who eat meat will have no problems choosing acid foods. Vegetarians will have to work at it a bit. Now, after eating only acid-forming foods for the entire day, the urine reading the following morning is very revealing. The very first voiding in the morning is the time to take this reading.

**Interpreting Part 3: Urine - Test B** (the next morning's urine test after eating *acid*-forming foods the day before): (Urine will reflect the excess acids taken in the night before, *if* the body has enough alkaline reserves to remove the acids via the urine.)

**7.5 or above** - Body has no alkaline minerals to draw upon. **This is serious. It is a sign that your life is in danger. The body has lost control and at any moment a coma could develop.** The liver may have lost its ability to convert ammonia into urea or the kidneys are forced to secret ammonia directly into the blood.[511] This is a state of alkalosis which is caused because of too much acid in the body, and normal metabolic function is failing.[512] Both conditions are serious and the odor of ammonia may be noticeable in the urine, which is proof that one of these conditions is present. Action should be taken immediately. **No strenuous exercise and no cleansing or fasting should be done.** Diet needs to be changed quickly and emotional stress must be solved.[513]

**6.8 - 7.4** - Serious depletion of alkaline minerals is indicated. This means that the body is unable to handle acids effectively and either the liver or kidneys are operating in an emergency mode. Fasting is prohibited, but doing the beginning phase (two meals per day) or the alternate beginning phase (2 1/2 meals per day) is OK, but not the final phase (no meals) or the intermediate phase (one meal per day). Check saliva pH before exercising strenuously. Health may be in a detrimental condition. Work on increasing alkaline-forming foods and decrease acid-forming foods. Light exercise is beneficial, but do not run or exercise vigorously unless saliva reading is above 6.1.

**6.2 - 6.7** - Depletion is indicated, but not dangerous, unless saliva pH is 6.1 or below. If the pH reading during Part 1: Saliva was 6.1 or higher and during Part 2: Saliva with Lemon was 7 or higher, it is OK to cleanse; but it is necessary to take an alkalizing supplement, or drink mineral broth and/or carrot/celery juice while on an ideal cleanse program. Water fasting and strenuous exercise is not advised. If the test readings were below 7 during the lemon test, it is not advisable to do the final phase, or the intermediate phase, or even the gentle phase until readings improve. The mildest phase is the only cleansing phase that should be used. This person should be on a crash program to bring the alkaline reserve back into balance.

---

[511] Guyton, pg. 837.

[512] Guyton, pg. 447.

[513] **See the end of this Appendix under "Rebuilding the Alkaline Reserve".**

**4.5 - 6.1** - Body is removing acids quickly and efficiently. No acids are being stored. There are plenty of electrolyte minerals. This is a good sign.

**Note**: For those with high urine pH the day after eating acid foods. After consistently eating alkaline-forming foods to bring the alkaline reserve back into balance, the urine pH will drop to about 5.5 pH. This means that the body finally has enough electrolytes to remove the acids it could not remove before. Once it removes the acids, it will then begin to store electrolytes and build a reserve. Then the urine pH will begin to rise. When it reaches 7.5, the full alkaline reserve has been reached. This may take several weeks to several months.

For the vegan vegetarian, a 6.0 or below = Passed the test.[514]
For the meat-eater, a 5.5 or below = Passed the test.

---

# Summary of pH Tests

**Indicators of possible serious mineral depletion and poor health regardless of how one feels are:**

1. Saliva pH between meals is below 6.1.
2. Saliva with Lemon test does not reveal a pH above 7.
3. After eating 100% alkaline-forming foods, the next morning's pH is below 7.0.
4. After eating 100% acid-forming foods, the next morning's pH is above 6.8

**Signs of good health - a full reserve of alkaline minerals are:**

1. Saliva pH between meals is 6.4 - 6.8.
2. Lemon test reveals 7.5 or above.
3. After eating alkaline-forming foods the next morning's urine pH is 7.5 or above.
4. After eating acid-forming foods, the next morning's urine pH is 6 or below.

**Explanation:** Urine can only be acid if alkaline minerals are available to combine with the acids and remove the acids through the kidneys. When a

---

[514] The reason for the difference here is that vegan vegetarians will have to eat grains to get an acid urine, and grains are not nearly as acid-forming as meat and dairy products. Therefore they will not be able to have such an acid urine.

person hasn't enough alkaline minerals to get rid of the acids, then the body will dilute the acids with liquid, mainly lymph, and store it in body tissue or gradually remove them via the skin and intestines. Otherwise, kidney damage may occur and many other things might be damaged by the acids before reaching the kidneys.

When we eat an acid meal for dinner, the next morning our urine pH should be about 4.5 to 6, depending upon how acid the meal was and how much of it was eaten. What we had for lunch could also affect the next morning's reading. If the body cannot obtain a low urine pH after acid meals the night before, it is because the body does not have any alkaline minerals to use to get rid of the acids. That means **the body may be stealing minerals from other parts of the body just to stay alive**. People in this category often gain weight, because the body is diluting the acids with lymph and storing them, or they may loose weight and often suffer noticeable digestive disorders. This does not mean a healthy-looking person is free of these conditions. Such persons could be depleting their bones of calcium, their joints, stomach, liver, bile and muscles of sodium, etc. even faster than either an obese or thin person, because they are unable to store acids in lymph or remove the acids out of the skin or bowel.

If the morning urine pH readings after an acid meal are above a 7, then this is the worst situation of all. It means that this person has no alkaline reserve left. It indicates that the body is rapidly extracting minerals from organs and tissues, further depleting the system; and the kidneys are producing ammonia to alkalize the body just to keep it alive. Ammonia is extremely toxic and is the last resort before a coma. People with these figures usually end up in the hospital and have serious chronic, and possibly degenerative, diseases.

**These people can feel sick when trying to alkalize their bodies.** They must take it more slowly and not try to alkalize too quickly. One exception: if they have AIDS, cancer, or some other degenerative disease, then they don't have time to alkalize gradually. They must act without delay, even though they will probably experience cleansing reactions. I recommend that these people find a doctor who understands the material in this book, and follow his or her advice. In any case, starting with the mildest phase (two and 1/2 meals per day) immediately is recommended. Drinking plenty of carrot/celery juice and taking an alkalizing supplement, as well as freshly made vegetable mineral broth, is required in these cases while using the mildest phase.

All those who did not pass the pH test, whether ill or not, should stop eating acid-forming foods, alkalize their bodies by eating mostly fruits and vegetables, and may start cleansing with the alternate beginning (mildest) phase. After alkalizing and passing these tests, then it is safe to cleanse more deeply.

# Miscellaneous Factors
# That Can Influence pH

- Kidneys help control pH. Kidney problems can cause a pH problem.
- Breathing affects pH. Habitual shallow breathing can cause acidosis and may indicate a problem with the medulla.[515]
- High altitude can cause a person to breathe at a faster rate, thereby increasing alkalinity.
- Lung damage can inhibit acids from being removed through the lungs.
- Stressful emotions create acids and cause increased acidity.[516]
- Parasite infections, fungal overgrowths, yeast infections, and bacterial overgrowths can create enough acidity to prevent a balanced pH.

# Rebuilding the Alkaline Reserve

The more alkaline-forming foods we eat[517], the faster we can obtain the needed electrolytes, provided the foods are organically grown and contain adequate minerals. The foods you eat must be organically grown. **Commercially grown foods, such as those available in most supermarkets, are mineral deficient**. Organically grown vegetable juice, especially carrot and celery juice, are very high in electrolytes. Electrolyte supplements containing dehydrated beet, celery, and carrot juices are excellent, especially if they contain goat milk whey. **Never use cow whey for any reason. It is mucus forming and toxic**. Drinking freshly made vegetable broth (with no table salt) is a very good way to build electrolyte reserves.

---

[515] Guyton, pg. 448.

[516] Guyton, pg. 448.

[517] **See Chart One, following the Appendices for a listing of alkaline-forming foods.**

# ESSENTIAL ELEMENTS FOR EFFECTIVE CLEANSING AND REBUILDING

## Critical Ingredients for Effective Cleansing*

### 1. Essential Herbs to Soften and Break Up Mucoid Plaque

Barberry Bark
Cascara Sagrada Bark
Fennel Seed
Ginger Root
Golden Seal Root
Lobelia Leaf
Myrrh Gum
Peppermint Leaf
Plantain Leaf
Red Raspberry Leaf
Turkey Rhubarb Root
Sheep Sorrel Leaf

---

*
  Note: DO NOT try to prepare your own herbs, using equal parts of the ingredients listed. Proper proportions of each ingredient are essential for each formula's effectiveness.

## 2. Essential Ingredients to Strengthen the Body While Cleansing, and Enhance the Action of the First Herbal Mix. (Both Are Needed For the Removal of Mucoid Plaque.)

Alfalfa Leaf
Dandelion Root
Atlantic Kelp
Rose Hips
Shavegrass
Yellow Dock Root
Chickweed Leaf
Hawthorne Berry
Irish Moss
Licorice Root
Marshmallow Root
Cellulase
Amylase

## 3. A Neutral Absorbing Agent

Hydrated Bentonite Clay - Extra Thick
Distilled Water

## 4. A Fibrous Bulking Agent

100% pure Psyllium Husks Powder - ground to 40 mesh for maximum effectiveness

## 5. A General Use (More Alkaline-forming) Probiotic Mix
### (Should Contain at Least These Items, and May Contain More)

*Bifidobacterium infantis*
*Bifidobacterium bifidum*
*Lactobacillus acidophilus*
*Lactobacillus casei*
*Lactobacillus plantarum*

## 6. pH Papers

5.5 to 8.0
(in increments of two tenths)

# Critical Ingredients for Rebuilding Vital Organs

All herbs should be wild-crafted or organically grown and should be harvested by a reliable, experienced herbalist. Most herbs are not, and it *does* make a significant difference.

## Liver Detox and Strengthen

Artichoke Leaf
Dandelion Root
Barberry Bark
Buplelurum
Oregon Grape Root
Milk Thistle Extract
Burdock Root
Black Walnut Hulls
Mandrake Root
Wild Yam Root
Milk Thistle Seed
Fennel Seed
Stillingia Root

## Rapid and Deep Liver Detox

Dandelion Root Extract
Milk Thistle Extract
Burdock Root Extract
Licorice Root Extract
American Ginseng Root
Burdock Root
Rhubarb Root
L-Cysteine
L-Methionine
L-Carnitine
L-Taurine
L-Glutamine
L-Arginine
Lipoic Acid
Glutathione
Choline (bitartrate)
Inositol
Magnesium citrate
Vitamin B-6
Stillingia Root
Zinc L-Monomethione
Folic Acid
Chromium
Selenium
(L-Selenomethionine)
Vitamin B-12
(Cyanocobalamin)

# Antioxidant Protection

We need a wide spectrum antioxidant formula. Many antioxidants support and feed each other. Formulas with only a half dozen antioxidants are, in my opinion, ineffective and a waste of money. The finest antioxidant formula should include major liver support elements. For taking care of the liver is essential for long term health.

Milk Thistle Extract (Silymarin standardized 80%)
Curcumin
Ginkgo Biloba Extract (24% ginkgo flavone glycoside)
Grape Seed Extract
Pine Bark Extract
Vitamin A (Beta Carotene from Dunaliella Salina)

Vitamin C (Ascorbic Acid from Ascorbyl
  Palmitate and beet sugar)
Vitamin E (Natural d-alpha tocopheryl succinate
Bioflavonoids (Vitamin P)
  Quercitin
  Hesperidin
  Rutin
  Lemon Bioflavonoids
Lipoic acid
Vitamin B-6
Co-Enzyme Q-10
Zinc L-Monomethione
Chromium (Amino acid chelate)
Selenium (L-Selenomethionine)
L-Cysteine, not NAC
Glutathione

# Kidneys - Detox and Strengthen

Gravel Root
Juniper Berries
Uva Ursi Leaf
Burdock Root
Hydrangea Root
Parsley Root
Marshmallow Root
Ginger Root
Lobelia Leaf

# A Bowel Preparation to Renew the Bowel Wall, Derived From Totally Natural Sources

Quercitin
Rutin
Lemon Bioflavonoid
L-Glutamine
L-Cysteine
L-Methionine
L-Glycine
L-Arginine
Glutathione
Vitamin A
Vitamin E
Selenium
Grape Seed Extract
Comfrey Root
Mullein Leaf
Golden Seal Root
Vitamin C
Vitamin B6
N-acetyl
L-glucosamine
Silica (young shavegrass extract)
Pantothenic Acid
Fructooligosaccharides
Zinc (Zinc L-Monomethione)

# An Herbal Mix for Building the Bowel, Complementary to the First Bowel Preparation

Marshmallow Root
White Oak Root Bark
Ginger Root
Chickweed Leaf
Red Raspberry leaf
Slippery Elm Bark
Kelp Leaf
Wakame
Apple Pectin
Bifidus
Goat whey
L-glutamine
Red Beet Root Juice Crystals

L-Glutamic Acid
L-Lysine

## Nutrients for the Brain

Osha Root
Ginkgo Biloba
Gotu Kola Nut
Plantain Leaf
Calamus Rhizomes
Schizandra Berries
Kelp Leaf
Bay Berry
Blessed Thistle Seed
Scullcap
Dong Quai Root
American Ginseng Root
Lobelia Leaf
L-Glutamine

## Support for the Eyes

Bay Berry Bark
Bilberry Fruit
Bilberry Fruit Extract
Cayenne Pepper
Eyebright Leaf
Eyebright Leaf Extract
Fennel Seed
Ginger Root
Golden Seal Root
Juniper Berries
Lobelia Leaf
Passion Flower
Red Raspberry Leaf
Rosemary Leaf

# Cayenne Pepper

90 Heat Units (HU) - extra potency

# Parasites

Use a *concentrated* **citrus seed extract** for most protozoa. What is found in most health food stores has been diluted.

Green Black Walnut Hulls tincture is used for parasites in blood and other parts of the body. Most black walnut tinctures are ineffective because they were not prepared properly and are weak.

### For Removing Roundworms

Green Black Walnut Hulls
Wormwood (Artemisia annua)
Cloves
Gentian Root
Ginger
Mandrake Root

### For Removing Flatworms Such as Tapes and Flukes

Male Fern
Pumpkin Seeds
Pink Root
Wood Betony
Camomile
Senna

# Bacteria Formulas

A more alkaline-forming bacteria formula sustains a healthy bowel environment.

### Probiotic for Cleansing and General Use
(critical ingredients, may include more)

*Bifidobacterium infantis*
*Bifidobacterium bifidum*
*Bifidobacterium longum*
*Lactobacillus acidophilus*
*Lactobacillus plantarum*
*Lactobacillus casei*

A more acid bacteria formula is more effective in removing pathogenic microorganisms, but is not healthy for the bowel on a long term basis. Enzymes in a formula like this can also attack bacteria and help break down mucus. Herbs for the immune system also help combat microorganisms and are highly effective against colds and sore throats. I have seen sore throats disappear in minutes after sucking on this bacteria formula. It depends, however, upon what is causing the sore throat.

### Probiotic Mix for Removal of Pathogenic Organisms

*L. acidophilus*
*S. faecium*
*L. casei*
*L. salivarius*
*L. plantarum*
*L. bulgaricus*
Protease
Amylase
Lipase
Cellulase
Echinacea angustifolia root extract
Astragalus root extract

# Notes for Hypersensitive Persons

## Preliminary Tests

For those who are extremely sensitive to foods, herbs, and practically everything else, who may be very weak, very ill, very old, or are just plain nervous about cleansing or trying new herbs, it would be good to do a few tests before using any herbs. For example:

1. Try only half (1/2) of a capsule or tablet of an herbal formula, one at a time. Wait a few minutes and see how you feel. The next time try one (1) and see. Then gradually increase. Do the same with any herb unfamiliar to you.

2. When you make your first shake, try it with only half (1/2) teaspoon of psyllium and no bentonite (with the normal 4 oz. juice and 8 oz. water). The next one use both psyllium and bentonite, but both in tiny portions.

3. Have only one or two (2) shakes per day (as per the alternate beginning phase), increasing portions gradually until you're up to normal.

Most people who ordinarily experience problems with various herbs, foods, etc., can adapt to new herbal formulas easily, if they start out very slowly with small quantities and gradually increase.

# Healthful Hints for Hypersensitive Persons

- Increase at your own speed. All of the herbs are very natural, gentle, and safe, but you'll have more confidence if you increase slowly.
- Be sure to remember that one of the herbal formulas has some laxative effects and the bentonite and psyllium have the opposite. So balance everything according to your own body needs.
- The intelligent use of the herbal formula with laxative properties and the bentonite control the consistency of the stool. It should be loose but not runny.
- Use the beginning phases for a few weeks, before going into the deeper phases.
- If your stomach is sensitive to the herbs, you can separate them by five minutes. That is, take one (1) of each, wait 5 minutes, then take one (1) of each again. Wait 5 minutes and repeat until you've taken the full amount.
- Ginger/fennel tea will help settle the stomach.
- If you are allergic to psyllium, use equal parts of psyllium husk powder, corn silk, and guar gum, or try my psyllium substitute formula.
- If the stomach is sensitive to cayenne, take it with meals only. Don't use it on the final phase.
- If you have never or rarely taken probiotic supplements before, begin taking the general use formula three to five days before starting to cleanse. Suggested intake: one capsule per day for the first three days; then two capsules per day on the fourth and fifth days.
- Continue taking the proper probiotics during and after the cleanse. Some people need to take large dosages for several months.
- People with a history of constipation should take a minimum of two probiotic capsules a day while cleansing. (Provided each capsule contains at least 2 billion bacteria.)
- People with a history of yeast problems, such as Candidiasis, should take one probiotic capsule approximately one-half hour after each set of herbs, one-half hour after each meal and two capsules at least one hour before bedtime.

**Note:** Whatever affects a part, affects the whole.

# HOW TO TAKE ENEMAS AND IMPLANTS

*Whatever affects a part, affects the whole.*

-Anonymous

## First Recorded Enema in History

"Think not that it is sufficient that the angel of water embrace you outwards only. I tell you truly, **the uncleanness within is greater by much than the uncleanness without**. And he who cleanses himself without, but within remains unclean, is like unto tombs that outwards are painted fair, but are within full of all manner of horrible uncleanness and abominations."

"Seek, therefore, a large trailing gourd, having a stalk the length of a man; take out its inwards and fill it with water from the river which the sun has warmed. Hang it upon a branch of a tree, and kneel upon the ground before the angel of water, and suffer the end of the stalk of the trailing gourd to enter your hinder parts, that the water may flow through all your bowels. Afterwards rest kneeling on the ground before the angel of water that he will free your body from every uncleanness and disease. Then let the water run out from your body, that it may carry away from within all the unclean and evil-smelling things of Satan. And you shall see with your eyes and smell with your nose all the abominations and uncleanness which defiled the temple of your body; even all the sins which abode in your body, tormenting you with all manner of pains." (*Gospel of Peace of Jesus Christ* by the Disciple John - reprinted as *The Essene Gospel of Peace*, translated by Edmond Bordeaux Szekely)

Here we have a striking description of taking an enema, as suggested by the Great Master Himself. Whether one believes these words as coming from Him or not, it is still great wisdom; and if we practiced this, we would indeed agree that it is wisdom to take enemas when we need them.   If we do, we will truly see the horrible abominations and uncleanliness which are making our bodies sick and causing disease.[518]

Let's learn to appreciate and enjoy enemas.   Nothing short of Divine Intervention (also known as miracles) **can come to our rescue more quickly to relieve us of pressure, headaches, constipation, various pains, gas, and massive accumulations of toxic mucus, pus, and poisonous waste.**[519]

Some people are downright afraid to take enemas.   This is generally due to either embarrassment or lack of knowledge.  **Anything this good for us should not be embarrassing.**  Taking enemas is wise and intelligent until one is completely pure inside.   They are fully constructive, lifting us to a higher level of existence through purification.   If we choose to be embarrassed, let us consider being embarrassed by the things we do which are destructive to our Temples - like drinking alcoholic beverages, coffee, pop; eating the flesh and muscles of innocent animals; eating sugar; drinking or eating liquid extracted from animals (dairy products); eating more than we need, swearing, or being overweight.

On the other hand, some people may simply not know how to take an enema. They should not let that stop them.   It's easy to learn. People, be brave! Consider it a new dimension of living yet to be explored. A vast, new frontier of experience awaits those who are daring enough!   I guarantee that it will become an enjoyable part of an ideal cleansing

---

[518] Earlier in this century, before medical science was completely taken over by money-mongers, enemas were common functions in all hospitals.  My mother was a nurse, and she used to tell me how they had to give enemas to their patients.

[519] There are a few doctors who do not believe in using enemas when fasting.  I absolutely disagree.  There is no logic to that concept at all.  I have seen people come close to death when fasting because they followed that kind of advice.  If these doctors understood what takes place in the bowels of one on a fast, I am sure they would change their views.  An important consideration, is the fact that most people do not have the healthy bacteria in their bowels.  During a fast, there is almost no bowel movement and the harmful bacteria, which was kept under some degree of control by food moving through, can become dominant.  This in itself, can cause a serious bacterial and protozoan infection.  The fermentation and other bi-products of these critters, could, under unusual conditions, even cause death during a water fast or at least cause serious harm to other internal organs.  Using enemas can keep the colon free of these accumulating conditions.  These facts about bacteria and parasites are only one of the reasons why it is important to thoroughly cleanse the alimentary canal, before fasting.

program - seeing the results of all those efforts - proof that we are getting stronger and healthier, and experiencing the increased energy - the feeling of improved health!

When on the final phase, taking enemas twice daily will usually help people rid their bodies of an extra ten feet of mucoid plaque in a seven-day period. White Crow was one who refused to take enemas during his cleanse. Being an herbalist, he figured that if he took extra herbs he could keep things moving and avoid enemas completely. It did work, but there were times when he did not feel as good as he could have - a clear indication that toxic substance was being stirred up and needed to be released. He would have had relief had he taken enemas. The next time he went on a cleanse, he decided to go with the enemas. He overcame his aversion to them very quickly when he saw the benefits. His cleansing went much easier and now he never fails to use them during a cleanse or when fasting. He recommends them to everyone doing the final phase. People will do better if they use them. If people get headaches, feel tired, or just don't feel good, and they refuse to take an enema, they should remember they would probably be just fine had they taken an enema.

# Equipment Needed

I recommend a douche bag instead of the regular enema bags, because they are easier and faster to use. They are also less expensive. If you get the douche bag, also get an enema tip to replace the douche tip, because it is smaller and easier to insert, although either will work.

Olive oil, vitamin E oil, coconut oil, or any natural lubricant is placed on the tip of the applicator and on the anus for easy injection. A gallon jug is useful to fill the enema bag. We can use any size container, but the gallon jug makes it easier and faster to use.

# What to Use for the Liquid

Use plain tap water, only when you know it is free of chlorine, fluoride and other toxic elements. In most areas of the country I would not use tap water. If the water has chlorine or fluoride, I would avoid it. There are not very many places where you can get good water right out of the tap. **Distilled water is the best**. Distilled water is what they call 'hungry water'. This means that it is so empty of minerals that it attracts things to itself, something like bentonite. Distilled water only pulls from the body that which is loose. It cannot pull out anything that is part of cell tissue. The only problem with distilled water is that in the process of being distilled, the life force is lost. You can replace that life force by adding some freshly-squeezed lemon, lime, or orange juice to it.  You could also completely rejuvenate the water by pumping purified air back into it.

If people cannot get good water which is free of chlorine, then they should at least boil the water.  Boiling will evaporate the chlorine. After it cools, it will be good for drinking and taking enemas.  But, if it has fluoride in it, then we need to obtain distilled water.  Fluoride is a deadly poison and will not dissipate by boiling.[520]

## Temperature of Enema Liquid

The hotter the liquid, the faster it is absorbed through the colon. The muscles will relax and this is not what you want.  I prefer the liquid to

---

[520] Why do they put sodium fluoride in the drinking water of large cities?  To prevent tooth decay? That is what they want us to believe.  Why is it that in every city that uses fluoride in their drinking water, tooth decay increases, births of  Mongoloid children increase, crime rate increases, and disease increases?  Calcium fluoride is what can help our teeth.  But they don't use calcium fluoride; they use sodium fluoride - a deadly poison.  It would be like saying that the air we breathe is a gas (which it is), so therefore breathing Mustard Gas must be good also.  Mustard Gas is good for killing just like sodium fluoride is good for killing.  Sodium fluoride is registered with the EPA as a rat poison, and is a by-product of the aluminum industry. They say it is used in such small amounts that it cannot hurt us.  But the FDA has just recently required that fluoride toothpaste carry a warning label saying: **WARNING: Keep out of reach of children under six years of age. If you accidentally swallow more than used for brushing, seek professional help or contact a poison control center immediately**.  This was reported in the Townsend Letter for Doctors and Patients in April of 1998, pg. 11.  Authorities also said mercury was OK in our teeth.  Yet mercury and chlorine are two of the most deadly poisons on the planet. They said the mercury in our teeth is not harmful.  Now after using it for almost century, we find out it is harmful.  Also, during this period, America dropped from the healthiest nation in the world to the sickest.  We know that sodium fluoride ends up in our brains.  Why did Nazi Germany use sodium fluoride in their drinking water prior to the W.W.II?  And why did Russia use it in their P.O.W. camps?  They said it kept the Germans "calm."  In countries that have used sodium fluoride in their water for long periods, their citizens become susceptible to suggestion, especially from their government. Source: Dr. Hans Moolenburgh, *Fluoride: The Freedom Flight,* available only in German.  May request from the National Library of Medicine through your local library. Practitioners of natural medicine have been saying for 25 years that sodium fluoride is bad for you, but not many listened. The same practitioners identified Candidiasis years ago, but conventional medicine denied its significance until recently.

be right at body temperature. The muscles will stay strong at this tepid temperature for maximum evacuation.

To awaken and bring strength to the peristaltic muscles in the colon, use cooler or cold water for your last gallon of enema liquid (it is best to do this after you feel you have gotten all of the loose matter out with a gallon or so of lukewarm water first). You will feel a wonderful stimulation in the colon that will strengthen the whole lower abdomen.

# Instructions

### Note: When putting liquid in an enema bag, be sure the valve is shut.

After you've sprayed your feet and the clean bathroom with an herbal tea enema the first time, you won't have to remind yourself of this anymore!

Place the filled enema bag on the shower or bathroom door handle, or on the towel rack. This is a comfortable height. After you get used to enemas, feel free to hang it higher - remember that the higher you hang the bag, the more pressure there is and the liquid will flow out more quickly. You can control the flow with the enema bag shut-off valve, which should be about two inches from the tip.

### Position

Some people prefer lying on the back - this way they are in a good position to be comfortable and massage the colon. Some like to be on their knees with their heads on the floor. In this position it feels like the liquid flows to the furthest end of the colon[521] much more easily than when on the back. (Some people take enemas in the bathtub for obvious reasons.) You will want to find a position that allows you to very thoroughly massage the colon (while the liquid is inside) before getting up to eliminate. While some may not choose to massage at all, you can realize that the more you massage the colon, the more material will be loosened.

---

[521] Some people are concerned about getting liquid past the ileocecal valve. This is a one-way valve and prevents substance from going into the small intestine. Maybe 1 out of 10,000 people have a defective illeocecal valve, and what do you think these people need to do? Remove the mucoid plaque from around the valve so that it will be free to function properly.

## Warning

Put the lubricant on the enema tip and on the anus. Place the tip over the toilet, sink, or bathtub, and open the valve, allowing the liquid to flow until the air bubbles are removed from the tube. (Air bubbles can hurt.) Then get into position (after shutting off the valve) and insert the tip. After insertion, open the valve gradually, allowing the liquid to flow into the colon slowly until you get used to it. Always keep your hand on the valve for quick shut-off when needed and to keep the tip from slipping out.

Do not allow too much pressure in the colon, as there is never a need for that. If there is a blockage and you can't get much water in, just put in as much as you can without too much pressure, massage the blocked area, and then try to get some more water in. If you can't, then sit on the toilet, release the liquid, and hopefully the blockage will be eliminated. If it isn't, start over, but don't put so much water in that you feel pain. That could stretch your intestines and possibly pull the ligaments. **Please do not ever let an enema be painful.**

## Massage

Starting with the descending colon (left side of the lower abdomen), work up to the transverse (just behind the lower rib cage, unless you have a prolapsus) and then down the ascending colon (right side). Work it well - get the liquid all the way down to the ileocecal. Lying on the right side (after all the water is in) is another way to help get the water to flow up to the ileocecal while you're massaging it. If you aren't sure where all these parts of the colon are, just massage the heck out of your lower abdomen. Then release the water and be prepared to be amazed and astounded at what will be eliminated. Now you will begin to enjoy enemas.

When the liquid has difficulty flowing up into the colon, it helps considerably to take deep breaths - all the way in and all the way out. Try this, and you may be surprised how well it works. This changes the pressure in the abdominal area and makes it easier for the liquid to pass through blockages.

## How Much Liquid

When beginning the enema, it may be possible to inject only a cup or so of liquid, depending upon how compacted a person is. That's okay - don't force it. As soon as the pressure gets uncomfortable, shut off the valve. Try to work the liquid past the congestion by massaging, as indicated above; then add more liquid. You will know when it's too much.

Then evacuate. You should pass some blockages. Let it all out, then do it again. This time you will get more in. Although you may never reach it, make a goal of continuing the procedure until you can hold the whole bag (2 quarts). Eliminate again and keep doing this until no more material is being eliminated. *I recommend going through two gallons for each enema, period.*[522] If you haven't enough time, remember that a shorter enema (at least one bag) is infinitely better than none, and you'll be a lot more comfortable wherever you're going if you take extra time for the enema before you go.

I would suggest that an enema be taken first thing in the morning after the first psyllium shake; and then another one in the evening, two to three hours before bed. If you take it just before bed, you may have to get up during the night, since the liquid left in the colon often seeps gradually into the bladder. If you are urinating too often, chew some juniper berries. You may want to take juniper berry powder instead. This will break up uric acid deposits and clean the urinary system, especially the kidneys. It will also help relax the bladder. After taking juniper for a few days, you will experience how much it assists in sleeping through the night. Juniper tea works even more quickly. The best of all is to use a good herbal formula for the kidneys[523]. This should cleanse the kidneys, bladder, and urinary tract, and will work for almost everyone except men with a swollen prostate. When the prostate is swollen, it puts pressure on the bladder and ureters. This makes it difficult to urinate and often there will be dripping. The greatest thing for the prostate is saw palmetto herbal extract. I have seen this work in just a few days. I have not seen anything else work like the extract.

# SPECIAL ENEMAS

## Herbal Tea Enemas

When I take an enema, I like to use herbal teas in the enema water. This is a good way to make things happen fast. For example, for many years I had a great deal of pain in my eyes. I began to use my formula for the eyes. I would make it into a tea and drink it, and also take enemas

---

[522] "Enema" refers to the whole cycle of injecting a bag of water in, eliminating, and repeating at least three more times. "Two gallons per enema" means to go through 4 of the 2-quart bags with eliminations after each bag.

[523] I recommend making a tea with a good kidney formula. Buying it in bulk will cost less and will not contain any fillers or flow agents.

with it. This, along with my cleanse program, has improved my eyesight to the point where I have now purchased my fourth pair of weaker specs.[524] When I wanted to improve my skin, I used a program I developed to remove toxins via the skin. You may contact my office on where to find this skin cleansing program. I also took enemas with it, and had some rather impressive results. I sometimes use a formula I made for the kidneys. Making a tea out this formula did more for me than anything else, except an entire cleanse program. I used a formula I developed for the brain in an enema to help get my brain working when I was sluggish in the mornings. I have experimented with many things.

The following herbs* make excellent enemas:

**\*Note: Always use high quality wild-crafted or organically grown herbs.** Do not settle for the average quality found in stores.

**CATNIP** has a soothing effect on the body; good for energy; improves circulation; excellent for colds, fever, gas, and especially good for children or those who have trouble taking enemas.

**BURDOCK ROOT** is one of the best blood purifiers you'll find; the best herb for the skin; improves kidney action, and helps eliminate calcium deposits.

**YARROW** is one of the better herbs; good for the liver, stomach, and glands; a blood purifier, it opens the pores of the skin (the body's largest elimination organ) for rapid elimination; good for colds, cramps, fever, and flu; also good for bathing.

**RED RASPBERRY** is excellent for all kinds of female problems; high in iron, it is good for the eyes and for elimination; it is very nutritious.

**WILD CHERRY BARK** is very effective for those who take an enema and have trouble expelling the water. Wild Cherry Bark tea will go in easily and come out with a rush. It is gentle in its action and really shortens the time it takes to do an enema.

**WHITE OAK BARK** is an astringent and after an ideal cleanse program, it helps to draw the flabby intestines back into shape. Taking an enema with it helps the colon. It also helps to remove pinworms from children. We need to take it orally with ginger root in order to reach the small intestines, but this is a good way to pull those overhangs back into shape

---

[524] After using a computer, my eyesight has become worse again. Was it worth it to me? Maybe I should stop using a computer.

once the mucoid plaque is removed. For shrinking the gut, take two or three capsules each of both white oak bark and ginger root, twice a day on an empty stomach.

**A BULK KIDNEY FORMULA,** as described in Appendix II is a combination of herbs to assist the kidneys. Use 1 level teaspoon in 1 quart of water, bring to a boil, keep the lid on, and let it steep for about 20 minutes. Then pour into a gallon jug and add enough cool water to bring it to body temperature. It not only helps the kidneys, but the eyes and energy. It also seems to help remove bad bacteria from the colon.

**GARLIC ENEMAS** are about the fastest way to stink up a house that there is. If you must take a garlic enema, take it outside - maybe it will help get rid of the mosquitoes! However, garlic is known to be a great medicinal herb. One of the main reasons people recommend garlic enemas is to kill worms. This would only be semi-effective in the colon which would soon be re-infected from the small intestine. So it is better to take garlic orally. Worms generally hide in the mucoid layers, so get rid of the mucoid plaque first, then "de-worm", and they'll have no place to hide. (Never use raw garlic for longer than a day. It can cause a hernia.)

For those unwilling to cleanse the guts - for heaven's sake, keep your worms! Some would explain it this way: gardeners love earthworms because they burrow holes which condition the soil for a healthy plantation. Constipated guts are assisted by worms because they burrow holes through the mucoid plaque, thereby breaking it apart for better assimilation of nutrients. It makes one wonder if a heavily-impacted person could absorb any nourishment were it not for worms.

**Note**: Unless you are an herbalist, I suggest caution about using various combinations of herbs.

# Coffee Enemas

Once, after receiving instructions on how to take a coffee enema, I proceeded to do so. Afterwards, I felt as though I had starch and cayenne pepper in my veins all at the same time. I therefore concluded that a coffee enema was bad for those who were fairly cleansed. A few years passed and some friends approached me about what I had said in my original book regarding coffee enemas. They were convinced that coffee enemas were very helpful in assisting the liver in eliminating toxic overloads. I told them my experience and how I was taught to do the coffee enema. "Ahh," they said, "that was not the correct method and no wonder you got into trouble." So then I started doing coffee enemas every day for 30 days to see what effect it would have. Not once did I have the problem I had the first time. I felt my liver do a few flip-flops, but other than that I never noticed any changes.

However, the coffee enema has been used successfully in helping to dump a great deal of toxins from the liver. I can't tell you enough how helpful it can be. Many people who do not feel good whether fasting, cleansing, or doing nothing at all, may find great relief if they take a coffee enema. It usually gets rid of headaches within 20 minutes after taking the coffee enema, most often, much sooner.

The coffee enema is used by Gerson Institute with life-saving results.[525]

**The coffee enema is very effective for the following conditions:**

| | | |
|---|---|---|
| severe pain | nausea | nervous tension |
| depression | spasms | precordial pain |
| sluggishness | weakness and headaches | |

# How To Take Coffee Enemas

Based upon Dr. Gerson's work. More information
is available in his book,
*A Cancer Therapy. Results of Fifty Cases*

Coffee enemas help remove toxins from the liver within 15 minutes. They often provide quick relief when fatigued, sleepy, having headaches, and when just feeling bad. They also help against spasms, precordial (heart, throat, chest) pain, and difficulties resulting from the sudden withdrawal of all intoxicating sedation.

A coffee enema, when done properly, causes the liver to produce more bile, opens the bile ducts, and causes the bile to flow. In this process, a toxic liver can dump many of its toxicants into the bile and get rid of them in just a few minutes. This can give great relief to all parts of the body, but especially the liver, and often makes the difference between feeling miserable and being active and alive.

With extremely toxic individuals, in the beginning of this treatment and during "flare-ups", the bile contains poisons, may produce

---

[525] Read Max Gerson, M.D., *A Cancer Therapy, Results of Fifty Cases and The Cure Of Advanced Cancer By Diet Therapy*, (Bonita, CA: Gerson Institute, 1990). It's found in most health food stores, or write to Gerson Institute, P.O. Box 430, Bonita, California 92002.

spasms in the duodenum and small intestines, and occasionally may cause some overflow into the stomach, with a resultant feeling of nausea or even vomiting of bile. In these cases, great amounts of peppermint tea are necessary to wash out bile from the stomach. Afterwards, patients feel much better. So if this happens, drink lots of peppermint tea.[526]

**Drinking a cup of coffee has an entirely different effect and we should not do it.** Drinking coffee causes the following problems: increases reflex response, lowers blood pressure, increases heart rate, causes insomnia, constipation, and heart palpitation, over-stimulates adrenals, irritates the stomach, and leaves a toxic residue in the body. A coffee enema when done properly will not produce these effects.

WARNING: Great care should be used with coffee enemas when water fasting. Coffee enemas cause bile to be excreted from the liver. The bile contains many valuable mineral salts. To lose these salts without replenishing them could be very harmful. **People using many coffee enemas a day must be on a good diet of broth and fresh juices that assures the replenishing of mineral salts.** However, I never recommend taking coffee enemas more than once a day at the most.

When doing intestinal cleansing, one or two coffee enemas a week should be fine if, before cleansing, the person passed the pH tests. Taking electrolyte supplements will also help in replenishing the bile salts lost through coffee enemas.

### Preparing the Coffee Enema

Take 3 tablespoons of ground coffee (organically grown coffee is absolutely essential[527]) to 1 quart of water (preferably distilled). Let it lightly boil for 3 minutes and then lightly simmer for 20 minutes. Strain and use at body temperature. The daily amount can be prepared at one time, but should not be kept overnight.

The body should be lying down on its right side, with both legs drawn close to the abdomen. Breathe deeply, in order to suck the greatest

---

[526] Peppermint Tea Preparation:
Add one tablespoon of dried peppermint leaves to 2 cups (one pint) of boiling water (preferably distilled water). Let it lightly simmer for 5 minutes and strain.

[527] The toxic sprays that are used on commercially grown coffee can be harmful to the liver and could produce severe toxic reactions. Don't use commercially grown coffee!!!

amount of fluid into the necessary parts of the colon. It also helps to let all the air out of the lungs and suck the gut in and out while in this position.

The fluid should be retained 10 to 15 minutes. It helps to have a clock in easy view. It may help to have something to read while lying there. Dr. Gerson found that all the caffeine is absorbed from the fluid within 10 to 12 minutes. The caffeine goes through the hemorrhoidal veins directly into the portal veins and into the liver.

## Colema Boards and Colonics

Is there anything that works better than an enema? Yes! Colema boards allow one to lay on your back, massage your bowels, and control the in and out flow without moving. Many people believe that they are the greatest thing ever invented. You can go through 5 or 6 gallons in about an hour or two. The only problem is that some people have difficulty in removing the liquids while on the back. I happen to be one of them. But the majority never have this problem and thousands swear by them. Dr. Jensen highly recommends them.

Is there anything that works better than a colema board? Yes! Colonics work even better than either and enema or colema board. With a colonic you can just sit back and relax. The colonic therapist will do all the work for you. About 30 gallons of water is used in a colonic. Massage and perhaps other tools to help you eliminate are at your disposal. Colonics have helped many, many people. It is the fastest method to quickly release toxic accumulations. Will the enema, colema or colonic remove mucoid plaque? Only if the mucoid plaque has already broken away from the colonic wall. Mucoid plaque adheres to the gut wall almost like glue. This is why we need herbs to condition the plaque so it will break off. When it breaks off, toxic particles are released and float around. These methods of washing out the colon help to move these toxins out before they can be re-absorbed into the bloodstream. What a blessing!

## Rectal Implants

Implants of friendly bacteria are not required when cleansing, as long as you take the recommended amounts of friendly bacteria each evening at least one hour before bedtime. However, if you are concerned about whether your bacteria levels are adequate, and you want to significantly boost your friendly bacteria, you may choose to do an implant.

# Implant Instructions

Approximately 48 hours before doing the implant, soak 6 to 8 capsules of the probiotic (friendly bacteria) formula in about 16 ounces of spring or mineral water - must be pure, unchlorinated, uncarbonated, and not distilled. Be sure to use a sanitized container. Stir and keep covered, and out of the light. Keep in a warm area nearest body temperature as possible. Up to 100 degrees. In this way it will grow very rapidly.

**Note**: if using the main probiotic formula in bulk, use about 2 level teaspoons.[528]

When the time comes for the implant, take a normal enema. After all the water from your enema is out, inject 8 ounces (half) of the probiotic formula in solution which you prepared as described above. Lie on right side with knees to chest. Retain the solution as long as you can. It may help to raise your hips with some pillows to keep the water from coming out. If the urge comes to release, raise your left leg and gently rub the sigmoid colon area to relax the muscles. The urge should pass within a few seconds. Try to keep the water in, but if you have to release, your body will still benefit. Now prepare your next implant by pouring eight ounces of your probiotic mixture into your enema bag, and then adding another eight ounces of clean water to your solution, and let it grow until your next implant the following day.

**Note**: Never take bacteria orally just before bed. When in the prone position, the bacteria may remain in the stomach and fail to enter the small intestines. This can cause discomfort and destroy many of the bacteria.

---

[528] These amounts are based upon capsules containing two billion bacteria per capsule.

## Appendix IV

# CHEMOTHERAPY DRUGS

Here is an example of what you will find in the PDR under chemotherapy drugs:

"ADRIAMYCIN RDF™. **Serious irreversible myocardia toxicity with delayed congestive failure, often unresponsive to any cardiac supportive therapy.... Acute life-threatening arrhythmias have been reported to occur during or within a few hours** after ADRIAMYCIN administration. There is a **high incidence of bone marrow depression**, primarily of leukocytes (white blood cells), requiring careful hematologic monitoring. **Ulceration and necrosis of the colon, especially the cecum, may occur, leading to bleeding or severe infections which can be fatal.**"

"ADRUCIL. Although **severe toxicity and fatalities are more likely to occur in poor risk patients, these effects have occasionally been encountered in patients in relatively good condition.** Should be discontinued when leukopenia[529] occurs. **Severe hematologic toxicity, gastrointestinal hemorrhage and even death may result** from use of Adrucil (Fluorouracil) injection. Adrucil (Fluorouracil) injection is **a highly toxic drug with a narrow margin of safety.**"

"METHOTREXATE. Because of the possibility of **fatal or severe toxic reactions**, the patient should be fully informed by ... If profound **leukopenia occurs during therapy, bacterial infection may occur or become a threat. The most common adverse reactions include ulcerative stomatitis, leukopenia, nausea and abdominal distress, bone marrow depression, thrombocytopenia, anemia, intestinal ulceration and bleeding, renal failure. Deaths have been reported and chronic interstitial obstructure pulmonary disease** has occasionally occurred. Found in Physicians Desk Reference, Edition 42, 1988."

If after reading this anyone decides to have chemotherapy, I suggest that this person has been drinking too much water containing sodium fluoride. There is evidence that sodium fluoride, which is extremely toxic, used as rat poison, and is being added to many U.S. municipal water systems, has an effect upon the brain that dulls the mind and makes the

---

[529] Leukopenia - Leuko = white blood cells. Penia = deficiency. Leukopenia means deficiency of white blood cells. It is a term indicating a serious problem with the immune system.

victim susceptible to suggestion. Prior to World War II, Nazi Germany added fluoride to the drinking water of German people.[530] Could that have been the reason that Hitler was able to pull the wool over the eyes of his gullible countrymen? Is this the reason that Communist Russia began to use it? Why is it happening in America? To stop tooth decay? No! Definitely not for dental reasons, for it has been proven that sodium fluoride in drinking water has increased dental decay as well as many other problems.

---

[530] Source: Dr. Hans Moolenburgh, *Fluoride: The Freedom Flight,* Available only in German. May request from the National Library of Medicine through your local library.

# *CHART*

## ALKALINE VS. ACID-FORMING FOODS

### ALKALINE-ASH FOODS

| | | |
|---|---|---|
| Alfalfa Sprouts | Apricots | |
| Beets & Greens | Apples | |
| Broccoli | Avocado | |
| Brussel Sprouts | Bananas | |
| Cabbage | Berries | |
| Carrots | Blackberries | |
| Cauliflower | Cantaloupe | |
| Celery | Cherries | |
| Collard Greens | Dates | |
| Fresh Corn | Figs | |
| Cucumbers | Grapefruit | |
| Dulse | Grapes | |
| Green Beans | Leeche Nuts | |
| Green Lima Beans | Lemons | |
| Green Peas | Limes | |
| Green Soy Beans | Mangoes | |
| Kale | Melons (all) | |
| Kelp | Oranges | |
| Leaf Lettuce | Peaches | |
| Mushrooms | Pears | |
| Mustard Greens | Pineapple | |
| Okra | Raisins | |
| Onions | Raspberries | |
| Parsley | Plums & Prunes | |
| Peppers | Cider Vinegar | |
| Potatoes* | Goat Whey | |
| Parsnips | Maple Syrup | |
| Radishes | Millet* | |
| Rhubarb | Quinoa* | |
| Rutabagas | Molasses* | |
| Sauerkraut | | |

### ACID-ASH FOODS

Alcohol
Aspirin
Barley, pearled
Bread
Cake
Cereals (all)
Chickpeas
Chocolate
Coffee
Corn
Corn Starch
Cranberries
Eggs
Grains except Millet
Honey
Legumes
Lentils
Niacin
Mustard
Nuts
Oatmeal
Pasta
Pepper, black
Rice
Seeds
Soda Crackers
Soft Drinks
Sugar
Tea, black
Vinegar, distilled
Vitamin C

## ALKALINE-ASH FOODS

Spinach
Sprouts
Squash
Turnip Greens
Tomatoes, ripe
Watercress
Yams

## ACID-ASH FOODS

Wheat Bran
Wheat Germ
Wheat
Canned Fruits, glazed,
sulfured
Dairy Products
(butter, milk,
cheese, yogurt, etc.)
All Animal, Mammal,
Foul, & Sea Animal
products, etc.)

**Foods with a * significantly slow the cleanse process, and can reduce the amount of plaque removed. It is suggested that, while cleansing, foods with a asterisk be limited to 2-3 servings per week.**

Note: All foods become acid when sugar is added.

# SUGGESTED READING LIST

## Raw Food Cookbooks

Christine Dreher, *The Cleanse Cookbook*. Christine's Cleanse Corner, P.O. Box 421423, San Diego, CA 92142. Phone/FAX: (877) 673-0224.

Marcia Madhuri Acciardo, *Light Eating For Survival*. 21st Century Publications, P. O. Box 702, Fairfield, LA 52556

Frances Kendall, *Sweet Temptations*. Garden City Park, NY: Avery Publishing Group, 1988.

Ann Wigmore, *Recipes for Longer Life*. Wayne, New Jersey: Avery Publishing Group, 1978.

Harvey and Marilyn Diamond, *Fit For Life*. New York, NY: Warner Books, 1985.

Dr. Abramowski, *Fruitarian Diet and Physical Rejuvenation, A Medical Doctor's Cure on a Fruit and Raw Diet*. Denver, Colorado: Nutri-Books, no longer in print. Check used book stores, and libraries.

Dr. and Elizabeth Baker, *The UNcook Book*. Indianola, WA: Drelwood Publications, 1980. (P.O. Box 149, Indianola, WA 98342)

George and Doris Fathman, *Live Foods-Nature's Perfect System of Human Nutrition*. Beaumont, CA: Sun Heaven Publisher, 1958. (No longer in print. Includes 192 raw food recipes).

Dr. Kirstine Nolfi, *The Raw Food Treatment of Cancer and Other Diseases*. Payson, Arizona: Leaves of Autumn Books, 1994.

Viktoras Kulvinskas, M.S., *Love Your Body - Live Food Recipes*. Woodstock Valley, CT: Omangod Press, 1972.

Leslie and Susannah Kenton, *Raw Energy*. New York, NY: Warner Books, 1984.

Dr. Bernard Jensen, Ph.D., *Juicing Therapy*. Escondido, CA: Bernard Jensen Publishing, 1992.

## Iridology

Dr. Bernard Jensen, *Iridology: The Science and Practice of the Healing Arts*, Volume II. Escondido, CA: Bernard Jensen, Pub., 1982.

Dr. Donald Banner, *Applied Iridology and Herbology*. Orem, Utah: Bi-World Publishers, 1982.

# Cleansing, Fasting, and Self-Healing

Dr. John R. Christopher, *Regenerative Diet.* Springville, Utah: Christopher Publications, 1982.

Professor Arnold Ehret, *Mucusless Diet Healing System.* Yonkers, NY: Ehret Literature Publishing Company, 1953.

Professor Arnold Ehret, *Rational Fasting.* Yonkers, NY: Ehret Literature Publishing Company, 1965.

Dr. Bernard Jensen, *Tissue Cleansing Through Bowel Management.* Escondido, CA: Bernard Jensen Publications, 1981.

Dr. Bernard Jensen, *Doctor-Patient Handbook.* Escondido, CA: Bernard Jensen Publishing, 1976.

Phillip Partee, *Fasting and Losing Weight.* Sarasota, FL: United Press, Inc., Publication, 1979.

Oswald/Shelton, *Fasting For The Health Of It.* Tampa FL: American Natural Hygiene Society, 1983.

Johanna Brandt, *The Grape Cure.* Yonkers, NY (soon to move to Ardsley, NY): Ehret Literature Publishing Co., 1930.

J. H. Tilden, *Toxemia Explained.* Denver, CO: World Press, 1926.

# Medical Conspiracy

Harvey, Diamond, *A Case Against Medicine.* Santa Monica, California: Golden Glow Publishers, 1979.

Edward Griffin, *World Without Cancer.* Denver, Colorado: Nutri-Books, 1976.

Dr. Robert Mendelsohn, *Confessions of a Medical Heretic.* New York, NY: Warner Books, 1980.

Paul Stitt, *Fighting the Food Giants.* Denver, Colorado: Nutri-Books, 1980.

Barry Lynes, *The Healing of Cancer, The Cures - the Cover-Up and the Solution Now!* Ontario, Canada: Marcus Books, 1989.

Eustace Mullins, *Murder By Injection, The Story of the Medical Conspiracy Against America.* Staunton, VA: The National Council for medical Research, 1988.

Elaine Feuer, *Innocent Casualties - The FDA's War Against Humanity.* Pittsburgh, PA: Dorrance Publishing Co., Inc., 1996.

Ralph W. Moss, *The Cancer Industry - Unraveling the Politics.* New York, NY: Paragon House, 1989.

Morris A. Bealle, *The Drug Story.* Spanish Fork, UT: The Hornets' Nest, 1976.

Robert Mendelsohn, M.D., *Confessions of a Medical Heretic.* New York, NY: Warner Books, 1980.

Robert Mendelsohn, M.D., *MAL E PRACTICE - How Doctors Manipulate Women*. Don Mills, Ontario, Canada: Beaverbooks, Ltd., 1981.

*The Price of Root Canals,* compiled by Hal A. Huggins, DDS, MS. Contact Dr. Hal Huggins' office in Colorado Springs, CO, for this book and more information about the root canals and all the studies done. (719) 522-0566.

Dr. John Yiamouyiannis, *Fluoride The Aging Factor*. Delaware, OH: Health Action Press, 1993.

Alan Cantwell Jr., M.D., *AIDS And The Doctors of Death*. Los Angeles, CA: Aries Rising Press, 1988.

Guylaine Lanctot, M.D., *The Medical Mafia*. Coaticook, QC, Canada: Here's The Key Inc., 1995.

Charles, B. Inlander President, People's Medical Society, Lowell S. Levin, Professor, Yale University School of Medicine, Ed Weiner Senior Editor, *People's Medical Society, Medicine On Trial - The Appalling Story of Ineptitude, Malfeasance, Neglect, and Arrogance*. New York, NY: Prentice Hall Press, 1988.

P.J. Lisa, *Are You A Target For Elimination*. Huntington Beach, CA: International Institute of Natural Health Sciences, Inc., 1984.

# Essenes

*The Essene Gospel Of Peace*. Arise & Shine, PO Box 901, Mt. Shasta, CA 96067, 800-688-2444.

*The Gospel Of The Holy Twelve - The Essene New Testament*. Translated from the original Aramaic. Published by Essene Church of Christ, P.O. Box 1113, Creswell, Oregon 97426.

For more information about the Essenes, contact Brother David Owen, P.O. Box 1113, Creswell, Oregon 97426.

# Healing and Nutrition

Dr. Edward Howell, *Enzyme Nutrition*. Wayne, New Jersey: Avery Publishing Group, Inc., 1985.

Yogi Ramacharaka, *The Hindu Yogi Practical Water Cure*. Chicago, Illinois: The Yoga Publication Society, 1935.

Beatrice Hunter, *Consumer Beware! Your Food and What's Been Done to It*. Denver, Colorado: Nutri-Books. No longer in print. Check your library or used book stores - some specialize in books no longer in print.

Dr. Bernard Jensen, *Food Healing for Man*. Escondido, California: Jensen Publishing Company, 1983.

William Duffy, *Sugar Blues*. Atlanta, Georgia: New Leaf Distributing Co., 1965.

Barbara Parham, *What's Wrong With Eating Meat?* Denver, Colorado: Ananda Marga Publications, 1979.

# Herbology

Jethro Kloss, *Back to Eden.* Santa Barbara, California: Lifeline Books, 1975.

Louise Tenney, *Today's Herbal Health.* Provo, Utah: Woodland Books, 1983.

Dr. John R. Christopher, *School of Natural Healing.* Springville, UT: Christopher Publications, 1976.

# Books About Vaccines

Harold E. Buttram, M.D, and J. C. Hoffman, *Vaccinations and Immune Malfunctions.* Quakertown, PA: Randolph Society, 1987.

Eleanor McBean, Ph.D., *Vaccinations Do Not Protect.* Manachaca, TX: Health Excellence Systems, 1991.

Robert S. Mendelsohn, M.D., *But Doctor, About That Shot... The Risks of Immunizations and How to Avoid Them.* Evanston, IL: "The People's Doctor Newsletter," 1988.

Isaac Golden, Ph.D., *Vaccination? A Review of Risks and Alternatives*, 4th edition. Geelong, Victoria, CAN: Aurum Healing Centre, 1993.

Neil Z. Miller, *Vaccines: Are They Really Safe and Effective? A Parent's Guide To Childhood Shots.* Santa Fe, NM: New Atlantean Press, 1993.

Hannah Allen, *Don't Get Stuck: The Case Against Vaccinations.* Tampa, Florida: American Natural Hygiene Society, 1985.

M. Beddow Bayly, *The Case Against Vaccination.* York Road, London: William H. Taylor and Sons, Ltd. Printers, 1936.

Harris L. Coulter, *Vaccination, Social Violence, and Criminality: The Medical Assault on the American Brain.* Berkeley, CA: Atlantic Books, 1990.

Harris L. Coulter, and Barbara Loe Fisher, *A Shot in the Dark: Why the P in DPT Vaccination May be Hazardous to Your Child's Health.* Garden City Park, NY: Avery Publishing Group, 1991.

James Walene. *Immunization: The Reality Behind the Myth.* South Hadley, MA: Bergin & Garvey, 1988.

Richard Moskowitz, M.D., *The Case Against Immunizations.* Washington D.C.: National Center for Homeopathy, 1983.

Eleanor McBean, *The Poisoned Needle.* Mokelumne Hill, CA: Health Research, 1974.

The Randolph Society, Inc. *The Dangers of Immunization.* Quakertown, PA: The Randolph Society, Inc., 1987.

Attorney Tom Finn, *Dangers of Compulsory Immunizations - How to Avoid Them Legally.* New Port Richey, Florida: Family Fitness Press, 1988.

Elben, *Vaccination Condemned - Book One.* Los Angeles, CA: Better Life Research, 1981.

## Books About Recovery from AIDS

Bob Owen, Ph.D., *Roger's Recovery From AIDS.* Malibu, CA: Davar Publisher, 1987.

Ed McCabe, *Oxygen Therapies.* Morrisville, NY: Energy Publications, 1988.

# BIBLIOGRAPHY

Akers, Keith. *A Vegetarian Sourcebook*. New York, NY: Putnam, 1983

Albert, M.J.; Mathan, V. I.; & Baker, S.J. "Vitamin B-12 Synthesis by Human Small Intestinal Bacteria." *Nature*, 1980; 283, pg. 781-782.

Allen, A.; Bell, A.; and McQueen, S. "Mechanisms of Mucosal Protection of the Upper Gastrointestinal Tract.*" Mucus and Mucosal Protection*. Philadelphia, PA: Raven Press, 1984.

Allen, A., et al. "Studies on Gastrointestinal Mucus." *Scandinavian Journal of Gastroenterology*, Supplements, 1984; 93, pg. 101-113.

Allen, Hannah. *Don't Get Stuck! The Case Against Vaccinations and Injections*. Tampa, Florida: American Natural Hygiene Society, 1985.

Allen, Ph.D., Lindsay H.; Oddoye, Ph.D., E.A.; and Margen, M.D., S. "Protein Induced Hypercalciuria: A Longer Term Study." *The American Journal of Clinical Nutrition,* 1979; April; Issue 32, pg. 741-749.

*Arizona Daily Star, The.* Tucson, Arizona, Wednesday, May 9th, 1990, pg.14 - Section A.

Bailes, Frederick. *Your Mind Can Heal You*. Marina del Ray, CA: DeVorss & Co. Inc., 1971.

Baron, Samuel. *Medical Microbiology*, 3rd Edition. New York, NY: Addison-Wesley Publishing, 1981.

Beddoe, D.D.S., Alexander F. *Biological Ionization*. Grass Valley, CA: Agro-Bio Systems, 1990.

Berkow, Robert, M.D., ed. *The Merck Manual,* 15th Edition. Rahway, NJ: Merck Sharp and Dohme Research Laboratories, Division of Merck and Company, 1987.

Bernet, M. F.; Brassart, D.; Nesser, J. R.; Servin, A. L. "Adhesion of Human Bifidobacterial Strains to Cultured Human Intestinal Epithelial Cells and Inhibition of Enteropathogen-cell Interactions." *Applied Environmental Microbiology*, 1993; Dec., 59 (12), pg. 4121-4128.

Besant, P.T.S., Annie; and Leadbeater, Charles W. *Occult Chemistry - Clairvoyant Observations on the Chemical Elements*. London: Theosophical Publishing House, 1919.

Bieler, M.D., Henry G. *Food Is Your Best Medicine*. New York, NY: Ballantine Books, 1965.

Brennan, T. A.; Leap, L.L.; Liard, N. M.; Herbert, L.; Localio, A. R.; Lawthers, A.G.; Newhouse, J. P.; Weiler, P.C.; Hiatt, H.H. "Incidence of Adverse Event and Negligence in Hospitalized Patients. Results of the Harvard Medical Practice Study." *New England Journal of Medicine*, 1991; Feb 7, pg. 370-376.

Callender, Sheila & Spray, G.H. "Latent Pernicious Anaemia." Oxford, England: Nuffield Dept. of Clinical Medicine, The Radcliffe Infirmary, Oxford, Br., *Journal of Haematology*, 1962; 8, pg. 230-240.

Cheadle and Levanthal. *Medical Parasitology*. Philadelphia, Pennsylvania: F.A. Davis Company, 1985.

Center for Disease Control's *Agency for Toxic Substances and Disease Registry*. See: http:\\atsdr1.atsdr.cdc.gov:8080\hazdat.html

"Chlorine, Human Health and the Environment: The Breast Cancer Warning." A Greenpeace report. 1436 U Street NW, Washington DC 20009, (202) 462-1177.

Chopra, M.D., Deepak . *Ageless Body, Timeless Mind*. New York, NY: Harmony Books, 1994.

Chopra, M.D., Deepak. *Quantum Healing, Exploring the Frontiers of Mind/Body Medicine*. New York, NY: Bantam Books, 1989.

"Chronic Mercury Toxicity - New Hope Against an Endemic Disease." (A topic of importance to doctors of every health specialty, as chronic mercury toxicity may be on the rise.) In *Counseling*, Volume 1. Colorado Springs, Colorado: Queen and Company Health Communications, Inc., 1968.

Cook, H. C. "Neutral Mucin Content of Gastric Carcinomas as a Diagnostic Aid In the Identification of Secondary Deposits." *Histopathology*, 1982; 6, pg. 591-599.

Corfield, A. P., et al. "Mucus Glycoproteins and Their Role in Colorectal Disease." *Journal of Pathology*, 1996; Sept.; 180(1), pg. 14.

Coulter, Harris L.; and Fisher, Barbara Loe. *A Shot In The Dark*. Garden City Park, New York: Avery Publishing Group Inc., 1991.

Culling, C. F. A.; Reid, P. E.; Burton, J. D.; and Dunn, W. I. "A Histochemical Method Of Differentiating Lower Gastrointestinal Tract Mucin From Other Mucins In Primary or Metastatic Tumors." *Journal of Clinical Pathology*, 1975; 28, pg. 656-658.

Davenport, H. W. *Physiology of the Digestive Tract*, Vol. 4. New York: Yearbook Medical Publisher, 1980, pg. 162 and *Digestive Disease and Sciences*, Vol. 25, No. 7, July 7,1980, pg. 513.

Degidio, D.O., M.D., Anthony James. *Everything You Need to Know About AIDS*. Burlingame, CA: New Additions Publishing, 1994.

DeMeo, Ph.D., James, Director of Research. "Anti-Constitutional Activities and Abuse of Police Power by the U.S. Food and Drug Administration and Other Federal Agencies." Ashland, OR: Orgone Biophysical Research Lab, 1998.

"End of Antibiotics, The." *Newsweek*, 1994; March 28.

Erasmus, Udo. *Fats and Oils*. Burnaby BC, Canada: Alive Books, 1986.

Edward Every, ed. *"Physician's Desk Reference."* Oradell, NJ: Edward Barnhart Publishers, 1988.

Exton-Smith, A. "Physiological Aspects of Aging: Relationship to Nutrition." *American Journal of Clinical Nutrition,* 1972; 25, pg. 853-59.

Filipe, M. L. "Transitional Mucosa." *Histopathology,* 1984; July; 8(4), pg. 707-708.

Finegold, Sydney M.; Attenbery, Howard R.; and Sutter, Vera L. "Effect of Diet on Human Fecal Flora: Comparison of Japanese and American

Diets." *The American Journal of Clinical Nutrition*, 1974; 27: Dec.; pg. 1456-1469.

Forstner, J. R. "Intestinal Mucins in Health and Disease." *Digestion,* 1978; 17(3), pg. 234-263.

Friberg, Lars; Nordberg, Gunnar F.; and Vouk, Velimir B. *Handbook on the Toxicology of Metals*, 1st Edition. Amsterdam and New York, NY: Elsevier/N. Holland Biomedical Press, 1979.

Friberg, Lars, and Vostal, Jaroslav, *Mercury in the Environment.* Cleveland, OH: Chemical Rubber Company (CRC) Press, 1972.

Fuhrman, Peter. "No Need for Valium." *Forbes*, 1994; Jan. 31, pg. 84-85.

Gerson, M.D., Max. *A Cancer Therapy, Results of Fifty Cases and The Cure of Advanced Cancer by Diet Therapy.* Bonita, CA: Gerson Institute, 1990.

Gibson, Glenn R.; and Macfarlane, George T., ed. *Human Colonic Bacteria, Role in Nutrition, Physiology, and Pathology.* Boca Raton, FL: CRC Press, 1995.

Go, V.L.W.; and Summerskill, W.H.J. "Digestion, Maldigestion, and the Gastrointestinal Hormones." *American Journal of Clinical Nutrition*, 1971; 24, pg. 160-167.

Gray, Dr. Robert. *The Colon Health Handbook.* Reno, NV: Emerald Publishing, 1986.

Griffin, G. Edward. *World without Cancer.* Denver, CO: Nutri-Books, 1974.

Gustafsson, B. E. "The Physiological Importance of the Colonic Microflora." *Scandinavian Journal of Gastroenterology.* Supplements. 1982; 77, pg. 117-121.

Guyton, A.C. *Textbook Medical Physiology,* 7th Edition. Philadelphia, PA, W.B. Saunders Company, 1986.

Guyton, A. C. and Hall, J. E. *Textbook of Medical Physiology*, 9th Edition. Philadelphia, PA: W.B. Saunders Company, 1996.

Heltman, Robert F. "Organic Food Is More Nutritious." *Townsend Letter for Doctors & Patients*, Issue # 172, 1997; Nov., pg. 12.

Henry, M.D., John Bernard. *Clinical Diagnosis & Management by Laboratory Methods.* Philadelphia, PA: W.B. Saunders Co., 1991.

Hensyl, W. R., ed. *Stedman's Medical Dictionary*, 25th Edition. Baltimore, MD: Williams & Wilkins, 1991.

Herbert, M.D., J. D., Victor. "Vitamin B-12: Plant Sources, Requirements, and Assay." In *American Journal of Clinical Nutrition,* 1988; Vol. 48, pg. 852-858.

Holland, J.; Bast, Jr., R.; Morton, D.; Freil III, E.; Kute, D.; Weichselbaum, R. *Cancer Medicine*, Volume 1, 4th Edition. Baltimore, MD: Williams & Wilkins, 1997, pg. 228

*Holy Bible, The.* King James version.

Holt, John G.; and Krieg, Noel R., ed. *Bergey's Manual of Systematic Bacteriology*, Vol. 2. Baltimore, MD: Williams & Wilkins, 1986.

Howell, Dr. Edward. *Enzyme Nutrition.* Wayne, New Jersey : Avery Publishing Group, Inc., 1985.

Huggins D.D.S., Dr. Hal. *It's All in Your Head.* New York, NY: Avery Press, 1993.

Huggins, D.D.S., M.S., Hal, ed. *The Price of Root Canals.* This book is available from Dr. Huggins office at (719) 522-0566 in Colorado Springs, CO.

Irons, Sr., Victor Earl. *The Destruction Of Your Own Natural Protective Mechanism.* Kansas City, MO: V.E. Irons, Inc., 1995.

Jass, J. R.; Filpe, M. I.; "Sulphomucins and Precancerous Lesions of the Human Stomach." *Histopathology,* 1980; 4, pg. 271-279.

Jelliffe, D.B. "Ascaris Lubricoides and Malnutrition in Young Children." *Documenta de Medicina Geographica et Tropica.* 1953; 5, pg. 314.

Jensen, D.C., N.D., Ph.D., Dr. Bernard. *Doctor-Patient Handbook.* Escondido, CA: Bernard Jensen Publishing, 1976.

Jensen, Bernard. *Food Healing for Man.* Escondido, CA: Bernard Jensen, Publisher, 1983.

Jensen, Ph.D., N.D., D.C., Dr. Bernard. *Iridology: The Science and Practice of the Healing Arts,* Vol. II. Escondido, CA: Bernard Jensen, Pub., 1982.

Jensen, Ph.D., N.D., D.C., Bernard. *The Chemistry of Man.* Escondido, California: Bernard Jensen, Publisher, 1984.

Jensen, Ph.D., N.D., D.C., M.H., Bernard. *Tissue Cleansing Through Bowel Management.* Escondido, CA: Bernard Jensen Publications, 1981.

Jones, Hardin. "Report on Cancer." March 7, 1969. Available at the University of California Bancroft Library. (510) 642-6481. Found in the Manuscript Collection: "Hardin Blair Jones Papers, 1937-1978." Request call number: BANC MSS 79/112 C. (Found in Carton #4.)

*Journal of Community Health,* 1980; Spring; Vol. 5, No. 3, pg. 149-158.

Kapit, Wynn; Macey, Robert I.; Meisami, Esmail. *The Physiology Coloring Book.* Cambridge, MA: Harper Collins Publishers, 1987.

Kauffman, Jr. and Ligumsky, "Role of Endogenous Prostaglandins in Gastric Mucosal Integrity." Found in: Allen, Bell and McQueen, "Mechanisms of Mucosal Protection of the Upper Gastrointestinal Tract." *Mucus and Mucosal Protection,* (Philadelphia, PA: Raven Press, 1984), pg. 317.

Kervran, Professor C. Louis. *Biological Transmutations.* Magalia, CA: Happiness Press, 1988.

Kirsner, Joseph B., M.D., Ph.D., D.Sc. (Hon.) and Shorter , Roy G., M.D., *Inflammatory Bowel Disease,* 4th Edition. Baltimore, MD: Williams and Wilkins, 1995.

Koch, Ph.D., M.D., William Frederick. *The Survival Factor In Neoplastic And Viral Diseases.* Detroit, MI, No publisher, 1961. Available through National Library of Medicine (800-272-4787) when requested by a local library.

Koenigsberg, Ruth, ed. *Churchill's Illustrated Medical Dictionary.* New York, NY: Churchill Livingstone, Inc., 1989.

Koivusalo, M.; Vartianinen, Rev. T. "Drinking Water Chlorination By-Products and Cancer." *Environmental Health,* 1997; Apr-Jun; 12(2), pg. 81-90.

Krohn, P. "Rapid Growth, Short Life." *Journal of the American Medical Association,* 1959; 171: pg. 461.

Kupsinel, M.D., Roy, ed. *Health Consciousness Magazine.* Dec. 1990.

Kurtz, M.D., Theodore W.; Al-Bander, M.D., Hamoundi A.; and Morris, Jr., M.D., R. Curtis. "Salt-Sensitive Essential Hypertension In Men." *New England Journal Of Medicine,* 1987; Vol. 317(17), pg. 1043-1048.

Larson, M.D., David, Editor-in-chief. *Mayo Clinic Family Health Book.* New York, NY: William Morrow and Co., 1990.

Lee, M.D., Richard; Bithell, M.D., Thomas; Forester, M.D., John; Athens, M.D., John; Lukens, M.D., John. *Wintrobe's Clinical Hematology.* Philadelphia, PA: Lea & Febiger, 1993.

Leventhal, Ruth; Cheadle, Russel F. *Medical Parasitology.* Philadelphia, Pennsylvania.: F. A. Davis Co., 1985.

Linkswiler, H. M.; Zemel, M. B.; Hegsted, M.; Schuette, S. "Protein-Induced Hypercalciuria." *Federal Proceedings,* 1981; 40: 2429.

Lynes, Barry. *The Healing of Cancer, The Cures - the Cover-Up and the Solution Now!* Ontario, Canada: Marcus Books, 1984.

Malstrom, N.D., M.T., Stan. "Your Colon - Its Character, Care and Therapy." Orem, Utah BiWorld Pub. Inc., 1981.

Mattman, Lida H. *Cell Wall Deficient Forms, Stealth Pathogens,* 2nd Edition. Ann Arbor, CRC Press, 1993, pg. 241.

McDougall, M.D., John A. & Mary A. *The McDougall Plan.* Clinton, NJ: New Win Publishing, Inc., 1983.

Mehlmauer, Dr. Leonard. *SCLEROLOGY, A New View of an Ancient Art.* Camarillo, CA: Grand Medicine, 1996.

Mendelsohn, M.D., Robert S. *Confessions of a Medical Heretic.* Chicago, Illinois: Contemporary Books, Inc., 1979.

Mendelsohn, M.D., Robert S. *Mal e Practice - How Doctors Manipulate Women.* Chicago, Illinois: Contemporary Books, Inc., 1982.

Mendelsohn, M.D., Robert S. *How to Raise a Healthy Child In Spite of Your Doctor.* New York, NY: Ballantine Books, and Toronto, Ontario, Canada: Random House, 1984.

*Merck Manual of Diagnosis and Therapy,* 15th Edition. Rahway, NJ: Merck Sharp and Dohme Research Laboratories, Division of Merck and Company, 1987.

Miller, Neil Z. *Vaccines: Are They Really Safe and Effective?* Santa Fe, NM: New Atlantean Press, 1993.

Mindell, Earl. *Vitamin Bible.* New York, NY: Warner Books, 1985.

Mindell, Earl. The Web page of.

Moolenburgh, Dr. Hans. *Fluoride: The Freedom Flight.* Available only in German. May request from the National Library of Medicine through your local library.

Morson, B. C. *Color Atlas of Gastrointestinal Pathology*. London, England: Harvey Miller Publishers/W.B. Saunders Co., 1988.

Morter, Jr. B.S., M.A., D.C., Ted M. *Correlative Urinalysis*. Rogers, AR: B.E.S.T. Research Inc., 1987.

Morter, Dr. Ted. *Your Health Choice*. Hollywood, FL: Fell Publishers and Company, Inc., 1990.

Mouridsen, S. E.; Nielsen, S. "Reversible Somatotrophin Deficiency (Psychological Dwarfism) Presenting as Conduct Disorder and Growth Hormone Deficiency." *Developmental Medicine and Child Neurology,* 1990; 32(12), pg. 1093-1098.

National Center for Health Statistics through the U.S. Dept. of Health and Human Services, Centers for Disease Control.

Netter, M.D., Frank H. "Digestive System, Part III, Upper Digestive Tract." In *The Ciba Collection of Medical Illustrations*, Volume 3. Summit, NJ: R.R. Donnelley & Sons Company, 1979.

Netter, M.D., Frank H. "Digestive System, Part II, Lower Digestive Tract." In *The Ciba Collection of Medical Illustrations*, Volume 3. Summit, NJ: R. R. Donnelley & Sons Company, 1979.

Neville, E. W. *The Resurrection*. Marina del Ray, CA: DeVorss & Co., 1966.

"Ozone In Medicine". In Volume 3, *Proceedings of the Ninth Ozone World Congress June 3-9, 1989*. New York, NY, USA: International Ozone Association Port City Press, Inc., 1989.

Pizzorno, N.D., Joseph E.; and Murray, N.D., Michael T. *A Textbook of Natural Medicine*. Seattle, WA: John Bastyr College Publications, 1991.

Poley, J. Rainer. "Loss of the Glycocalyx of Enterocytes in Small Intestine: A Feature Detected by Scanning Electron Microscopy in Children with Gastrointestinal Intolerance to Dietary Protein." *Journal of Pediatric Gastroenterology and Nutrition*, 1988; 7, pg. 836-394.

Poley, J. R. "Scanning Electron Microscopy of Soy Protein-Induced Damage of Small Bowel Mucosa in Infants." *Journal of Pediatric Gastroenterology and Nutrition,* 1983; May; 2 (2), pg. 271-278.

Poley, J. Rainier. "The Scanning Electron Microscope: How Valuable In The Evaluation of Small Bowel Mucosal Pathology In Chronic Childhood Diarrhea?" *Journal of Pediatric Gastroenterology and Nutrition*, 1991; May-June; 7(3), pg. 386-394.

Pottenger, Jr., M.D., Francis M. *Pottenger's Cats*. La Mesa, CA: The Price-Pottenger Nutrition Foundation, 1983.

Pounder, R. E.; Allison, M.C.; Dhillon, A. P. *Color Atlas of the Digestive Tract*. Chicago, IL: Year Book Medical Publisher Inc., 1989.

"Protein, Calories and Life Expectancy." *Federation Proceedings,* 1959; 18, pg. 1190-1207.

Rangavajhyala, N.; Shahani, K.M.; Sridevi, G.; and Srikumaran, S. "Nonlippolysaccaharide Components of Lactobacillus acidophilus Stimulate the Production of Interleukin-a and Tumor Necrosis Factor q by Murine Macrophages." *Nutrition and Cancer*, Vol. 27 or 28(2), pg. 130-134.

Robbins, John. *Diet For A New America*. Walpole, New Hampshire: Stillpoint Publishing, 1987. (See especially pages 187, 188).

Roitt, Ivan; Brosoff, Jonathan; Male, David. *Immunology*. Philadelphia, PA: J.B. Lippincott Co., 1989.

Rona M.D., M.Sc., Zoltan P. The Web page of.

Schmidt, Gerald K.; Roberts, Larry S. *Foundations of Parasitology*. St. Louis, MO: Times Mirror/Mosby College Publishing, 1985.

Shahani, Ph.D., Khem. "Antibiotic Acidophilin and Process of Preparing the Same." U.S. Patent 3,689,640 - Lincoln, NE: University of Nebraska, 1972.

Shahani, Ph.D., K.M.; Vakil, J. R.; Kilara, A. Natural Antibiotic Activity of Lactobacillus Acidophilus and Bulgaricus. Department of Food Sciences and Technology, University of Nebraska, Lincoln, NE 68583.

Shahani, Dr. Khem M., Professor, Food Science and Technology. *Facts and Fallacies About Probiotics*. University of Nebraska, Lincoln, NE 68583-0919.

Shaw, Ph.D., William. *Autism and Microorganisms*. Videotape Series: Tape 1. Great Plains Laboratory, Overland Park, KS. Phone 913-341-8949.

Sherman, H. *Chemistry of Food and Nutrition*. New York: H. Macmillan Co., 1952.

Sherman, H. *The Science of Nutrition*. New York: Columbia University Press, 1943.

Shils, Maunce E. and Young, Vernon R. *Modern Nutrition in Health and Disease*, 7th Edition. Philadelphia, PA: Lea & Febiger, , 1988.

Siegel, M.D., Bernie. *Love, Medicine and Miracles*. New York, NY: Harper and Row Publishers, 1986.

Simonton, M.D., O. Carl; Matthews-Simonton, Stephanie; and Creighton, James L. *Getting Well Again*. New York, NY: Bantam Books, 1978.

Sipponen, P.; Seppala, K.; Varis, E. et al. "Intestinal Metaplasia With Colonic-Type Sulphomucins In the Gastric Mucosa, Its Association With Gastric Carcinoma." Acta Pathologica Microbiologica Scandinavica, 1980; 88, pg. 217-224.

Skuse, D.; Albanese, A.; Stanhope, R.; Gilmore, J.; Voss, L. "A New Stress-related Syndrome of Growth Failure and Hyperphagia in Children, Associated with Reversibility of Growth Hormone Insufficiency." *Lancet*, 1996; Vol. 348(9024), pg. 353-356.

Spiro, Howard M. "Composition of Gallstones." In *Clinical Gastroenterology*, 4th Edition. New York, NY: McGraw Hill, 1993, pg. 873-888.

Spiro, Howard M. *Clinical Gastroenterology*, 4th Edition. New York, NY: McGraw Hill, 1983.

Stitt, Paul A. *Fighting the Food Giants*. Manitowoc, WI: Natural Press, 1981.

Stolberg, Lawrence; Rolfe, Rial; Gitlin, Norman; Merritt, Jeffrey; Mann, Jr., Lewis; Linder, Jean; Finegold, Sydney. "D-lactic Acidosis Due To Abnormal Gut Flora." *The New England Journal Of Medicine*, 1982; June 3, pg. 1347.

Strasinger D.A, M.T. (A.S.C.P.), Susan King. *Urinalysis And Body Fluids*. Philadelphia, Pennsylvania F.A. Davis Company, 1989.

Szekely, Edmond Bordeaux (translator). *The Essene Gospel of Peace*. United States: International Biogenic Society, 1981.

Thiru, S.; Devereux, G.; King, A. "Abnormal Fucosylation of Ileal Mucus In Cystic Fibrosis: I. A Histochemical Study Using Peroxidase Labeled Lectins." *Journal of Clinical Pathology*, 1990; 43, pg. 1014-1018.

*Tibetan Medicine*. May be ordered (or special ordered) from Greenleaf - (800) 905-8367. They must order from the wholesaler: New Leaf.

Tortora, Gerard J.; Funke, Berdell R.; Case, Christine L. *Microbiology, An Introduction*, 3rd Edition. New York: The Benjamin/Cummings Publisher, 1989.

Tortora, Gerard J.; and Grabowski. *Principles of Anatomy and Physiology*, 7th Edition. New York, NY: Harper Collins College Publishers, 1993.

Thurn, Joseph T.; Pierpont, Gordon L.; Ludvigsen, Carl W.; Eckfeldt, John H. "D-Lactate Encephalopathy." *The American Journal of Medicine*, 1985; Dec.; Vol:79, pg. 720.

Trowbridge, M.D., John Parks; and Walker, D.P.M., Morton. *The Yeast Syndrome*. Toronto, CAN: Bantam Books, 1988.

*Tucson Citizen, The*. Friday, October 4, 1991, Front page headline.

Vincenzio, J. V. "Trends in Medical Care Cost - Revisited." *Statistical Bulletin of Metropolitan Insurance Company*, 1997; July, Vol. 78, Issue (3), pg. 10-16.

Vital Statistics http:\\www.cdc.gov\nchswww\

Walker, D.P.M., Norton. "Medical Journalist Report of Innovative Biologics." *Townsend Letter for Doctors and Patients*, 1977; October, pg. 86.

Walzer, Peter D. and Genta, Robert M. *Parasitic Infections in the Compromised Host*. New York, New York : Marcel Dekker, Inc., 1989.

Welsh, Jack D.; Poley, J. Rainer; Hensley, Jess; and Bhatia, Mira. "Intestinal Disaccharidase and Alkaline Phosphatase Activity in Giardiasis." *Journal of Pediatric Gastroenterology and Nutrition*, 1984; 3(1), pg. 37-40.

West, John B. *Physiological Basis of Medical Practice*, Twelfth Edition. Baltimore, MD: Williams & Wilkins, 1990.

Whitehead, R., ed. *Gastrointestinal and Oesophageal Pathology*, 2nd Edition. New York, NY: Churchill Livingstone, 1995.

Yamada, T., ed. *Textbook of Gastroenterology*. Philadelphia, PA: J.P. Lippincott Co., 1991.

Yeung, Stadler J.; Furrer, R.; Marcon, N.; Himal, H. S.; Ruce, W. R. "Proliferative Activity of Rectal Mucosa and Soluble Fecal Bile Acids." *Cancer Letter,* 1988; Vol. 38: pg. 315.

*Your Health, Your Choice.* B.E.S.T. Research, Inc. Rogers, Arkansas 72756, 1-800-874-1478.

# INDEX

# —B—

*Bach Flower Remedies, 1-11*
bacteria, 1-24, 2-33, 2-37, 2-40, 2-43, 2-46, 4-97, 4-99, 5-108, 5-115, 5-116, 6-130, 6-131, 6-133, 6-134, 6-137, 6-140, 6-141, 6-145, 7-171, 7-178, 8-182, 9-199, 9-205, 9-217, 11-246, 11-251, 11-252, 11-254, 12-258, 12-267, 12-268, 12-269, 13-275, 13-277
  Acidophilus, 14-336
  B. Breve, 14-336
  B. Infantis, 14-336
  Bifidobacteria, 14-336
  E. Coli, 14-336
  friendly, 5-115, 6-131, 6-134, 6-150, 13-275
  Salmonella, 14-336
bad breath, 6-141, 8-182, 12-262
Bainbridge, 4-99
Basic Food Groups, The 12, 5-115
Basic Food Groups, The 4, 5-115
bath, 7-172, 9-210, 11-255
Belief creates biology, 1-16
bentonite, 9-206, 9-217, 11-251, 11-254
Bernard Jensen, 4-96, 4-97, 410
Bernie Siegel, 1-16
*bifidobacteria, 14-341*
Bifidobacterium Infantis, 9-218, 14-336, *14-341*
bile, 2-33, 2-34, 2-38, 2-39, 2-40, 6-147, 12-258, 12-260, 13-277
bladder, 7-165, 7-179, 12-262, 12-265, 12-267
blame, 1-20, 10-231
blind, 9-203, 9-211, 10-244, 12-262
bliss, 1-2
blood, 1-4, 1-14, 1-22, 1-28, 2-33, 2-34, 2-35, 2-38, 2-41, 2-43, 4-96, 4-97, 4-99, 5-113, 5-113, 6-131, 6-135, 6-139, 6-141, 6-148, 7-166, 7-173, 7-178, 9-197, 9-204, 9-205, 10-227, 11-253, 11-256, 12-260, 12-265, 12-266, 12-268, 12-269, 13-277, 14-345, 14-347
blood pressure, 2-35

bone, v, 1-4, 2-38, 5-106, 13-276
bones, 5-106
bowel, 1-5, 1-23, 2-33, 2-40, 2-41, 2-44, 2-45, 4-95, 4-96, 4-97, 4-98, 4-99, 4-100, 5-104, 5-107, 5-115, 6-130, 6-132, 6-135, 6-136, 6-137, 6-139, 6-140, 6-141, 6-145, 6-146, 6-148, 6-150, 7-164, 7-165, 7-166, 7-167, 7-171, 7-177, 7-178, 8-182, 8-186, 9-207, 9-212, 9-217, 9-223, 11-247, 11-248, 12-260, 12-261, 12-266, 12-267, 12-268, 12-269, 12-270, 13-277, 14-345, 14-346
brain, 1-2, 4-95, 4-100, 5-106, 5-108, 5-110, 5-116, 6-141, 6-147, 7-168, 7-170, 7-175, 9-192, 9-205, 11-251, 12-259, 13-275, 14-327
bread, 12-269
breast, 5-106
breath, 1-4, 2-43, 6-149
breath practice, [10-225]
breathing, 6-149
bronchitis, 12-262
buck, 13-293, 13-294, 13-295
Buddha, 14-343

# —C—

cadmium, 14-349, 14-350
calcium, 2-33, 2-35, 2-36, 2-38, 6-131, 9-210, 11-250, 12-260, 13-276, 13-279, 13-281, 13-282, 13-289, 14-338, 14-339, 14-340, 374, 388, 392
cancer, v, 1-4, 1-14, 1-15, 1-16, 1-23, 1-24, 1-25, 1-27, 1-28, 1-29, 2-38, 2-44, 2-45, 2-47, 5-106, 5-116, 5-118, 6-134, 6-135, 6-151, 7-165, 7-168, 7-170, 9-197, 10-240, 11-250, 11-253, 12-259, 12-262, 13-277, 13-283, 13-287, 13-288, 13-289, 13-290, 13-298, 13-299, 14-327, 14-330, 14-333, 14-336, 14-338, 14-344, 14-346, 14-356, A1-374
  bladder, 7-165
  bone, 7-165, 9-197
  breast, 1-14, 1-15, 1-16

225, 10-226, 10-229, 10-233, 10-234, 10-238, 10-239, 10-242, 11-245, 11-246, 11-247, 11-249, 11-251, 11-252, 11-255, 11-256, 12-257, 12-258, 12-260, 12-263, 14-316, 14-345, 14-346
co-creator, 4-101
Coenzyme Q-10, 14-333
coffee enema, 9-192, 9-207, 11-248, 14-346
colema, 11-247
colitis, 1-5, 2-44, 2-45, 5-110, 12-268, 13-277
colon, 1-8, 2-44, 2-45, 2-46, 4-96, 4-97, 4-98, 5-106, 5-110, 6-133, 6-135, 6-139, 6-146, 6-150, 7-164, 7-167, 7-168, 7-169, 7-178, 8-183, 8-186, 9-189, 9-190, 9-201, 9-202, 9-207, 9-212, 9-223, 11-247, 11-251, 11-252
colonic, 11-247, 11-252
colonics, 4-97
commercially grown produce, 1-27, 2-41
completely loving acts, 1-9
condemnation, 1-20
Conflict, 1-11
congested bowel, 7-178
congestion, 1-21, 1-22, 1-23, 7-178, 8-183, 9-197, 9-209, 9-210, 12-262, 12-267, 12-268, 13-277, 14-318, 14-319, 14-321, 14-328, 14-345, 390
consciousness, iv, 1-2, 1-7, 1-8, 1-12, 1-15, 1-17, 1-18, 1-19, 1-21, 1-30, 5-108, 13-304, 14-316, 14-317
constipation, 1-5, 2-41, 4-97, 4-98, 7-166, 7-171, 7-176, 7-178, 8-182, 12-267, 13-299, 13-301, 13-302, 14-338, 14-339, 386, 395
control over food, 7-167
conventional medicine, 1-24, 2-47, 6-148
cooked food, 6-134, 13-304
cough, 9-205, 9-209
courage, iii, iv, 1-30, 5-104, 5-109, 5-110, 5-115
creative power, 1-6

Crile, 4-98
criticism, 1-11, 1-20
Crone's disease, 13-277
Cysteine, 12-260, 14-333

## —D—

dairy, 1-25, 1-27, 5-105, 5-106, 5-108, 5-115, 6-134, 6-139
dairy products, 13-276, 13-279, 13-282, 13-288, 13-302, 14-335, 373, 386
death, v, 1-1, 1-3, 1-4, 1-5, 1-6, 1-9, 1-10, 1-29, 2-33, 2-44, 4-98, 4-100, 4-101, 5-111, 6-144, 6-145, 7-162, 7-162, 7-164, 7-174, 8-181, 9-190, 9-201, 10-230, 10-235, 11-255, 14-327, 14-333, 14-345, 14-346, 14-348
decreased appetite, 14-350
decreased growth, 14-350
deep inner joy, 7-165
Deepak Chopra, 1-15
deer, 13-292, 13-293, 13-294, 13-295, 13-296
degenerative disease, v, 1-1, 5-104
depressed immune function, 14-350
depression, 1-13, 1-14, 1-20, 2-38, 7-163, 7-170, 14-339, 14-348, 14-353, 14-355, 394, 398
determination, 7-155
diabetes, 7-163, 7-173, 7-174, 11-253, 12-259, 12-262, 12-266, 13-283, 13-287, 14-344
diabetic, 11-250
diarrhea, 2-41, 5-110
diet, v, 5-106, 5-107, 5-108, 5-109, 5-114, 5-115, 5-116, 5-117, 5-118, 5-123, 6-139, 6-145, 7-167, 7-170, 7-174, 7-176, 7-179, 9-204, 9-208, 9-209, 9-210, 9-211, 9-212, 11-246, 11-252, 11-253, 11-255, 11-256, 12-258, 12-260, 12-262, 12-266, 13-276, 13-278, 14-316, 14-330, 14-343
digestion, 2-37, 2-38, 2-40, 2-42, 6-130, 6-131, 6-133, 11-246, 12-260, 12-262, 12-267

# —F—

# —M—

poor absorption of iron, cooper
and manganese, 14-350
poor milk production, 14-350
positive attitude, 9-208
potassium, 2-33, 2-38, 2-39, 6-
135
power, i, iv, 1-1, 1-4, 1-6, 1-11, 1-
14, 1-18, 1-19, 2-46, 2-47, 4-
101, 5-104, 5-112, 5-116, 5-
123, 6-149
power of the mind, 5-104
prayer, 7-173, 10-236
pregnant, 7-176, 11-251
probiotics, 14-334, 14-335, 384
processed food, 5-105, 5-108, 5-
112, 5-115, 6-146
processed foods, 1-25, 1-27, 2-41,
5-112
programmed, 1-19, 1-24, 5-108, 5-
114
prolapsus, 6-150, 7-178, 11-247
prophecy, 1-4, 1-5
prostate, 7-179
protect, 1-3, 1-10, 1-27, 2-37, 2-
40, 5-116, 6-145, 13-277
protein, 1-25, 2-34, 2-35, 2-39, 5-
115, 5-116, 6-131, 6-134, 6-
146, 9-197, 9-202, 9-205, 9-
206, 11-246, 12-259, 12-260,
12-265, 12-266, 12-268, 13-
279, 13-281, 13-283, 13-284,
13-286, 13-287, 13-288, 13-
289, 13-291, 13-307, 14-318,
14-322, 14-323, 14-338, 14-
344, 14-345
psychological dwarfism, 1-13
psychological methods, 7-156
psyllium, 7-179, 9-206, 9-207, 9-
215, 9-216, 9-217, 11-245, 11-
251, 11-254
psyllium shake, 11-245
purification, 7-166, 10-235, 11-
248, 12-262
purify, iv, 1-2, 1-6, 1-21, 1-26, 6-
149

—Q—

quickening, 14-316, 14-317

—R—

radiation, 1-23, 1-26, 1-27, 1-28,
1-29, 1-30, 5-105, 5-110, 5-
112, 5-114, 5-118, 5-123, 10-
240, 14-327, 14-330
rage, iii, iv, 1-11, 2-43, 5-104, 5-
105, 5-109, 5-110, 5-113, 5-
115
rash, 1-5, 5-108, 6-141, 7-166, 7-
167, 7-175, 11-251
rattlesnake, 1-11, 5-110
raw food, 7-169, 7-171, 7-175, 7-
176, 9-204, 11-252
raw food diet, 14-316
raw foods, 12-258, 13-278, 14-316
raw fruits and vegetables, 8-181, 9-
209
rebuild, 1-23, 5-118, 12-258
rectum, 2-44, 6-148
reflex points, 7-179, 8-186
research, iv, 1-16, 1-17, 1-28, 2-
36, 5-107
resentment, 1-4, 1-9, 1-14, 1-18,
1-20
responsibility, 1-19, 1-25, 4-101
revitalizing, 4-98
rheumatism, 4-96
rheumatoid arthritis, 1-15
Richard Bach, 10-242

—S—

saliva, 1-11, 2-40, 12-260
salmonella, 9-218
salt, 1-25, 1-27, 2-35, 2-40, 2-44,
6-147, 9-219, 9-220, 9-222, 11-
254, 12-266, 12-269, 13-275
salt water, 9-219
Satan, 1-6
schizophrenic, 5-116
sciatica, 7-169
science, 5-107
scientific, 1-1, 1-18, 5-107, 7-162
seizure, 4-99
seizures, 14-352, 14-353
selenium, 14-330
self-control, 10-236
self-pity, 1-4, 1-20
separation, 10-228, 10-229
Seven Steps, 1-20, 1-24

—T—

# —U—

# —V—

# —W—

12-260, 12-262, 12-268, 14-344, 14-345, 14-346

weakness, 2-32, 2-38, 2-41, 2-44, 5-110, 9-205, 9-208, 10-238, 11-248, 12-260, 12-266

weight, 7-168, 7-170, 7-174, 7-178, 8-182, 9-222, 11-246, 14-350

Whatsoever we do to the least of our brethren, 10-240

wheat, 12-267, 12-269

white oak bark, 9-223, 11-247

will, 7-154, 7-155, 7-156, 7-157, 7-160, 7-162, 7-163, 7-164, 7-167, 7-173, 7-178, 7-179, 8-186, 9-190, 9-193, 9-200, 9-201, 9-202, 9-203, 9-205, 9-207, 9-208, 9-210, 9-211, 9-212, 9-213, 10-226, 10-234, 10-235, 10-236, 10-237, 10-238, 10-239, 10-242, 10-244, 11-248, 11-250, 11-251, 11-252, 11-253, 11-254, 11-255,

12-261, 12-269, 14-327, 14-343, 14-345

willingness, 1-9, 4-100, 10-240

wisdom, 1-3, 1-4, 1-29, 4-95, 4-101, 5-118, 7-154, 8-186, 12-257, 13-285, 13-286, 13-308, 13-309, 14-324, 15-361, 15-362, 385

worms, 2-46, 6-140, 6-144, 6-145, 6-146, 6-147

## —Y—

yeast, 2-33, 2-37, 5-108, 5-113, 5-116, 6-130, 6-140, 6-141, 8-182, 9-217, 12-259, 12-268, 13-275

yoga, 7-169

## —Z—

zinc deficiencies, 14-350